smog ALERT

'As many as 1.6 billion people may be at risk from poor air quality in urban areas throughout the world'

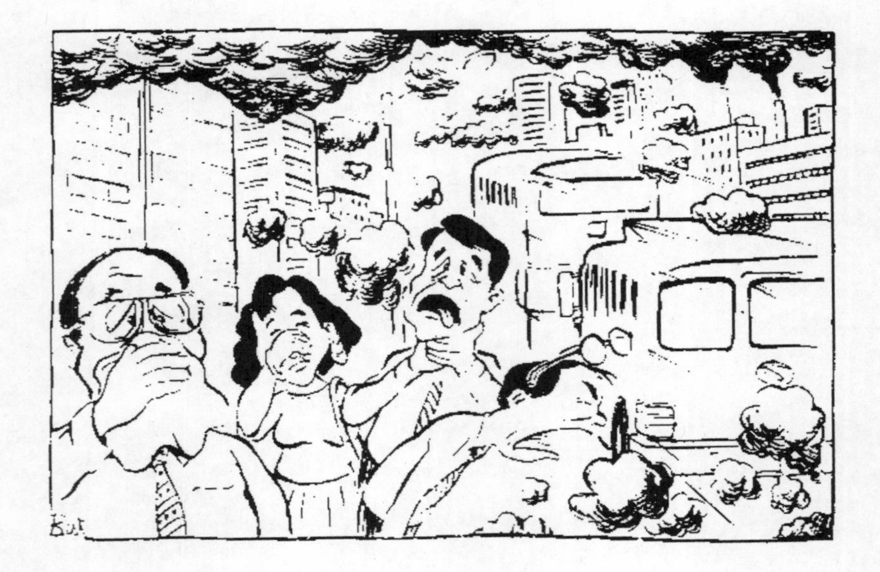

Cartoonist Paul Best, usage courtesy of the Hong Kong Government, Environmental Protection Department

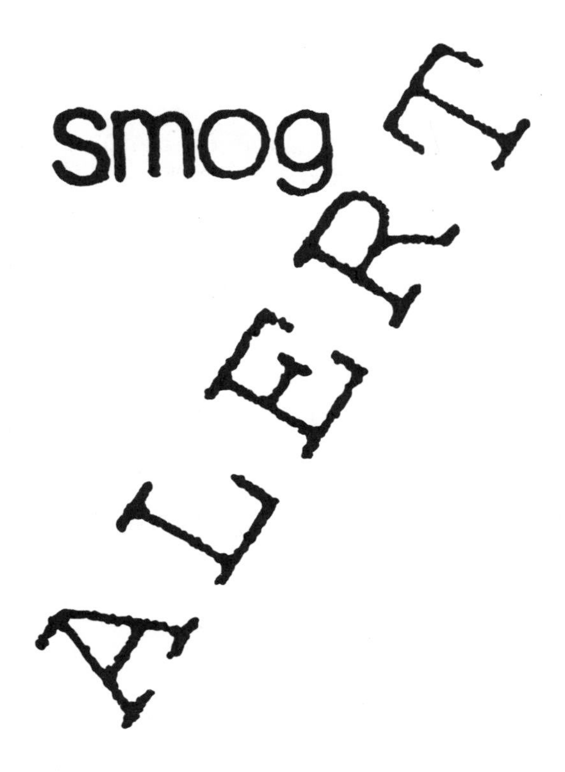

MANAGING URBAN AIR QUALITY

DEREK ELSOM

EARTHSCAN
Earthscan Publications Ltd, London

First published in the UK in 1996 by
Earthscan Publications Limited

A catalogue record for this book is available from the British Library

ISBN 1 85383 192 1 Paperback

Typeset by JS Typesetting, Wellingborough, Northants
Printed and bound by Biddles Ltd, Guildford and King's Lynn

For a full list of publications please contact:

Earthscan Publications Limited
120 Pentonville Road
London N1 9JN
Tel: 0171 278 0433
Fax: 0171 278 1142

Earthscan is an editorially independent subsidiary of Kogan Page Limited and publishes in association with WWF-UK and the International Institute for Environment and Development.

Contents

List of Figures

List of Tables

To my wife, Elizabeth,
our daughters, Sally and Clare,
and our Godchildren,
Nicola Jacks and Elise Hart

Preface and Acknowledgements

Urban air pollution is one of several major atmospheric pollution problems currently confronting the world's population. When it is realised that the health of 1.6 billion people may be at risk from poor urban air quality, then it is clear that urban air pollution ranks alongside such problems as acid rain, stratospheric ozone depletion and even global warming. *Smog Alert* examines the seriousness and causes of air pollution problems in the world's cities. It explains who is most at risk from poor air quality and what health threats each pollutant poses. A framework for the effective management of urban air quality is then outlined. Once such a framework has been established, national and city authorities can then consider what pollution control policies and measures are needed to deliver healthy urban air quality and to sustain it through the twenty-first century. Case studies of Athens, London, Los Angeles and Mexico City illustrate the difficulties facing the major world cities in reaching the goal of healthy air quality.

Smog Alert examines alternative policies and measures which can halt and eventually reverse declining air quality. Inevitably, many of the policies and measures are concerned with reducing emissions from cars, but the need to curb emissions from industry power stations and homes is also examined. Attention is given to the problem of tackling short-term smogs and to achieving long-term improvement in air quality. Recent examples of smogs suffered by cities throughout the world are given. These smogs generate widespread public concern and have resulted in many city authorities developing procedures to warn the public of unhealthy air quality, to give advice about what the public can do to minimise risks to their health, and to implement voluntary and enforced emission-reduction measures such as temporary traffic bans and cutbacks in industrial activity. The air quality effectiveness of such measures is examined. Consideration is given to whether more urban areas should introduce smog alert procedures or whether such developments divert resources away from the ultimate goal of achieving and sustaining healthy urban air quality.

Smog Alert was first conceived during the final stages of completing *Atmospheric Pollution: a Global Problem* (second edition, Blackwell, Oxford, 1992). I realised that air pollution problems in urban areas had become such a serious worldwide problem that they needed an entire book to be devoted to them rather than just a chapter or two. Many individuals and organisations have supplied information, stimulated ideas and encouraged the writing of this book. Particular thanks go to Helen Crabbe, Oxford Brookes University, who has supplied a seemingly endless stream of copies of relevant publications and provided me with many opportunities to discuss aspects of urban air quality management. I am grateful to Jonathan Sinclair Wilson, Publishing Director of Earthscan, for his patience and support while he awaited the final manuscript. There are too many other people who have helped me during the preparation and writing of *Smog Alert* to mention them all by name, but I am very grateful to every one of them. A large number of organisations have been helpful in responding to my requests both by post and in person. These include the Pollution Control Agencies of Athens, Beijing, Birmingham, Denver, Helsinki, Hong Kong, London, Los Angeles, Mexico City, Paris, San Diego, São Paulo and Toronto. In the UK, the National Society for Clean Air and Environmental Protection (NSCA) has provided a series of seminars, workshops and conferences in the past few years which I have found very productive occasions during which to reflect on and discuss urban air quality issues. I have been fortunate to have been a member of NSCA's air quality management working group at a time when this organisation played a key part in persuading the government to introduce legislation giving local authorities the responsibility and powers for assessing air quality within their local areas and setting out what policies and measures are needed to deal with any air quality problems.

In the years following the completion of my doctorate in urban air pollution meteorology in the mid-1970s, supervised by Professor Tony J Chandler and sponsored by Warren Spring Laboratory, relatively little interest was shown in UK urban air pollution issues by the public, politicians or the media. Acid rain, the ozone hole, ionising radiation from nuclear power stations such as Chernobyl, and global warming became the focuses of attention instead. Many people considered that local air pollution problems had been solved. However, by the late 1980s, the problems caused by rising levels of traffic emissions resulting in urban smogs could be ignored no longer. During the past few years attention on urban air quality issues has been growing at a phenomenal rate. The UK Environment Act 1995 setting out a National Air Quality Strategy marks the beginning of a new phase of close attention being given to local air pollution problems in the UK. However, *Smog Alert* is aimed at a much wider readership than the UK. It is intended to provide a stimulating read and a useful source of information and ideas for people concerned about poor air quality in towns and cities throughout the world.

Finally, there are few occasions when anyone can express gratitude in print to their family, so I take this opportunity to thank my wife, Elizabeth, and our daughters, Sally and Clare, who have been so very supportive while

Smog Alert was being researched and written. I also thank my parents, Joy and Edgar, for all their encouragement.

Derek M Elsom
Professor of Climatology
Oxford Brookes University

Chapter 1

Polluted Cities: A Worldwide Problem

Urban Air Pollution

Breathing in urban areas may endanger your health. Poor urban air quality in developed and developing countries threatens the health and well-being of about one-half of the world's urban population.[1] In Europe alone, the European Environment Agency has estimated that in 70–80 per cent of the 105 European cities with more than 500,000 inhabitants examined, levels of one or more pollutants exceed the World Health Organisation (WHO) air

1 An assessment of Global Environment Monitoring System (GEMS) data for a sample of about 50 cities in the mid-1980s indicated that about 1.3 billion people – mostly in The South – lived in towns or cities of more than 250,000 population which did not meet World Health Organisation (WHO) guidelines for suspended particulates. For sulphur dioxide in the late 1980s the figure was 1.0 billion, with another 600 million living in areas of marginal sulphur dioxide air quality; World Bank (1992) *World Development Report 1992: Development and the Environment*, Oxford University Press, New York, pp 51–52. According to the United Nations Environment Programme (UNEP) and WHO, about 1.2 billion people worldwide may be exposed to levels of sulphur dioxide above WHO guidelines and 1.4 billion people to levels of suspended particulates and smoke above WHO guidelines; UNEP/WHO (1993) *City Air Quality Trends (GEMS/AIR Data)*, vol 2, UNEP, Nairobi, p 3. According to Dietrich H. Schwela, when expanding on his paper 'Public health implications of urban air pollution in developing countries' in the *Proceedings of the 10th World Clean Air Congress, Espoo, Finland*, May–June 1995, vol 3, Finnish Air Pollution Prevention Society, Helsinki, paper 617, a revised analysis of GEMS data by the WHO suggests that 1.6 billion people are at risk from air pollution and that without effective pollution control measures this number is expected to increase due to urban migration and high birth rates. Many estimates of the number of people at risk worldwide limit their assessments to suspended particulates and sulphur dioxide so that the actual number at risk from all pollutants may be much higher.

quality guidelines at least once in a typical year.[2] The situation in cities in The South is even worse. Worldwide as many as 1.6 billion people may be at risk from poor air quality. Hundreds of millions of people throughout the world live in cities where air pollution is so severe that several hundred thousand die prematurely every year and many tens of thousands become acutely or chronically ill.[3] Air pollution is a growing problem because of rapidly increasing urban populations, unchecked urban and industrial expansion, and the phenomenal surge in the number and use of motor vehicles. In many cities around the world new sources of pollution are being added at a rate which exceeds the ability of authorities to control them. Many city authorities are losing the struggle to ensure that urban residents breathe air which is safe.

Root Causes of the Problem

Population growth is at the heart of the pollution problem as nations attempt to provide the energy, food, products, fresh water, sanitation, housing and transport needed and desired by the growing urban populations. Currently, the global population is increasing by over 95 million every year, or about 260,000 each day. In trying to satisfy the demands made by the increasing numbers of people in urban areas, vast amounts of air pollutants are being added to urban atmospheres. If the growth in demand for transport and electricity were to be met with the techniques currently in use, emissions of the main pollutants derived from these sources would increase five-fold and 11-fold, respectively, by about 2030.[4] In 1970 the world population was 3.7 billion, with 37 per cent concentrated within urban areas. By 1990 the world's population had reached 5.3 billion, of which 43 per cent lived in urban areas.[5] Eighteen cities exceed 9 million people, 29 cities have more than 6 million and 69 have over 3 million (Figure 1.1). Of the 69 largest cities,

---

2 Stanners, D and Bourdeau, P (1995) *Europe's Environment: the Dobris Assessment*, European Environment Agency, Copenhagen, pp 27–56

3 Estimates suggest that if unhealthy levels of suspended particulate matter were brought down to the annual average level that the WHO considers safe, between 300,000 and 700,000 premature deaths a year could be averted in The South. This is equivalent to 2–5 per cent of all the deaths in urban areas that have excessive levels of particulates. Many of these averted deaths would be in China and India; World Bank (1992) op cit, p 52. Schwela (1995) op cit suggests unhealthy levels of suspended particulates and sulphur dioxide lead to around 464,000 and 370,000 excess deaths each year in urban areas. Some urban areas experience high levels of both pollutants so these two totals of excess deaths should not be added together. Further, high levels of suspended particulates do not necessarily mean high levels of fine particulates (PM_{10}), which can penetrate deep into the lungs and tend to be more toxic than larger particles, because a high proportion of the particulates in some cities is made up of large soil particles.

4 World Bank (1992) op cit, p 50

5 In Northern countries in 1990, 73 per cent of the population resided in cities, whereas the figure was only 34 per cent for Southern countries. However, the trend for urbanisation has been accelerating in The South. By 2025 the urban population

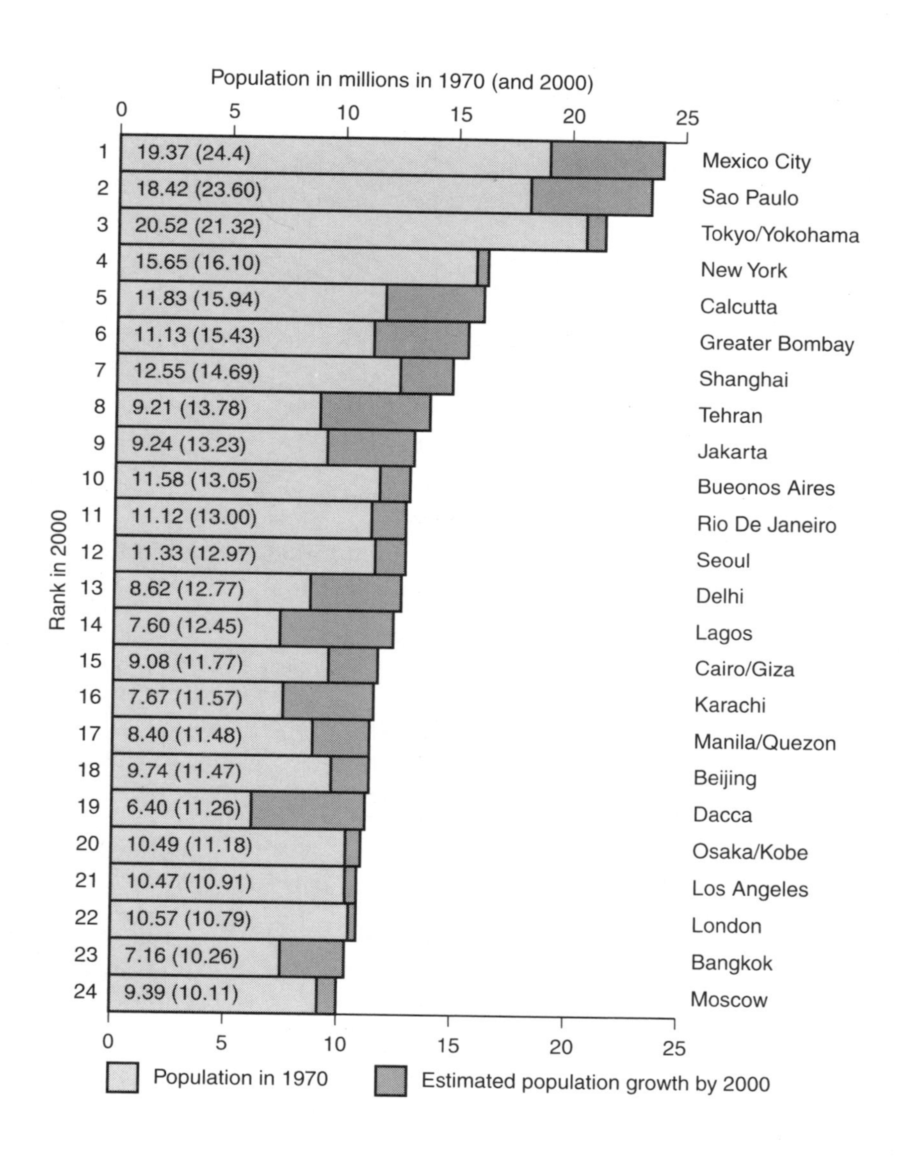

Figure 1.1 *World cities expected to reach a population exceeding 10 million in 2000.*

Source: compiled from information given in United Nations (1989) *Prospects of World Urbanization 1988*, Population Studies No 112, UN Department of International Economic and Social Affairs, New York

45 are in The South. These developing cities act as magnets, drawing in tens of thousands of migrants into squatter settlements each year. Overcrowding is much worse in cities in The South than in European or North American cities and countries in The North have more resources to cope. Whereas Chicago supports 2500 people per square kilometre and London 4000, the density in Buenos Aires is 15,000, Santiago 17,000, Cairo 24,000, Lima 29,000, Mexico City 34,000, Manila 43,000 and Calcutta 88,000 people per square kilometre.

As these congested cities in The South progress industrially, many lack the economic and technical resources needed to cope with, let alone reduce, the massive amounts of pollutants being discharged into the atmosphere by expanding industries. Weak economies, not only in The South but also in The North, such as in eastern Europe, often lead to minimal investment in pollution control equipment and a reliance on cheap but highly polluting fuels such as coal or lignite (brown coal). Consequently, increasing numbers of people in many of the world's cities are being exposed to ever worsening air quality. By the year 2000, the United Nations estimates that the world's population will reach 6.25 billion, and half that number will live in urban areas, with the bulk of urban growth occurring in The South. Looking further ahead, the United Nations suggests that it may take two centuries or more before the world's population may eventually stabilise at around 11.6 billion.[6] As many as 25 megacities will accommodate 9 million people, requiring vast amounts of energy and industrially produced products as well as transport facilities in the form of millions of cars, buses, taxis and trucks.

Countries in The South currently account for only 10 per cent of the world's vehicles, including 20 per cent of the buses. As their need and desire for transport grows, together with their ability to manufacture these vehicles, there will be a phenomenal increase in the number of motor vehicles worldwide. Although annual average rates of growth in vehicle numbers in the 1980s in Northern countries such as the UK and US were only 2 to 3 per cent, the rates were much higher in The South. Pakistan experienced a vehicle growth rate of 9 per cent, Brazil 11 per cent, China 14 per cent, Kenya 26 per cent and both the Republic of Korea and Thailand 30 per cent. Generally southeast Asia has one of the fastest growing car markets in the world. These rates are increasing to such an extent that the number of motor vehicles worldwide may increase from 650–675 million

---

in The South may reach 57 per cent, compared with around 80 per cent in The North. In absolute terms it is estimated that from 1990 to 2025, 2904 million people will be added to the world's urban population, of which 2609 million will be in cities in The South; UNEP (1993) *Environmental Data Report 1993–94*, UNEP/Blackwell, Oxford, p 206; World Resources Institute (1994) *World Resources 1994–5*, WRI/UNEP, Oxford University Press, Oxford

6 Brown, L R, Kane H and Roodman, D M (1994) *Vital Signs: the Trends That Are Shaping Our Future 1994–95*, Worldwatch Institute/Earthscan, London, pp 98–99; UNEP (1993) op cit, p 202

motor vehicles in 1990 to 1 billion by 2030, a rate of increase exceeding that of world population growth.[7]

The potential for growth in the number of vehicles is truly immense. For example, China, with 1.2 billion people, possessed about 400 million bicycles in 1990 but only 700,000 private cars and about 5 million other motor vehicles – less than the number of vehicles in Los Angeles alone. With a high priority given to expanding their domestic motor vehicle manufacturing industries, countries such as China and India will add to the world's total number of vehicles considerably. China intends to increase its car production to about 3 million a year by 2003.[8]

Currently, 34 million cars are produced each year worldwide, which represents more than one new car every second.[9] Spend the night in bed and when you wake up the next morning 30,000 new vehicles will be driving along already congested urban roads, adding their burden of pollutants to the air we breathe. National transport policies which build new roads to cope with traffic congestion simply encourage more vehicles to use the roads. It almost seems to be an immutable law that traffic increases faster than the ability of roads to handle it or pollution control authorities to check the rise in the annual total emissions from motor vehicles.

Motor vehicles in Southern countries tend to be less fuel-efficient and more polluting than those in Northern countries because of a lack of access to new technologies, a greater proportion of older vehicles, poorly surfaced or badly maintained roads, weaker environmental legislation or weak enforcement of the regulations, poor vehicle maintenance (as vehicle emission inspections are less rigorous or non-existent), and the dominance of low quality fuels (eg diesel with a high sulphur content). Even in richer, Northern countries where cars are more fuel-efficient, the total amount of pollutant emissions from vehicles may be increasing or is forecast to do so in the coming decades. This arises because of the current rapid increase in the number of vehicles and the distances they are being driven, which is outweighing the emission improvements gained from the application of improved technology (eg fitting catalytic converters, increasing fuel efficiency) to individual vehicles. For example, as long as urban areas continue to expand, the distance that commuters have to travel to work or into city centres from the suburbs increases. Concurrently, as long as commuters and shoppers opt for the comfort and convenience of personal

---

7 Faiz, A, Sinha, K, Walsh, M and Varma, A (1990) *Automotive Air Pollution: Issues and Options for Developing Countries*, Working Paper Transport WPS 492, World Bank, Washington DC; Organization for Economic Cooperation and Development (OECD) (1995) *Motor Vehicle Pollution*, OECD, Paris; Tolba, M F and El-Kholy, O A (1992) *The World Environment 1972–92*, UNEP/Chapman and Hall; 'Car laws won't curb Far East's transport pollution', *The Environmental Digest*, vol 61, Jul 1992, p 14

8 Brown, L R *et al* (1995) *State of the World 1995*, Earthscan, London

9 Op cit, pp 88–89

mobility rather than using public transport, so the demand for cars will continue to escalate.

Links with Other Atmospheric Pollution Problems

Urban air pollution is one of several major atmospheric pollution problems currently confronting the world's population: global warming, stratospheric ozone depletion and acid deposition are also serious problems. They all stem from our failure to recognise that the atmosphere is not an infinite sink into which we can dump waste products without adverse consequences for our own health and well-being as well as those of our planet. For too long we have held a blinkered view of the short-term gains resulting from our activities, ignoring the long-term losses. Fortunately, during the past few years we have begun to recognise the potential value of sustainable economic development and it is the widespread adoption of this approach that many people hope will create a less polluted urban, regional and global atmosphere.

Global warming due to an increase in the atmospheric concentrations of greenhouse gases such as carbon dioxide, methane and nitrous oxide has the potential to affect the urban air pollution problem, although it is unclear whether the weather and climate changes associated with global warming will favour an improvement or a worsening of urban air pollution in the coming decades. An increase or decrease in the frequency, intensity and relative position of blocking anticyclones, which are characterised by light or calm winds and temperature inversions, will increase or reduce the frequency of smogs, respectively. Milder winters in some high-latitude areas may lessen the need for heating of homes and offices, so reducing pollutant emissions. In contrast, higher summer temperatures and more sunshine in the middle and lower latitudes will favour increased evaporative emissions of volatile organic compounds (VOCs) as well as more intense photochemical smog reactions, perhaps increasing ozone levels by up to 10 per cent. Changing water vapour levels (relative humidity) will affect the solubility of pollutants and the rate of chemical reactions, especially the oxidation of VOCs, sulphur dioxide and nitrogen oxides in the atmosphere. Drier conditions will lead to greater amounts of particulates being raised by moving traffic and where areas surrounding a city become arid, this will provide a source for large amounts of suspended particulates to be blown into the city. Stratospheric ozone depletion due to chlorine compounds such as chlorofluorocarbons (CFCs) is expected to remain a problem until the year 2030. During that time the increased ultraviolet radiation reaching ground level is likely to speed up photochemical reaction rates in the lower atmosphere, increasing the concentrations of photochemical oxidants such as ozone and nitrogen dioxide.[10]

---

10 Intergovernmental Panel on Climate Change (IPCC) (1990) *Potential Impacts of Climate Change*, Report from Working Group 2, IPCC, Geneva

One hope as far as urban pollution problems are concerned is that measures to limit global warming by reducing carbon dioxide emissions from combustion processes will also reduce emissions of health-threatening pollutants. However, actions taken to deal with the potential consequences of global warming may compete for the financial resources needed for urban pollution control policies. Rising sea levels and an increased frequency of devastating hurricanes, cyclones and typhoons triggered by warming the oceans are likely to threaten many cities in low-lying coastal areas throughout the tropics. The need to improve coastal defences and to introduce relocation policies will demand increasing national expenditure, which will compete for limited funds with attempts to tackle urban pollution problems in some cities and countries. Between 250 and 300 million people are threatened by rising sea levels due to global warming, including the cities of Bombay, Dacca, Rio de Janeiro and Shanghai.

Health-threatening Pollutants

Data collected by the Global Environment Monitoring System (GEMS), which monitors air pollution levels in major cities around the world, indicate that as many as 1.6 billion people worldwide may experience unhealthy air due to the high levels of sulphur dioxide and/or suspended particulates (including soot, smoke, PM_{10} and dust).[11] In addition, areas adjacent to congested roads suffer high levels of traffic-generated pollutants such as carbon monoxide, nitrogen dioxide, VOCs (hydrocarbons including carcinogenic substances such as benzene) and airborne lead. Toxic chemicals and metals produced by industrial plants and waste incinerators add to this urban cocktail of pollutants. Many of these pollutants drift downwind from urban areas to affect rural communities. Indeed, as polluted air masses drift over the surrounding countryside, photochemical reactions lead to increased concentrations of pollutants such as ozone reaching higher levels than they do in urban areas.

On several days it is not unusual for levels of one or more pollutants in many cities and even in adjacent rural areas to exceed levels defined by the WHO as being detrimental to the health and well-being of the population. It is not uncommon for cities such as Athens, Bangkok, Beijing, Calcutta, Delhi, Los Angeles, Mexico City, Seoul, Shenyang and Tehran to experience 30 days, or even more than 100 days in some cases, of poor air quality throughout the year (Figure 1.2). Simply breathing in such cities may indeed

11 Refer to notes 1 and 2. GEMS is a monitoring agency co-ordinated by the WHO and funded by the UNEP. The GEMS air programme has been in operation since 1974. Currently, it collects and analyses air quality data for sulphur dioxide, suspended particulate matter, fine particulates (PM_{10}), nitrogen oxides, ozone, carbon monoxide and lead from more than 80 cities in about 40 countries. Most cities report data from two or three types of site (eg city centre, suburban and industrial).

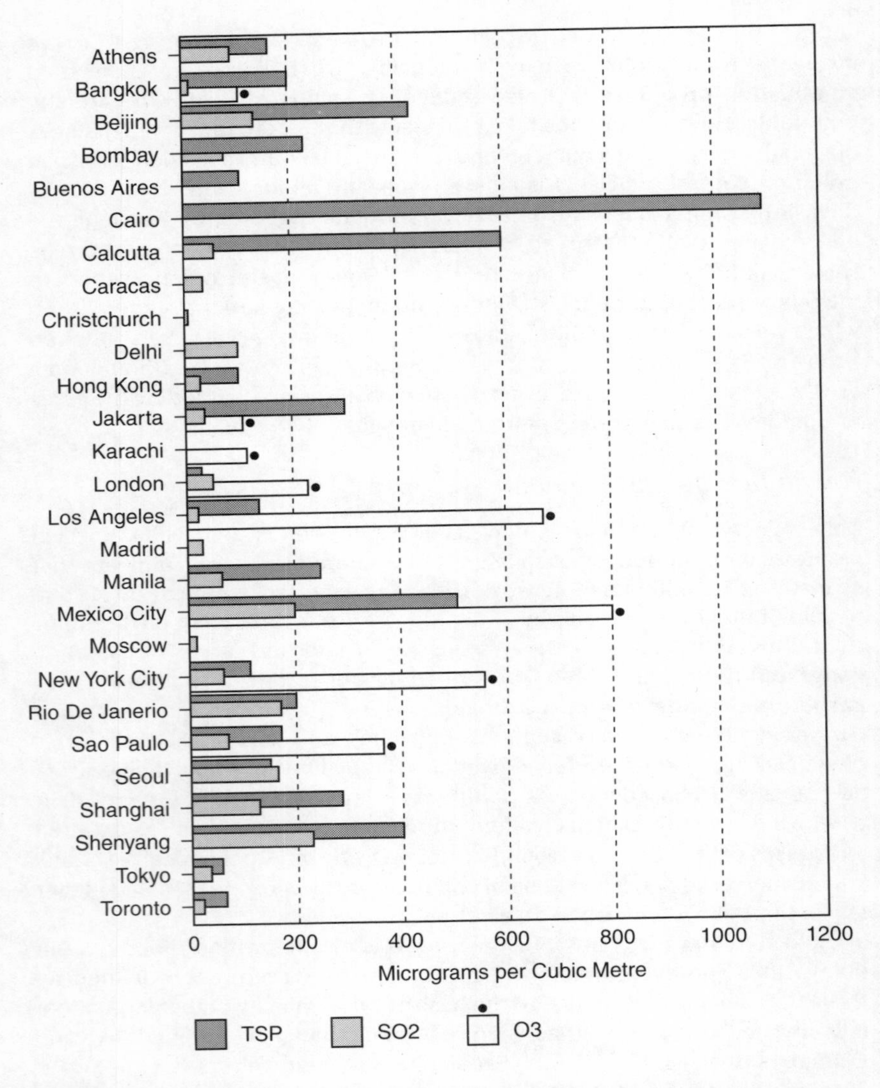

Figure 1.2 *Comparison of ambient levels of annual second daily maximum one-hour ozone, annual average total suspended particulate matter (TSP) and sulphur dioxide among selected world cities, 1988–1992. The highest TSPs occurred in Cairo, Calcutta and Mexico City. Sulphur dioxide was highest in Mexico City, Rio de Janeiro, Seoul, Beijing and Shanghai. Highest ozone levels occurred in Mexico City, Los Angeles, New York City and São Paulo (but data were available for only eight of the 20 cities studied).*

Source: US Environmental Protection Agency (1994) *National Air Quality and Emissions Trends Report, 1993*, USEPA, Report EPA 454/R-94-026, Research Triangle Park, NC, p 136

be hazardous to health. With such serious air pollution problems existing in so many urban areas of the world, it is clear that the pursuit of healthy urban atmospheres must gain a place on the world's agenda of priorities.

Summer and Winter Smogs

Poor air quality usually occurs during spells of several days during which the peak concentrations of one or more pollutants reach health-threatening levels. Such air pollution episodes or smogs are triggered by periods of stable weather conditions associated with the presence of an anticyclone (high air pressure). In some climates such as the west coast sub-tropical (Mediterranean) type, stable weather conditions prevail for an entire season, producing almost continuous photochemical smog conditions for months on end. Typically, smog occurs either during warm and sunny stable weather conditions or during cold and foggy stable conditions. These are sometimes described as summer and winter smog types, respectively. However, such descriptions are more appropriate to mid- and high-latitude climates than the tropics, where it is the dry season that triggers the smogs. It should be stressed that although stable weather conditions cause pollution levels to increase, smogs would not occur if pollutant emissions were not too high to begin with. In other words, it is human activities producing the pollutant emissions that are to blame for the smogs, not the weather conditions.

Summer smog occurs on warm sunny days when winds are calm or light and when photochemical activity encourages ozone formation. Ozone is created when nitrogen oxides and VOCs emitted by traffic, power stations and other polluting activities react chemically in the presence of sunlight. Other compounds are formed such as aldehydes, peroxyacetyl nitrate (PAN), hydrogen peroxide and acid aerosols such as sulphates, sulphuric acid, nitrates and nitric acid, but ozone is often used as the indicator pollutant for assessing the severity of a photochemical smog. Given that ozone formation needs an hour or two – even several hours – of sunlight for the chemical reactions to take effect on the precursor emissions, ozone increases in concentration as pollutants drift downwind of urban areas. This can lead to ozone pollution being a problem not only for nearby rural villages, but for more distant locations including areas across state or national borders.

Motor vehicles emit nitrogen oxides in two forms: nitric oxide (about 90 per cent) and nitrogen dioxide (about 10 per cent). The nitric oxide (a harmless pollutant at the ambient concentrations experienced) is oxidised to nitrogen dioxide (the health-threatening pollutant) slowly by reactions with oxygen and rapidly by reactions with ozone. Consequently, the latter reaction depletes ozone levels in traffic-congested city centres, causing levels of ozone to be relatively low compared with the suburbs and surrounding rural areas. Consequently, nitrogen dioxide rather than ozone is the gaseous pollutant that may pose the serious health threat in city centres.

Winter smogs usually occur during cold anticyclonic conditions when a low-level temperature inversion acts as a thermal lid, hindering vertical dilution and dispersion of emissions. Low temperatures lead to increased energy consumption for heating of homes and offices and so boost the emissions of sulphur dioxide and suspended particulates. Cold conditions cause motor vehicle engines to operate less efficiently, leading to increased emissions of carbon monoxide and hydrocarbons. The severity of this problem is made worse because catalytic converters take several minutes to reach their operating temperature from a cold start and during that time exhaust emissions are uncontrolled.

During winter smogs, hourly and daily concentrations of benzene, carbon monoxide, nitrogen dioxide, sulphur dioxide and suspended particulates reach many times their average winter values. Urban areas located in basins and valleys are particularly at risk from winter smogs because dense cold air flowing down slopes (katabatic winds) strengthens the temperature inversion (thermal lid), reducing the vertical dispersion of contaminants. At the same time, the surrounding hills prevent the pollution escaping from the basin or valley.

One city's pollution can add to another city's smog problems as pollutants drift across the intervening countryside to reach a neighbouring urban area. Some scavenging of the pollutants takes place en route, but this is not always the case. If the ground is covered by snow, dry deposition of sulphur dioxide onto the smooth snow-covered surfaces is markedly reduced, perhaps to one-eighth of its usual rate of deposition. In regions where high-sulphur fuels are burned, such as lignite in parts of eastern Europe, this situation can result in high concentrations of sulphur dioxide lingering in the atmosphere and drifting across national boundaries, creating regional-scale pollution episodes. Tall industrial stacks of coal-fired power stations, metal-processing plants and oil refineries can contribute significantly to the long-range transport of pollutants. Such stacks emit pollutants well above surface and low-level inversions, when they are present, causing little or no pollution locally. However, these well-defined pollution plumes may travel hundreds of kilometres to locations where thermal mixing may bring down the pollutants to the surface. Alternatively, orographic precipitation washes out the pollutants as 'acid rain' over hilly and mountainous regions.

Pollutants such as nitrogen dioxide, suspended particulates and benzene may pose health threats during winter or summer. In the past few years the adverse health effects of very fine particulates, less than 10 μm (PM_{10}), which are small enough to penetrate deep into the lungs, are increasingly being recognised. American research suggests that an increase of 10 $\mu g/m^3$ in PM_{10} in urban areas is associated with a daily rise in the death rate of 1 per cent, such that PM_{10} pollution may cause 60,000 premature deaths a year in the US, mainly among the elderly and those with pneumonia and chronic lung disease.[12] In the UK alone this figure may reach 10,000 deaths

12 The Harvard Six Cities Study showed a direct relationship between adjusted mortality ratios and levels of fine particulates ($PM_{2.5}$); Dockery, D W *et al* (1993)

a year.[13] Cities with large numbers of diesel-powered vehicles, especially where they are poorly maintained, can experience very high concentrations of PM_{10}, which is worrying if there is no safe health level for these pollutants. Airborne lead may be a problem during episodes at any time of the year in those cities where the content of lead in petrol is still relatively high.

North America

In the US 60 million people (120 million people during the smoggy summer heatwave in 1988) breathe city air which has failed to attain federal air quality standards even though the original intention was to ensure that these standards would be reached by the mid-1970s.[14] The 14 million residents of the Los Angeles basin suffer some of the worst summer air quality in the world, with air quality levels exceeding federal standards on more than 130 days each year (226 days in 1988). Ozone is the worst offender in the Los Angeles Basin, accounting for more than 100 (165 days in 1988) of those 'unhealthful' days. It is created when nitrogen oxides and VOCs from 9 million motor vehicles and 40,000 industrial sources react in sunlight. Ozone causes stinging eyes, running noses, coughing, headaches, chest pains, nausea and shortness of breath in healthy people, whereas people with asthma may experience severe breathing problems when ozone concentrations are high. Smog alerts have to be issued to warn people with asthma and those with chronic respiratory diseases to stay indoors and for healthy people not to participate in vigorous exercise as this increases the uptake of pollutants. During the smog the authorities attempt to curb emissions from traffic and industry to prevent air quality from deteriorating further. For people who were born and who have lived in Los Angeles all their lives, their long-term exposure to elevated levels of ozone may be breaking down their body's immune system, increasing their chances of suffering respiratory illness and harming their lungs in later life. Air pollution in Los Angeles is so bad that a radical lifestyle-changing plan is being adopted in an attempt to create healthy air in the city by the year 2010. Many doubt that even this drastic plan will be successful.

Ozone pollution problems are also serious outside California in Baltimore, Houston, New York City, Philadelphia and Washington, whereas Denver suffers from carbon monoxide pollution. Carbon monoxide emissions from

---

'An association between air pollution and mortality in six US cities', *New England Journal of Medicine*, vol 329, pp 1753–1759; Pope, C A, Schwartz, J and Ransom, M R (1992) 'Daily mortality and PM_{10} pollution in Utah Valley', *Archives of Environmental Health*, vol 47 (3), pp 211–17. The health effects of fine particulates are discussed further in Chapter 3.

13 Brown, W (1994) 'Dying from too much dust', *New Scientist*, 12 March 1994, pp 12–13

14 US Environmental Protection Agency (1994) *National Air Quality and Emissions Trends Report, 1993*, USEPA Report 454/R-94-026, Research Triangle Park, NC

motor vehicles increase in high-altitude cities such as Denver because there is less oxygen available. In recent winters, violations of the carbon monoxide air quality standard became so frequent in this 'mile-high city' that cars are now required to run on oxygenated fuel or 'gasohol', which contains, say, 10 per cent oxygen-rich ethers or alcohols and improves fuel combustion, especially at low temperatures. In 1992 oxygenated fuel began to be sold between November and February in 28 metropolitan areas across the country. Carbon monoxide emissions are reduced by about 10–15 per cent, but whether this is enough to offset the emissions being added by the increase in vehicle numbers and usage remains to be seen. If improvements are inadequate in Denver, requests to motorists not to drive on one working day a week may have to change from a voluntary system to a legal requirement.

The Windsor–Toronto–Quebec Corridor in Canada suffers especially poor air quality throughout its congested cities which will require radical control measures if air quality is to be improved. In 1990, Canada identified 14 urban areas with serious smog problems. More than one-half of all Canadians are exposed regularly each summer to ozone levels above the 'maximum acceptable' air quality standard. Tackling poor air quality is likely to require a smog control strategy capable of reducing smog-causing emissions by 40 per cent or more by the year 2000. Vehicle emissions tend to be the greatest concern and tighter emission standards will be needed, but an added problem in parts of the Windsor–Toronto–Quebec Corridor is that some of the pollution is imported from the US.[15]

Central and South America

Most South American cities suffer severe air pollution due to the rapid increase in the number of motor vehicles and in energy production and industrial processing, often concentrated in the cities. Some of the worst affected cities include Buenos Aires in Argentina, Bogota in Colombia, Caracas in Venezuela, Lima in Peru, Santiago in Chile, and São Paulo–Santos–Cubatao and Rio de Janeiro in Brazil. Santiago, the high-altitude capital of Chile containing 4.5 million people, is encircled by the snow-capped mountains of the Andes which trap the air pollutants. It suffers frequent pollution episodes in winter caused by emissions from 8000 poorly maintained and highly-polluting diesel buses and other vehicles as well as

15 Ministere de l'Environnement du Quebec (1992) 'La pollution atmospherique par l'ozone au Quebec: aspects de la problematique', Ministere de l'Environnement du Quebec, 161 pp; Murley, L (1991) *Clean Air Around the World*, second edition, International Union of Air Pollution Prevention Associations, Brighton, pp 109–121; Orchard, D (1991) 'The Green Plan: a national challenge for Canada' *JAPCA – Journal of Air and Waste Management Association*, vol 41, pp 268–271; Yap, D, Ning, D T and Dong, W (1988) 'An assessment of source contributions to the ozone concentrations in southern Ontario 1979–1985' *Atmospheric Environment*, vol 22, pp 1161–1168

132 polluting industries in and around the city. During the thick brown smog of June 1991, the city authorities closed schools, reduced the number of cars and buses entering the city centre by 40–50 per cent and shut down half the polluting factories. The smogs resulted in hospitals reporting a 30–60 per cent increase in the number of patients treated for respiratory ailments.[16]

In many of the expanding cities of South America migrant workers seeking a better life exchange rural poverty for unhealthy shantytown poverty and the search for work amidst smog-ridden capitals. Many migrants have little choice but to find accommodation adjacent to factory sites and to endure unhealthy emissions from foreign-owned industrial plants which spew forth toxic chemical emissions with little or no control. Symbolic of such industrial areas is Cubatao in Brazil, 40 km (25 miles) from São Paulo. This industrial city of 110,000 people became Brazil's largest industrial estate in the 1970s and it gained the unwelcome description of being the most polluted place on earth. This city developed as Brazil's response to the belief that 'poverty is the worst pollution'. The result was the rapid development of industry with few pollution control measures being incorporated. Industrial plants producing petrochemicals, steel, fertilisers, paper, cement and diverse chemicals poured out pollutants with little or no control throughout the 1970s. Infant mortality and cases of respiratory disease reached such excessive levels that the world's media labelled Cubatao the 'valley of death'. A 1983 survey of Vila Paris, a crowded Cubatao slum of 15,000 residents, found that 44 per cent had some kind of lung disease.

Stung into action by worldwide criticism of what was happening in Cubatao, the São Paulo State, backed by World Bank funding, introduced a long-term programme to tackle pollution in 1981. Industrial plants began installing pollution control equipment with the result that the number of smogs decreased markedly from 16 smog alerts in 1984 to only once or twice a year by the end of the decade. In 1989, 249 of 320 industrial plants were under control. However, pollution still remains a problem in Cubatao: in July 1991 pollution levels reached four times the acceptable limit, which required 24 industrial plants near the city to shut down for several days – but in the future the city may become symbolic of what can be done to remedy even the worst urban–industrial pollution problems. Ironically, one of the main polluters is the government-owned steel plant which is unable to invest in pollution control equipment because of restrictions imposed by a government facing a debt crisis.[17]

---

16 'Smog shuts schools', *Guardian*, 15 June 1991

17 Environmental Sanitation Technology Company (1990) *Cubatao: a Change of Air*, Environmental Sanitation Technology Company, São Paulo, 10 pp; Romieu, I, Weitzenfeld, H and Finkelman, J (1991) 'Urban air pollution in Latin America and the Caribbean', *JAPCA – Journal of Air and Waste Management Association*, vol 41, pp 1166–1171; World Resources Institute (1990) *World Resources 1990–91*, World Resources Institute/Basic Books, New York, p 41; 'State of pollution emergency in Brazil' *The Environmental Digest*, Jul/Aug, 49/50, 1991, p 14

Air pollution levels in the Central American capitals of Guatemala, Honduras and Costa Rica exceed WHO guidelines for carbon monoxide, nitrogen dioxide and particulates, with vehicles contributing 70 per cent of total emissions.[18] The 20 million residents of Mexico City suffer some of the worst air quality in the world. This city is encircled by mountains and subjected to prolonged periods of light winds and strong temperature inversions which trap the pollutants over the city. Smogs are common throughout the megalopolis between November and May. In 1991, hourly ozone levels exceeded the WHO guideline of 100 parts per billion (ppb) or 200 micrograms per cubic metre of air (μg/m^3) on 192 days – a situation much worse than even Los Angeles. In November 1992 ozone concentrations reached 600 ppb (1200 μg/m^3) in the southern parts of the city – a level not reached in Los Angeles since the 1950s. Smogs can be so severe that schoolchildren are given the month off and industrial plants are ordered to cut production by 50–75 per cent. Mexican environmental groups claim that, even without exceptional weather conditions to trap the smog, as many as 3000 people die each year from the pollution – a number similar to the number of migrants who stream into the city every day from the Mexican countryside. The young and elderly and those suffering from chest and lung illness are particularly at risk. By the year 2010, the population of Mexico City may have reached 30–40 million. With a massive national foreign debt, the government will be hard pressed to find the resources to tackle air pollution problems quickly and effectively without international assistance.[19]

Western Europe

During some warm summers, ozone reaches exceptional concentrations across many parts of Europe. Ground level ozone concentrations have been increasing by 1–2 per cent annually in Europe in the past few decades.[20] Summer ozone pollution episodes began to be recorded in the Rhine river basin cities of Cologne, Karlsruhe and Mannheim as early as the mid-1970s. This suggests that ozone was contributing to the increasing acid rain damage experienced by German forests during the 1970s. Today, Germany experiences 10–50 days each year when ozone levels exceed the national air quality guideline of 60 ppb (120 μg/m^3) and this frequency increases with altitude such that forested mountain slopes suffer lengthy periods of damaging ozone levels.[21]

---

18 'Central American smog' *The Environmental Digest*, 89/90, Nov/Dec, 1994, p 13

19 References are provided in Chapter 9, where Mexico City's pollution problems are discussed more fully.

20 Lefohn, A S, Shadwick, D S, Fiester, U and Mohnen, V A (1992) 'Surface-level ozone: climate change and evidence for trends' *JAPCA – Journal of Air and Waste Management Association*, vol 42, pp 136–144; UNEP (1993) op cit, pp 17–19

21 Wagner, H M (1990) *Photochemical Smog in Europe: an Overview*, Air Hygiene Report 2, WHO Collaborating Centre for Air Quality Management and Air Pollution Control, Langen, Germany

Like many large cities in the Mediterranean region, Athens, Greece, suffers from severe photochemical pollution episodes (Table 1.1). These smogs have become a worsening problem in the Athens basin since the late 1970s as its population expanded to 4 million. The rising trend in ozone levels of 20 per cent per year in the mid-1980s was among the largest recorded in Europe. In Athens many hundreds of people have been admitted to hospital for heart and respiratory problems during recent smogs when the 'nephos'

Table 1.1 *Indices describing air pollution conditions in selected large European cities*

City	Emission of smog-forming pollutants[a]		Exposure[b]
	Summer smog	Winter smog	City background: SO_2 + SPM
Amsterdam	3*	2*	2
Athens	4	2*	3
Belfast	2*	5	4
Berlin	5	5	4
Brussels	4*	3*	1
Budapest	4*	5*	4
Copenhagen	4	3	n/a
Dresden	2	4*	3
Dublin	2	2	4
Katowice	2	5*	4
Kraków	2	4*	3*
Leipzig	3*	5*	4
London	5*	2	n/a
Lyon	3*	3*	3
Moscow	4	2	2*
Munich	4*	2*	1
Oslo	2	1	2
Paris	5*	3	2
Prague	2	3*	4
Rome	4*	5*	3*
Sofia	3	5	3
Turin	4*	4*	4

* Uncertain data; n/a, data not available.

[a] The emission indices have been ranked in five classes from 'least favourable conditions' (1) to 'most favourable conditions' (5), relative to the average emission conditions in 105 selected European cities for compounds with summer (volatile organic compounds and nitrogen oxides) and winter (sulphur dioxide and suspended particulate matter; SPM) smog-forming potential.

[b] Exposure: 1 = 0–5 per cent population; 2 = 5–33 per cent population; 3 = 33–66 per cent population; and 4 = exceeding 66 per cent.

Source: Data selected from Table 4.4 in Stanners, D and Bourdeau, P (1995) *Europe's Environment: The Dobris Assessment*, European Environment Agency, Copenhagen, p 31

(literally meaning 'cloud') covers the city. At its worst, the nephos is believed to claim six lives a day in Greater Athens, but it is difficult to separate out deaths due to smog and those due to the high temperatures experienced at the same time (eg 43°C during a smog in August 1993). Ozone and nitrogen dioxide from petrol-driven vehicles, together with tiny black smoke particles from diesels, are the worst constituents of the smogs in this city, ringed by mountains on three sides and the Saronikos Bay on the fourth side. The city has become choked with fumes from 800,000 cars and trucks as well as 15,000 antiquated diesel-powered taxis, 5000 poorly maintained buses and 230,000 motorcycles. The acidic pollutants corrode the ancient buildings such as the Acropolis. Many Greeks and foreign tourists flee the capital to avoid the smog. Nitrogen dioxide arising from vehicle emissions creates a particularly serious problem in Athens, with hourly nitrogen dioxide concentrations frequently reaching two or nearly three times the European Union air quality standard of 105 ppb (200 $\mu g/m^3$). Temporary city centre traffic bans (permanent from April 1995), cutbacks in industrial emissions and flexible working hours have had to be introduced during smog alerts as city officials ponder on the best long-term strategy to tackle their air pollution problems.[22]

In Greater London, UK, there have been many spring and summer days since 1988 when ozone levels have exceeded WHO advisory hourly ozone levels of 76–100 ppb (150–200 $\mu g/m^3$). The number of exceedances has been even higher in the suburbs and in rural areas of southern and eastern England than in London's city centre. Nearly one-third of the UK's population is exposed to ozone levels exceeding 90 ppb (180 $\mu g/m^3$) – the level at which the public are required to be informed in accordance with the European Union's Ozone Directive – for at least 20 hours in a year.[23] Pollutants that lead to ozone formation not only drift downwind of London, but may also stream in from continental Europe, as on the hot sunny day of 22 July 1989. On this date, hourly ozone levels reached 112 ppb (224 $\mu g/m^3$) in London, but the highest concentration nationally of 122 ppb (244 $\mu g/m^3$) occurred on the east coast of England exposed to the polluted air arriving from continental Europe. A significant contribution to the UK's ozone problems comes from continental Europe. Contributions from other countries to ozone levels recorded at southern England coastal locations were estimated at about 20 per cent from France, 18 per cent from Germany and 6 per cent from the Netherlands. On some days of high ozone levels the imported contribution can be considerable, as on 6 May 1995 when 48 per cent was estimated to come from France and 26 per cent from Germany.[24]

---

22 References are provided in Chapter 9, where the pollution problems of Athens are examined in detail.

23 UK Photochemical Oxidants Review Group (1993) *Ozone in the UK*, Third Report, Department of the Environment, London

24 Stedman, J R and Williams, M L (1992) 'A trajectory model of the relationship between ozone and precursor emissions', *Atmospheric Environment*, vol 26A, pp 1271–1281

London, once infamous for its winter 'pea soupers' which culminated in the lethal acidic smogs of 1952, 1956, 1957 and 1962, had for some time believed mistakenly that it was free from winter smogs. Certainly, the dense smoky sulphurous fogs of earlier decades caused primarily by open-fire coal burning in residential areas have not returned. Instead increased traffic is to blame for the emergence of cold season smogs of a different kind, namely unhealthy episodes of high levels of nitrogen dioxide, carbon monoxide, fine particulates and benzene. During the cold foggy period of 12–15 December 1991, one-hour levels of nitrogen dioxide peaked at 423 ppb (809 $\mu g/m^3$), greatly exceeding the WHO air quality guideline of 209 ppb (400 $\mu g/m^3$). At the same time levels of benzene, a carcinogenic pollutant released from petrol-engined vehicles, increased by six to seven times its typical value.[25] Subsequently it was shown that 160 extra deaths could be attributed to the smog.[26] Not surprisingly, the leaders of the traffic wardens' union urged in 1991 that members should be given smog masks and shorter times on traffic duty. It is estimated that 8.5 million people live in areas in the UK where the European Union health-based one-hour air quality standard for nitrogen dioxide of 105 ppb (200 $\mu g/m^3$) may be exceeded.[27] Traffic-generated smogs are not restricted to Britain's capital city and on 22–23 December 1992 Manchester experienced a similar smog with hourly nitrogen dioxide and eight-hour carbon monoxide concentrations exceeding air quality guidelines.[28] On 22 December 1994 winter smogs occurred again, with hourly nitrogen dioxide concentrations reaching 288 ppb (551 $\mu g/m^3$) at London Victoria, 198 ppb (379 $\mu g/m^3$) in Birmingham and 170 ppb (325 $\mu g/m^3$) in Manchester.[29]

25 Bower, J (1992) *Initial Analysis of NO_2 Pollution Episode*, December 1991, Warren Spring Laboratory, Stevenage; Quality of Urban Air Review Group (1993) *Urban Air Quality in the UK*, First Report, Department of the Environment, London

26 There were about 1700 deaths in London during the week of 12–16 December 1991, so that the number of deaths caused by the smog was probably about 160. The number of deaths from respiratory diseases, including asthma and severe lung disease, was 22 per cent higher and cardiovascular disease 14 per cent higher than expected during the smog. Brown, W (1994) 'Deaths linked to London smog', *New Scientist*, 25 Jun, p 4

27 Campbell, G W, Cox, J, Downing C E H, Stedman, J R and Stevenson, K (1992) *A Survey of NO_2 Concentrations in the UK Using Diffusion Tubes: July to December 1991*, Report LR 893 (AP), Warren Spring Laboratory, Stevenage; Rowell, A, Holman, C and Soho, S (1992) *Population at Risk from Ambient Air Pollution in England*, Earth Resources Research, London

28 Broughton, G F J (1993) *Initial Analysis of NO_2 Pollution Episode*, December 1992, Warren Spring Laboratory, Stevenage

29 Association of London Government and South East Institute of Public Health (1995) *Air Quality in London 1994*, Second Report of the London Air Quality Network, SEIPH, Tunbridge Wells; 'UK suffers worst smog for three years', *The Environmental Digest*, 89/90, Nov/Dec 1994, p 13; 'Gummer launches air quality initiative', *The Environmental Digest*, 1995/1, Jan, p 12

Sulphur dioxide and smoke pollution arising from domestic coal burning has been largely eliminated as a problem from most British towns as natural gas and electricity have replaced coal as the primary domestic fuel. The exception is Belfast in Northern Ireland which continues to experience relatively high winter sulphur dioxide levels because of the domestic reliance on coal. More than 70 per cent of Belfast householders use coal as their main fuel compared with 12 per cent in Britain as a whole. This situation arises because Belfast householders have little alternative but to use coal. The province has no pipeline supplying natural gas, unlike other areas of Britain, and the production of town gas ceased in the mid-1980s. Current attempts to tackle the problem involve an intensive investment programme to designate the entire city a smokeless zone, to increase the availability of suitable smokeless fuels and to construct a natural gas pipeline from Scotland to Northern Ireland (opening in the spring of 1996).[30] Similar problems exist in Dublin, Ireland. When oil prices were high in the 1970s, the Irish Government encouraged people to switch to solid fuels but failed to foresee the air quality effects of a surge in the number of people burning coal and peat briquettes in their homes. The result has been an increase in winter pollution, with warnings broadcast to people with respiratory diseases to stay indoors during smogs. A costly programme to introduce smokeless zones throughout Dublin has now begun.[31]

The trend towards the greater use of diesel-engined vehicles in Europe has halted and even begun to reverse the downward trend in annual average levels of fine particulates (PM_{10}) in the air of some cities (cities in south east Asia as well as in other parts of The South are already experiencing very poor air quality due to diesel vehicle emissions). The growing sales of diesel vehicles in Europe during the late 1980s and 1990s occurred because of their greater fuel economy and reduced maintenance requirements. They were also promoted as less polluting vehicles by the motor industry and have received favourable encouragement from some governments (eg lower taxes on diesels than petrol-powered vehicles in France). Concern about diesels is now growing because of the fine black smoke they emit, frequently less than 1 μm in diameter. This means the particulates can penetrate deep into the lungs. These particles are recognised carriers of a group of chemical

30 In the UK in 1990–1991, the only exceedance of the European Union sulphur dioxide air quality limit took place in Belfast, where the 98th centile of daily means was 141 ppb (374 μg/m^3). Hourly values of sulphur dioxide reached 550 ppb (1462 μg/m^3) in December 1991. Quality of Urban Air Review Group (1993) *Urban Air Quality in the UK*, First Report, Department of the Environment, London, p 66

31 Cooke, K (1988) 'Dubliners depressed under a descending curtain of smog', *Financial Times*, 1 Dec; Nijkamp, P and Perrels, A (1994) *Sustainable Cities in Europe*, Earthscan, London, pp 76–78; Meskill, D (1989) 'Severe smog problems in Dublin', *Journal of Meteorology, UK*, vol 14 (136), p 64; 'Not such a fair city' *Clean Air*, vol 18 (4), 1988, pp 195–196; 'Dublin smog' *Clean Air*, vol 19 (4), 1989, p 188

compounds known as polyaromatic hydrocarbons (PAHs), including benzene. Rising levels of fine particulates may be increasing the incidence of cancer in urban areas.

Summer or winter smogs can occur in many European cities at the same time if an anticyclone covering the entire continent traps pollutants below a low-level temperature inversion, causing the air to stagnate and pollution levels to escalate. During the summers of 1994 and 1995 smog alerts were issued in many cities across Europe. On 1 July 1994, the UK Government's Department of the Environment suggested the ozone pollution episode was the worst since 1990 and people were asked not to drive unless they had to.[32] The European Union requires a public health warning to be issued if hourly ozone concentrations exceed 180 ppb (360 $\mu g/m^3$) and in Paris during 1994 this occurred 16 times.[33] (More than 70 cities in western Europe were subjected to one or more ozone pollution episodes between May and August in 1995.) In late January and early February 1989, at the same time that Paris suffered several days of an 'alerte du smog' as the temperature inversion trapped car exhaust pollutants, similar smogs occurred in Geneva, Milan, Madrid and London. In Milan, levels of sulphur dioxide and nitrogen dioxide reached such unhealthy levels that the mayor appealed for residents to turn down their central heating systems and avoid using their cars unless it was essential to do so. Smog conditions even extended as far east as Bursa, in Turkey, where industrial plants, many burning low-grade lignite, and schools were closed and traffic restricted in an attempt to lessen the smog which had already caused a rise in the number of deaths due to respiratory disease.[34] December 1992 and January 1993 produced further European-wide smogs, with vehicle restrictions enforced in Athens, 11 Italian cities and Madrid (where restrictions on the number of hours when central heating could be switched on were imposed).[35]

Several times during cold winters in the mid- and late 1980s, the worst occurring in January 1985, February 1987 and November/December 1989, many German cities were blanketed for several days by a dense smog which triggered alerts, requiring schools to be closed, traffic to be banned from city centres and industry to reduce emissions. Although German cars and factories contributed to the smog, the main blame focused on eastern Europe, where power stations burned highly polluting lignite and where

32 'Smog alerts across Europe', *The Environmental Digest*, 83/84, May/Jun 1994, p 16

33 Patel, T (1995) 'Paris chokes while officials fiddle', *New Scientist*, 29 Jul, p 9

34 Eskikaya, T, Kural, O and Ekinci, E (1989) 'Fluidised bed combustion systems reached commercial applications in Turkey', in Brasser, L J and Mulder W C (eds) *Man and His Ecosystem, Proceedings of the 8th World Clean Air Congress 1989*, The Hague, The Netherlands, Sep 1989, vol 5, pp 147–151; 'Foggy days, everywhere but in London town', *The Times*, 7 Feb 1989; 'Smog cloud: Ankara', *The Independent*, 21 Jan 1989

35 'European cities' action on traffic pollution', *The Environmental Digest*, 67, Jan 1993, p 13

industry lacked even the most basic pollution control technology. It was shown that pollution had drifted slowly westwards from eastern Europe, causing severe smogs throughout German cities. Countries such as Belgium, France and the Netherlands also suffered a rapid deterioration of their air quality as the smog cloud, laden with pollutants from eastern Europe and the highly urban–industrialized Ruhr, drifted across their countries. As much as 70 per cent of the sulphur dioxide pollution to which the Belgian population was subjected during such episodes came from outside its borders. This highlights the ineffectiveness of one's own national pollution control policies when faced with a massive influx of pollution from neighbouring countries. In this situation Belgium failed to meet European Union air quality standards through no fault of its own.[36]

Eastern Europe

After the introduction of glasnost (openness) in the former Soviet Union in the mid-1980s and the widespread political changes in eastern Europe in 1989 and 1990, socialist countries began to admit to experiencing horrendous environmental problems. The previous decades of secrecy, during which the governments made frequent claims that it was the western world's capitalist mode of production rather than the socialist approach that created pollution, had concealed the truth about air pollution problems. Today, 110 million Russians breathe air laden with five times, sometimes even ten times, as much pollution as the country's regulations permit. Pollution is particularly bad in Aleksandrovsk–Sakhalinsky, St Petersburg, Volvograd, Moscow, Vyborg and Magnitogorsk. In Kiev, Ukraine, high levels of industrial and traffic pollutants are blamed for the rising trend of lung

---

36 Laxen, D (1989) 'Winter smogs return to London?', *London Environmental Bulletin*, autumn, pp 6–7; Lubkert, B (1989) 'Characteristics of the mid-January 1985 sulphur dioxide smog episode in central Europe', *Atmospheric Environment*, vol 23, pp 611–623; Simpson, D, Davies, S, Gooriah, B D and McInnes, G (1987) 'Pollution levels in the UK during 14–22 January 1985', *Atmospheric Environment*, vol 21, pp 2495–2503. During the bitterly cold January 1985 episode, daily concentrations of sulphur dioxide exceeded 376 ppb (1000 μg/m^3) and suspended particulates exceeded 500 μg/m^3 in some German locations. Interestingly, air quality levels in the UK were not as bad as elsewhere in Europe during this episode. This was due not only to being more distant from the eastern European sources producing the pollution which drifted across western Europe, but because coal burning in the UK was exceptionally low during this period of subfreezing temperatures. Coal burning was reduced because the National Union of Miners were on strike and the government switched electricity generation, using the national electricity grid, from the coal-burning power stations located near the coalfields to remote oil-burning power stations using fuel oil which had a lower sulphur content than coal. Inadvertently, this action highlighted the national air quality benefits to be gained from generating electricity by fuel switching. Since that episode the contraction of the coal industry due to the preference among privatised electricity-generating companies for cheaper and cleaner natural gas has demonstrated further the air quality improvements resulting from fuel switching.

disease, allergies and cancer, whereas deaths among children have risen between 1.3 and 2.2 times in the past decade.[37] However, the worst pollution legacy of socialism is surely the region ominously known as the 'black triangle' ('sulphur triangle' or even 'death triangle'), composed of the northern Czech Republic, southern Poland and the southern part of former East Germany. Massive deposits of poor quality, highly polluting lignite (soft brown coal) are exploited for energy production and industrial processing with almost no effective pollution controls. The air pollution problems are exceptionally severe at times, with the population living in close proximity to a wide range of dirty factories, power stations and chemical plants which use obsolete technology and processes.

Lignite is characterised by having a high sulphur and ash content and is of such low calorific value that vast quantities have to be burned compared with, say, anthracite or bituminous coal. Some cities in the 'black triangle' suffer dangerously high sulphur dioxide concentrations throughout the entire winter, with several days experiencing 24-hour values exceeding 188 ppb (500 $\mu g/m^3$). In December 1989, daily sulphur dioxide levels reached 414–940 ppb (1100–2500 $\mu g/m^3$) in four cities in the southern part of eastern Germany (the WHO suggests 38–56 ppb or 100–150 $\mu g/m^3$ as an air quality guideline). Similar or worse concentrations of sulphur dioxide and suspended particulates are endured in southern Poland and the northern Czech Republic. Such extreme smogs are comparable with those which took place in London and New York in the 1950s and 1960s, causing large increases in mortality and morbidity.

In Kraków, in Poland, the vast Nowa Huta (now Sedzimir) steelworks built in the 1950s lies in the suburbs of this historical city. Vegetables grown in and around the city are so contaminated by heavy metals such as cadmium released from industrial plants (and arsenic released when lignite is burned) and lead from motor vehicles that residents are told not to eat them. However, Poland's food distribution system is so poor that residents have little choice but to do so. The problem extends to many areas of Poland. A study of vegetables from Warsaw's Ochota district showed they contained 16 mg of lead per kg – eight times higher than the maximum safety level specified by the WHO. Even a decline in industrial production and the recent closures of outdated polluting industrial plants in Poland cannot solve the problem of contaminated foods as the soils retain heavy metals for a long time. In 1993 the government declared the city of Kraków a 'disaster zone'.[38]

---

37 Feshback, M and Friendly, A (1992) *Ecocide in the USSR*, Aurum; Shahgedanova, M and Burt, T P (1994) 'New data on air pollution in the former Soviet Union', *Global Environmental Change*, vol 4, pp 201–207; 'Russian pollution records', *The Environmental Digest*, 71, May 1993, p 13; 'Kiev health problems', *The Environmental Digest*, 74, Aug 1993, p 12

38 Fischhoff, B (1991) 'Report from Poland' *Environment*, vol 33, pp 12–17 & 37; 'Polish lead pollution revealed', *The Environmental Digest*, 57, Mar 1992, p 12; 'Krakow appeals for help', *The Environmental Digest*, 71, May 1993, p 13

In 1991 Poland adopted a national pollution control strategy for the next 30 years, initially aimed at tackling the worst industrial polluters through higher emission charges and fines for exceeding permitted levels. This would then progress to adopting cleaner technologies such as coal-cleaning, flue-gas scrubbers and fluidised bed combustion systems to reduce sulphur dioxide and suspended particulates emitted from the burning of lignite and poor quality coals, for which there is no realistic alternative fuel in the country. There are some signs of improvement, with concentrations of suspended particulates decreasing by more than half between 1992 and 1994 and those of sulphur dioxide by more than 40 per cent. Even so, levels of most pollutants remain unacceptably high, and some of the improvements are due to industrial recession and may be lost when industrial output recovers. Poland faces a formidable problem. Without substantial international assistance, Poland's goal of healthy air quality is likely to take more than the target time-scale of 30 years.[39]

Prague, the capital of the Czech Republic, is another eastern European city that has been declared a 'disaster zone', with 20 times the permitted levels of sulphur dioxide in the atmosphere in winter. The children of Prague are sent to the country for at least one month every year, whereas doctors recommend expectant mothers to evacuate the city for the duration of their pregnancy. At Most, 80 km (50 miles) north of Prague in northern Bohemia, the authorities resorted to the desperate measure of distributing 20,000 smog masks to children in December 1990 to help them survive the occurrence of severe air pollution in this heavily industrialized city. In the city of Decin, northern Bohemia, where sulphur dioxide levels sometimes reach ten times WHO guidelines, child mortality is twice the national average and the daily number of children admitted to hospital with serious respiratory problems simply reflects the changing daily levels of sulphur dioxide concentrations. During a smog episode in northern Bohemia in February 1993, daily average sulphur dioxide levels exceeded 150 ppb (400 $\mu g/m^3$) at Most and Chomutov, 226 ppb (600 $\mu g/m^3$) at Usti n Labem and over 300 ppb (800 $\mu g/m^3$) near Teplice – more than six times the WHO (European) guidelines. As has happened in Poland, pollution problems have improved slightly in recent years due to a fall in industrial output and some measures to tackle pollution (eg fitting flue-gas scrubbers, use of natural gas instead of lignite). This gives hope to the residents of Teplice that days such as occurred during the late 1980s when sulphur dioxide levels reached 1128 ppb (3000 $\mu g/m^3$) will not happen again.[40]

39 Andersson, M (1992) 'Poland: radical policy reform' *Acid News*, 3, Jun, pp 1, 3–4; Bates, R, Cofala, J and Toman, M (1994) *Alternative Policies for the Control of Air Pollution in Poland*, World Bank Environment Paper 7, World Bank, Washington DC, 84 pp; Hlawiczka, S (1995) 'Poland: positive trends now appearing', *Acid News*, 3, Jun, pp 12–13

40 Kiernan, V (1994) 'US trades green points in Bohemia', *New Scientist*, 7 May, p 5 (includes a graph highlighting the relationship between hospital admissions and sulphur dioxide levels); Plaminkova, J (1995) 'North Bohemia: after five years',

In Chomutov, Czech Republic, smog alerts are regularly issued each winter. Schools keep children indoors and the children are given vitamin tablets to fortify them against the poisonous air, told to walk home slowly and not to play outdoors after school. A total of 20,000 smog masks was distributed to children in an attempt to offer some protection. In recent years there has been a 50 per cent increase in bronchitis and lung infections among babies and young children. Many other northern Bohemian industrialized cities suffer similar pollution problems, especially aggravated by being located in the bottoms of valleys. When a temperature inversion occurs, in which warm air lies above cold air, it acts as a lid to the vertical movement of pollutants and traps the pollutants in the valley below it, allowing a rapid build-up of pollution concentrations. At weekends the city residents escape into the mountains to enjoy the sunshine, while only a few hundred metres below lies their city encased in a cold, highly polluted fog. Payments are made to anyone who moves to the region and remains there for ten years. The government calls it 'stabilizing payment', but the locals call it 'burial money' as the life expectancy of residents in the cities of northern Bohemia is estimated to be 3–4 years less than the rest of the country.[41] During the Chomutov sulphurous smog of February 1993 the local authorities threatened to close the town to all traffic and call a general strike unless the government agreed to fit all power stations in the region with flue-gas desulphurisation equipment within two years. Children were told not to go to school and pregnant women were evacuated. Power stations were ordered to reduce output by about half, with electricity being imported from elsewhere in eastern Europe to meet demand.[42]

It is recognised that pollution levels could be drastically reduced if power stations used hard coal rather than lignite, but the Czech Electricity Company has resisted because of its higher cost. Nuclear power offers an alternative, albeit an expensive one, but the Chernobyl nuclear reactor fire and the resulting radioactive contamination of most European countries in April 1986 has shaken the public's confidence in the safety of nuclear reactors. Nevertheless, the 2000 MW Temelin reactor received the go-ahead in 1993 because of the severe pollution problems posed by emissions from the fossil-fuelled power stations.

Ironically, one part of eastern Europe has received massive financial help in tackling its pollution problems: the former East Germany. The reunification of Germany in October 1990 has meant that the strict emission

---

Acid News, 1, Feb, pp 1, 3–4; Stanners, D and Bourdeau, P (1995) *Europe's Environment: the Dobris Assessment*, European Environment Agency, Copenhagen (Figure 4.4 presents the spatial pattern of average daily sulphur dioxide levels during the February 1993 episode in northern Bohemia).

41 Glenny, M (1987) 'Czechoslovakia: living in a smog', *Acid News*, 4, Dec, pp 9–11; Havlicek, P (1993) 'The environmental situation in the Czech and Slovak Republics', *Environmental Policy Review*, 7, 42–56

42 'Bohemian pollution national disaster', *The Environmental Digest*, 68, Feb 1993, p 13

and air quality standards of the former West Germany and the European Union have been applied. This has resulted in a major reduction in pollution emissions through the closure of outdated inefficient industrial plants, together with a huge investment in pollution control equipment for existing industry. Generally, the changeover of eastern Europe from state socialism to free market economies has doubtless improved the chances of better air quality. Previous negligence of pollution problems and the suppression of public complaints about those problems is being replaced by positive actions to deal with them. The situation in Poland and the Czech Republic remains dire, but a serious commitment to improving air quality has now been made. In 1995, Poland, the Czech Republic and Hungary decided to work towards bringing their environmental legislation into compliance with that of the European Union by 2000, the year by which they hope to have formalised their accession.

Africa

Only five African cities rank in the list of 69 cities with populations exceeding 3 million. These are Alexandria and Cairo in Egypt, Algiers in Algeria, Casablanca in Morocco and Lagos in Nigeria. Cairo, with 9 million people, is the largest city in Africa and it experiences severe sulphur dioxide pollution with levels reaching five times the WHO annual mean guidelines in the city centre. The causes of this problem are the large emissions from the city's power stations (burning heavy fuel oil), the chemical and motor vehicle manufacturing industries, and the diesel-engined buses and cars which congest the city centre. Levels of suspended particulates are also a problem (in October 1993, smoke alarms in the Spanish Embassy were claimed to have been triggered by outdoor pollution). Particulates are emitted from poorly maintained diesel-engined vehicles, cement factories, iron and steel works, construction activities and from the open burning of rubbish. The dry desert climate leads to large amounts of wind-blown dust being added to the urban atmosphere.[43]

Many African towns and cities, like other cities in The South, are growing in a rapid and uncontrolled way. Only limited controls are applied to new and expanding industrial sources of pollution, many of them relatively small scale and energy-inefficient. The number of motor vehicles is increasing greatly and exhaust emission limits are often absent, weak or poorly enforced. The haphazard way in which shantytowns become established and expand usually means electricity supplies to homes are absent or inadequate. This results in poor quality fuels being used for household cooking and heating, so creating severe localised air pollution. The growing

43 UNEP (1992) *Urban Air Pollution in Megacities of the World*, WHO/UNEP, Blackwell, Oxford, pp 19, 81–90; UNEP/WHO (1993) *City Air Quality Trends (GEMS/AIR Data)*, vol 2, UNEP, Nairobi, pp 13–16; 'Cairo pollution triggers alarm', *The Environmental Digest*, 76, Oct 1993, p 14

size of shantytowns is illustrated by Soweto (an acronymic contraction of SOuth WEst TOwnship), not far from Johannesburg in South Africa, which has a population of around 3.5 million – with a newborn child arriving every five minutes. As they are located in tropical and sub-tropical climates, most African cities receive high amounts of insolation, which means that as vehicle emissions increase rapidly in the future the potential to create photochemical smog is great.[44]

Australasia

Photochemical smog arising from traffic-generated pollutant emissions is a significant problem in the largest cities of Australia and New Zealand. Sydney, Australia, with a population of nearly 4 million, began to suffer photochemical smogs as early as the 1970s. Since then it has been necessary to warn the public when high ozone levels are present as this pollutant causes irritation of the eyes, nose and throat as well as affecting the lung function. Sydney suffers the highest nitrogen dioxide and suspended particulate levels of any Australian city and its air quality is now considered worse than New York or Tokyo. The air quality situation in some cities is aggravated by diurnal sea breeze circulations which transport precursor pollutants offshore during the night and bring them back over the city the next morning to add to that day's pollution load. Adelaide and Melbourne in Australia suffer occasional episodes of high levels of suspended particulates due to dust storms and bushfires. Christchurch, New Zealand, a city of around a third of a million people, no longer suffers from serious pollution from industrial and domestic sources, but its lack of attention to the rise in vehicle emissions has resulted in a growing problem of carbon monoxide and other vehicle pollutants in its city centre streets.[45]

Asia

Some cities in the People's Republic of China are so thickly covered with air pollution that they are not visible on satellite photographs. The cities of Beijing, Guangzhou, Shanghai, Shenyang and Xian are among the world's ten worst cities for air pollution. Smogs occur on almost two out of every three days in the city of Shenyang, a city of 3 million people, due to

44 Dutkiewicz, R K, Ballard, R H and Loewenheim, L (1989) 'Photochemical smog potential in South Africa', in Brasser, L J and Mulder W C (eds) *Man and His Ecosystem, Proceedings of the 8th World Clean Air Congress 1989*, The Hague, The Netherlands, Sep 1989, vol 5, pp 413–417; Murley, L (1995) *Clean Air Around the World*, third edition, International Union of Air Pollution Prevention Associations, Brighton, pp 307–314

45 Bridgman, H (1990) *Global Air Pollution*, Belhaven, London, pp 204–208; Hess, G D (1989) 'Simulation of photochemical smog in the Melbourne airshed: worst case studies' *Atmospheric Environment*, vol 23, pp 661–669; Murley, L (1995) op cit, pp 1–41, 257–261; UNEP/WHO (1993) op cit, pp 21–24; 'As an air of malaise settles on the cities', *New Scientist*, 26 Sep 1992, p 10

uncontrolled industrial emissions arising from burning poor quality coal and from the growing numbers of highly polluting vehicles. It is claimed that relatively few industrial plants are fitted with pollution control systems and that many of those that have such controls operate them only when inspectors call to save on energy costs. In 1990, 2000 deaths were attributed to air pollution and over 3500 working years were lost in Shenyang due to illness. Pollution is implicated in a recent surge in birth defects and a life expectancy that is ten years less than the national average. Beijing, Shenyang and Xian experience an average of over 200 days each year when suspended particulate levels pose a risk to health. In 1991 in Shenyang, annual levels of suspended particulates in the city centre were over four times the WHO guidelines and sulphur dioxide more than three times. In January 1991, daily sulphur dioxide levels exceeded 338 ppb (900 $\mu g/m^3$) – six times the WHO guidelines. The most common cause of death in China as a whole is now respiratory illness brought on by air pollution.[46]

Bangkok, Thailand, is a city of over 7 million people and expanding rapidly. It is one of the world's fastest growing markets for cars. With 2 million vehicles the city is suffering severe air pollution, with smoke from vehicles so bad that reductions in visibility are a driving hazard. The authorities estimated in 1990 that 900,000 of the city's inhabitants suffered chronic respiratory problems and other illnesses caused by air pollution and that air pollution causes 1400 deaths each year. The World Bank estimated that the average child in the city has lost four IQ points by the age of seven because of elevated exposure to lead.[47] Seoul, Republic of Korea, a city with over 11 million people, faces serious pollution problems arising from the dominance of coal briquettes for household heating and cooking and because of pollutant emissions from nearly 3 million motor vehicles. Half of all motor vehicles are fuelled by diesel, which results in substantial emissions of fine particulates. Sulphur dioxide and suspended particulates in the city regularly exceed the WHO annual mean air quality guidelines.[48]

Traffic pollution is a growing problem in many Asian cities. In Tehran, Iran, in February 1991 a state of emergency was declared due to smog and people were asked to stop using their cars and to stay at home as nitrogen dioxide

---

46 Leijonhufvud, G (1994) 'China: heavily polluted air in steel city', *Acid News*, 2, Apr, p 11; UNEP (1988) *Assessment of Urban Air Quality*, UNEP/WHO, Monitoring and Assessment Research Centre, London; UNEP/WHO (1993) op cit, pp 43–47 (Shenyang); 'Health costs of Chinese pollution', *The Environmental Digest*, 56, Feb 1992, p 12; 'China choking on industrial waste', *The Environmental Digest*, 1995/1, p 12; 'Chinese pollution rather serious', *The Environmental Digest*, 1995/3, pp 12–13

47 Hunt, P (1992) 'Catalysts make converts in the Far East' *New Scientist*, 11 Jul, p 9; Hunt, P (1992) 'Far East: catalyzers making converts in four cities', *Acid News*, 4, Oct, p 10; Mallet, V (1993) 'Asian city pollution at danger levels', *Financial Times*, 25 Oct; 'Bangkok faces serious pollution', *The Environmental Digest*, 57, Mar 1992, p 11; 'Thailand attempts to limit cars', *The Environmental Digest*, 86, Aug 1994, p 15

48 UNEP (1992) op cit, pp 32, 195–202

levels rose to 23 times the permissible levels.[49] Tehran faces enormous problems in tackling air pollution and they may become worse as population growth indicates it may become the world's seventh largest city by 2010. In Istanbul, Turkey, sulphur dioxide levels reached seven times WHO guidelines in January 1994, requiring the imposition of 'anti-smog' restrictions, as also happened in December 1994.[50]

Cities in Bangladesh, India and Pakistan bustle with people and traffic. Delhi, the capital of India, suffers the problems of overcrowding and traffic congestion from 9 million people and nearly 2 million vehicles, three-quarters of which are two- or three-wheeled vehicles. Half the buses and trucks and all the three-wheeled vehicles (called tempoes), many of them old and poorly maintained, exceeded the recommended exhaust emission standards in 1988. With the government admitting to 5000 noxious industries in the capital, 868 of which are within the walled city itself, industrial emissions affect most of the residents, including emissions of chlorine from 28 large industries. The rapid industrial expansion taking place in and around the city suggests that air quality is likely to deteriorate markedly during the next decade unless strict pollution controls are enforced. Similar situations apply in Calcutta (where it is estimated that 60 per cent of residents suffer from respiratory diseases related to air pollution) and Bombay, whereas three more cities, Dacca, Karachi and Bangalore, are expected to expand to more than 8 million people by the start of the twenty-first century.[51] Air pollution is damaging India's most famous monument, the Taj Mahal at Agra. Nearby cities contain more than 2000 polluting industries ranging from brick kilns to an oil refinery, as well as traffic using high-sulphur diesel fuel. Acidic emissions of sulphur dioxide and nitrogen dioxide are eroding and dissolving the marble monument. Environmentalists argued that polluting industries should be moved out of the area, but this was rejected by the government who opted for introducing the use of cleaner fuels (eg natural gas for industry and low-sulphur fuel for diesel vehicles) in the vicinity instead.[52]

---

49 'Pollution brings Tehran to a standstill', *The Environmental Digest*, 44, Feb 1991, p 13

50 'Restrictions placed after Istanbul smog', *The Environmental Digest*, 79, Jan 1994, p 12; 'Smog alert in Turkey', *The Environmental Digest*, 89/90, Nov/Dec 1994, p 13 (chapter note 34 refers to the smog in Turkey in 1989)

51 Hardoy, J E, Mitlin, D and Satterthwaite, D (1992) *Environmental Problems in Third World Cities*, Earthscan, London, pp 84 and 85; Mangla, B (1988) 'Environmental problems of Delhi: mounting concern', *Ambio*, vol 17, pp 350–351; Singh, M P, Goyal, P, Basu, S, Agarwal, P, Nigam, S, Kumari, M and Panwar, T S (1990) 'Predicted and measured concentrations of traffic carbon monoxide over Delhi' *Atmospheric Environment*, 24A, pp 801–810; Sinha, R J (1993) 'Automotive pollution in India and its human impact', *The Environmentalist*, vol 13, pp 111–115; UNEP (1992) op cit (refers to Bombay, Calcutta, Delhi and Karachi); UNEP/WHO (1992) op cit, pp 17–20 (Bombay)

52 'Plan to limit Taj Mahal damage', *The Environmental Digest*, 1995/2, p 12; 'Taj Mahal rescue plan', *The Environmental Digest*, 1995/3, p 13

Residents of some Asian cities and in those elsewhere in The South may also be exposed to many hazardous industrial pollutants. The worst situation occurs when city authorities fail to segregate potentially dangerous industrial plants from residential areas or, if they do designate a safe (unpopulated) zone around the plant, then fail to prevent the encroachment of shantytowns. This leads to the population adjacent to industrial plants facing the risk of being exposed to accidental leaks of toxic emissions such as ammonia, chlorine and hydrogen sulphide as well as to the effects of a fire or explosion within the plant. When these industrial plants are owned by foreign companies, often attracted by lax or ineffectively applied environmental and safety standards, the possibilities of an air pollution disaster increase. Nowhere was this more evident than in Bhopal in India in December 1984. A leakage from the Union Carbide plant manufacturing pesticides created a lethal cloud of methyl isocyanate gas which crept across a densely populated area, initially causing stinging eyes followed by breathing difficulties and suffocation due to the lungs becoming full of liquid (pulmonary oedema). The Bhopal disaster left 3300 people dead, 30,000 with permanent injuries, mainly to eyes, lungs and stomach, and more than 150,000 with minor or short-term illnesses. The death and injury toll continues to rise a decade afterwards as lung diseases worsen and as new illnesses develop, such as mouth cancer, kidney and liver damage, cataracts and the breakdown of immune systems, which increases the susceptibility to common diseases such as tuberculosis and influenza.[53]

Some Asian cities and countries have made great strides in improving air quality, although only after air pollution problems reached disastrous levels. With the industry and economy of Japan in ruins in 1945, the country set about securing rapid economic growth with little thought given to the environmental consequences. Following a series of water and air pollution disasters in the 1960s and early 1970s, the government finally accepted the need to tackle pollution by the mid-1970s. Tokyo's air pollution problems had become so serious that schoolchildren were collapsing in playgrounds and coin-operated oxygen machines were installed on pavements for pedestrians. Soon after, pollution became a 'social crime' and air quality has improved greatly due to strictly applied policies of switching fuels from coal to low-sulphur oil, the widespread installation of pollution control equipment in industry, an efficient network of electric railways and subways, the reduction in the maximum lead content of petrol and the introduction of unleaded petrol in 1975. Dramatic decreases in sulphur dioxide, suspended particulates and airborne lead concentrations have been

---

53 Kayastha, S L and Nag, P (1989) 'The Bhopal disaster', in Clarke, J I, Curson, P, Kayastha, S L and Nag, P (eds) *Population and Disaster*, Blackwell, Oxford, pp 206–218; Shrivastava, P (1992) *Bhopal: Anatomy of a Crisis*, second edition, Paul Chapman, London; Marshall, V C (1987) *Major Chemical Hazards*, Ellis Horwood, Chichester, pp 372–379; Walker, G (1990) 'Bhopal: five years on', *Geography*, vol 75 (2), pp 158–160

achieved in this city of over 20 million people. Today, the main air quality problems are high levels of nitrogen dioxide and ozone due to an increase in the number and use of vehicles, especially diesel-powered trucks. Consequently, it remains necessary to operate a smog alert system to warn the public and to apply short-term measures to reduce industrial and traffic emissions during stable weather conditions.[54]

Conclusions: a Cocktail of Pollutant Threats

This brief world survey highlights the fact that far too many of the world's urban areas are experiencing serious air pollution problems. The polluted urban atmospheres that most of us breathe are cocktails of many different pollutants. The threat that each pollutant (or combination of pollutants) poses to our health and well-being depends on the type and concentration of the pollutants present, the length of time we are exposed to the pollutants and the state of our own health. The next two chapters examine and explain the degree of risk to health that pollutants pose.

54 Komeiji, T, Aoki, K, Koyama, I and Okita, T (1990) 'Trends of air quality and atmospheric deposition in Tokyo', *Atmospheric Environment*, 24A, 2099–2103; Murley, L (1995) op cit, pp 193–210; UNEP (1992) op cit, pp 34, 211–218; UNEP/WHO (1992) op cit, pp 37–40 (Tokyo)

Chapter 2

People at Risk: Setting Protective Air Quality Standards

Breathing Polluted Air

Inhalation of Pollutants An active person typically inhales 10,000 to 20,000 litres of air each day – approximately 7 to 14 litres every minute – drawing in life-giving oxygen. This intake increases with vigorous exercise such that a jogger may inhale up to 3000 litres per hour. As air is taken into the body, so too are particulate and gaseous pollutants. During inhalation and exhalation these pollutants can inflame, sensitise and even scar the lungs and tissues. If the pollutants reach the 300 million tiny air sacs deep inside the lungs called alveoli which create a surface area the size of a tennis court across which respiratory gas exchange takes place, then they may enter the bloodstream, thus affecting organs other than the lungs and they can take up permanent residence. At rest a child under 3 years of age inhales twice as much air per unit body weight than an adult and as their airways are narrower any constriction due to irritation by air pollutants is likely to result in breathing problems. As their lungs are still developing, long-term effects are likely to be worse, causing life-long problems.[1]

Severity of Effects Pollutants affect health in varying degrees of severity, ranging from minor irritation through serious illness to premature death in extreme cases. Health effects depend on the type and amount of pollutants present, the duration of exposure, and the state of health, age and level of activity of the person exposed. Pollutants may produce immediate (acute) symptoms as well as longer term (chronic) effects. Serious acute illnesses

---

1 In addition to the health effects caused by inhaling pollutants, some air pollutants affect health through direct contact with the skin and through ingestion of food and drink contaminated by pollutants.

may be reversible, whereas chronic illness implies a continuing state of ill health which might be moderated but not easily cured. Chronic illness may predispose a person to acute morbidity. Poor air quality affects health in many different ways. Some pollutants can cause headaches, tiredness, nausea and irritation of the eyes, nose and throat. They can sensitise the respiratory tract to asthma and hay fever, with the symptoms being triggered by common allergens such as pollens. Pollutants can worsen heart and lung disease and contribute to the development of such diseases as bronchitis, emphysema and cancer. They can add stress to the cardiovascular system, forcing the heart and lungs to work harder for the same effect. Some pollutants can damage the cells of the airways of the respiratory system, reducing the ability to clear foreign bodies, including bacteria, from the lungs, so weakening their defences against infection. They can reduce the lungs' ability to exhale air, which in terms of loss of lung capacity is part of the body's natural ageing process, but exposure to air pollution speeds up this process.

Air Pollution and Asthma There is current concern that worsening air quality may be causing an increase in both the incidence and severity of allergies in children in that the lungs of children exposed to high levels of pollution become sensitised to react to hay fever and to asthma triggers (allergens). Pollutants may cause a direct irritant effect on the respiratory airways, a toxic effect aggravating existing asthma, and may modify and weaken the immune response to inhaled allergens, so lowering the body's threshold to other irritants. The death rate from asthma has increased 40–60 per cent during the past ten years in countries such as Australia, Canada, France, the UK and the US.[2] Asthma is regarded as the most common disease in the western world. It is often the most common cause of hospital admission among 1–4 year olds and is responsible for about a quarter of school days lost through illness. One in seven children in the UK now suffer persistent wheezing and a wide range of indicators, such as the number of cases of asthma reported to doctors, the total cost of prescriptions for asthma (eg drugs to widen the airways during attacks) and the number of hospital treatments for asthma, have all shown a rising trend since the end of the 1970s which cannot be explained entirely by better diagnosis or greater public awareness of the disease.[3]

---

2 For example, according to the US Centre for Disease Control, deaths from asthma increased by 40 per cent in the US between 1982 and 1991. In 1991, 63 per cent of Americans who had asthma lived in areas that failed federal air quality standards. This implicates air pollution as a possible cause of the increase, but making buildings more airtight may also have played a part as such buildings seal in dust mites and other allergens; 'Asthma alert', *New Scientist*, 14 Jan 1995, p 11

3 House of Commons Transport Committee (1994) *Transport-related Air Pollution in London*, vol 2, HMSO, London, pp 131–142; Parliamentary Office of Science and Technology (POST) (1994) *Breathing in Our Cities*, POST, House of Commons, London

Pollutants believed to sensitise people to asthma include sulphur dioxide, ozone, acid aerosols, fine particulates (PM_{10}) and nitrogen dioxide.[4] There are many compounding factors involved in outbreaks of asthma. For example, the UK asthma outbreak of 24 June 1994, described by one doctor as 'equivalent of an air crash near every hospital', occurred during a day of exceptional thunderstorms across the country. A possible scenario was that high pollution levels in previous weeks sensitised people's lungs to high pollen and fungal spore counts stirred up by the gusty wind conditions.[5] The recent realisation that air pollution plays a major part in exacerbating asthma has profound implications for earlier studies. It is possible that early epidemiological studies of pollution–health relationships which attributed increased mortality during, say, the London 1952 smog to the deaths of patients with bronchitis may have failed to recognise that a large proportion of these patients were actually suffering from asthma.

Problems of Causality and Which Pollutants Are to Blame It is not always clear which pollutants are to blame for an adverse health response in an individual or group of people as the ambient urban atmosphere contains many different pollutants in varying amounts. For example, a study of 944 bridge and tunnel workers in New York City showed that tunnel workers had a significantly worse lung function and increased incidence of respiratory illness than bridge workers. Although this suggested that vehicle pollutants were damaging the health of the workers, it was not possible to conclude which pollutant (or specific combination of pollutants) and which concentrations were responsible. In Naples in December 1993, 130 people sought hospital treatment for breathing problems, coughs, irritated eyes and asthma-like symptoms. Nitrogen dioxide from car exhausts was believed to be the culprit, causing Naples to be closed to most private transport for one day. Subsequently, it was then found that the health problems were more likely to have been triggered by dust containing fungi from a shipload of soybeans being unloaded at the port at the time. However, the elevated nitrogen dioxide levels may have sensitised people to the soybean dust.[6] American research has suggested that nitrogen dioxide and ozone may work in combination on a diurnal basis to irritate the lungs of sensitive people. Nitrogen dioxide is highest during the morning rush hour and this initiates the irritation of the respiratory organs. Later in the day the increased level of ozone has a stronger effect on the mucous membranes of the respiratory

4 Devalia, J L, Wang, J H, Rusznak, C, Calderon, M and Davies, R J (1994) 'Does air pollution enhance the human airway response to allergies?' *ACI News*, vol 6 (3), pp 80–84; Rusznak, C, Devalia, J I and Davies, R J (1994) 'The impact of pollution on allergic disease', *Allergy*, vol 49, pp 21–27

5 'UK pollution outbreaks raise asthma concern', *The Environmental Digest*, 85, Jul 1994, pp 12–13

6 'Soybean dust causes Naples air pollution', *The Environmental Digest*, 77/78, Nov/Dec 1993, p 16

system and so accelerates the inflammation. Such people are then very sensitised to pollen and other allergens.[7]

Cost of Health Effects of Pollutants The direct health care costs of treating people affected by air pollution and the decreased work productivity due to illness is enormous. The American Lung Association estimated that the health care costs in the US amounted to $16 billion and decreased work productivity added another $24 billion, to make a total cost of $40 billion for exposure to the six atmospheric pollutants for which national air quality standards have been set.[8] Assessments of the health benefits to be gained through an improvement in air quality can provide powerful support for those advocating the need for costly pollution control policies and measures. For example, a World Bank study of Bangkok, Thailand, in 1994 showed that a 20 per cent reduction in levels of lead, particulates, ozone and sulphur dioxide would bring health benefits estimated at between $96 and $402 per capita.[9] Air pollution in Prague, Czech Republic, causes economic losses due to accelerated corrosion of buildings and materials, increased occurrence of diseases and damage to vegetation estimated to be almost $70 million each year.[10]

Monetary costs are invaluable when justifying actions to tackle air pollution problems, but to gain the support of the public for pollution control policies estimates of the number of people made ill or who die prematurely can be as persuasive. For example, in Europe alone the WHO estimates that exceedances of its daily sulphur dioxide guideline value are currently responsible for 6000–13,000 extra deaths a year among people aged over 65 years as well as 89,000–203,000 people suffering intensified chronic respiratory trouble. Exceedances of the WHO daily nitrogen dioxide guide value produces 58,000–99,000 extra cases of disease in the lower respiratory organs of children annually. Short episodes of high concentrations of ozone, especially in the Benelux countries and adjacent parts of France and Germany, give rise to between 220,000 and 1.9 million children suffering from coughs and eye irritation every year (the wide range reflecting years with differing weather conditions conducive to ozone formation). Long-term exposure to elevated levels of sulphur dioxide, especially in eastern Europe, reduces the average lung capacity of 9.7 million

---

7 Elvingson, P (1994) 'Allergies and air pollutants', *Acid News*, 3, Jun, p 15

8 Cannon, J S (1985) *The Health Costs of Air Pollution*, American Lung Association, New York; Cannon, J S (1990) *The Health Costs of Air Pollution: a Survey of Studies Published 1984–1989*, American Lung Association, Washington DC

9 Wijetilleke, L and Karunaratne, A R (1995) *Air Quality Management: Considerations for Developing Countries*, World Bank Technical Paper 278, World Bank, Washington DC, pp 77–79

10 Stanners, D and Bourdeau, P (1995) *Europe's Environment: the Dobris Assessment*, European Environment Agency, Copenhagen, pp 278–280

people by 5 per cent, and long-term exposure to elevated nitrogen dioxide reduces the lung function of 60 million people by 2–5 per cent.[11]

Sources of Pollutants

Diversity of Sources Contamination of the atmosphere by pollutants is due to many activities including the operation of motor vehicles and power stations, the manufacture of consumer goods and products, the processing of metals, petroleum and chemicals, heating and cooking in homes, the construction and repair of buildings and roads, and the incineration of wastes (Table 2.1). In most cases the type and amount of pollutants emitted are a function of the fuel being burned or the type of raw materials being processed to produce a product such as in the manufacture of steel, plastics and cement. High-sulphur coal, lignite and oil are regarded as the most polluting fuels and natural gas as one of the cleanest. Natural sources can contribute significantly to atmospheric contamination in the form of wind-blown dust from surrounding desert or dry areas as well as from bushfires. For example, dust storms have long contributed about 60 per cent of the suspended particulate concentrations recorded in Beijing during the summer, although this problem is being reduced by the planting of 30 million trees along the edge of the nearby desert.

Principal Pollutants of Concern The main urban air pollutants affecting health are sulphur dioxide (and its oxidation products, sulphates), suspended particulates (smoke, dust, PM_{10}), nitrogen oxides, carbon monoxide, VOCs (hydrocarbons and oxygenates), ozone, lead and other toxic metals (Table 2.1). In 1990, worldwide emissions of sulphur dioxide from human activities amounted to 99 million tonnes (Mt), suspended particulates 57 MT, nitrogen oxides 68 Mt and carbon monoxide 177 Mt. Chemical plants can create localised problems involving pollutants such as fluoride, chlorine, hydrogen fluoride and hydrogen sulphide and can give rise to odour pollution problems.

In addition, though not considered in detail in this study, there are other pollutants which directly or indirectly affect health such as noise and ionising radiation. Nuclear reactors produce health risks from accidental releases of radionuclides, whereas radon, a radioactive gas, may affect some homes where they are built on uranium-containing rocks and soils. Emissions of greenhouse gases such as carbon dioxide, methane and CFCs together with anthropogenic heat may indirectly affect the well-being of the urban community by modifying a city's weather and climate.

Motor Vehicles as Major Pollution Sources in Cities The relative contribution of each source type (e.g. transportation, power generation,

11 WHO (1995) *Concern for Tomorrow*, WHO Regional Office for Europe, Copenhagen; 'The effects of bad air on health', *Acid News*, 3, Jun 1995, p 3

Table 2.1 *Key air pollutants and their anthropogenic sources*

Pollutant	Anthropogenic sources
Sulphur dioxide	Coal- and oil-fired power stations, industrial boilers, waste incinerators, domestic heating, diesel vehicles, metal smelters, paper manufacturing
Particulates (dust, smoke, PM_{10})	Coal- and oil-fired power stations, industrial boilers, waste incinerators, domestic heating, many industrial plants, diesel vehicles, construction, mining, quarrying, cement manufacturing
Nitrogen oxides	Coal-, oil- and gas-fired power stations, industrial boilers, waste incinerators, motor vehicles
Carbon monoxide	Motor vehicles, fuel combustion
Volatile organic compounds (VOCs), eg benzene	Petrol-engined vehicle exhausts, leakage at petrol stations, paint manufacturing
Toxic organic micropollutants, eg polynuclear aromatic hydrocarbons, polychlorinated biphenyls, dioxins	Waste incinerators, coke production, coal combustion
Toxic metals, eg lead, cadmium	Vehicle exhausts (leaded petrol), metal processing, waste incinerators, oil and coal combustion, battery manufacturing, cement and fertiliser production
Toxic chemicals, eg chlorine, ammonia, fluoride	Chemical plants, metal processing, fertiliser manufacturing
Greenhouse gases, eg carbon dioxide, methane	Carbon dioxide: fuel combustion, especially power stations. Methane: coal mining, gas leakage, landfill sites
Ozone	Secondary pollutant formed from VOCs and nitrogen oxides
Ionising radiation (radionuclides)	Nuclear reactors, nuclear waste storage
Odours	Sewage treatment works, landfill sites, chemical plants, oil refineries, food processing, paintworks, brickworks, plastics manufacturing

Source: Elsom, D M (1995) 'Air and climate', in Morris, P and Therivel, R (eds) *Methods of Environmental Impact Assessment*, UCL Press, London, p 129

industrial processing) to each pollutant varies from city to city and from country to country, but it is clear that changes in urban–industrial development and technology have altered the relative importance of some source types. Road transport in urban areas, especially in the core of cities, is fast becoming the dominant source of many of the key pollutants affecting the health of urban residents.[12] More than 1 billion vehicles may be using the world's roads by 2030, emitting carbon monoxide, nitrogen oxides and VOCs (e.g. benzene), the latter two being the precursor emissions for producing the secondary pollutant, ozone. Lead is an important pollutant emitted by vehicles powered by leaded petrol, whereas in cities where diesel-engined vehicles constitute a sizeable proportion of the vehicle fleet, sulphur dioxide and fine suspended particulates (PM_{10}) are emitted in large amounts. Emissions from individual vehicles depend on the constituents of the fuel, the design and size of the engine, the external conditions in which it is being driven (road surface, air temperature, etc), the speed (and whether accelerating/decelerating or under stress due to load), its age and level of maintenance.[13]

Air Quality Standards and the Groups of People Most at Risk

Searching for Health-effect Thresholds Research into the effects of air pollutants on health indicate that many, though not all, pollutants have a threshold above which the health of some people may be affected adversely. Epidemiological studies of community groups and laboratory-based toxicological experiments using human volunteers or animals provide assessments of the health effects of pollutants. Epidemiological studies correlate pollutant concentrations with indicators of the health of the population as provided in doctors' consultation records, hospital admission

12 Transport emissions, of which road transport is the largest contributor, in France accounted for about 76 per cent of total carbon monoxide emissions, 69 per cent of VOCs, 56 per cent of nitrogen oxides, 30 per cent of suspended particulates, 21 per cent of sulphur dioxide and 80 per cent of lead. Figures for other countries are given in Wijetilleke and Karunaratne (1995) op cit, pp 64–66 and in Faiz, A (1993) 'Automotive emissions in developing countries: relative implications for global warming, acidification and urban air quality', *Transportation Research*, vol 27A (3), pp 167–186. Transport usually contributes higher percentages in urban areas. For example, in Budapest, Hungary, transport accounts for 98 per cent of total carbon monoxide emissions, 97 per cent of VOCs, 93 per cent of nitrogen oxides, 60 per cent of sulphur dioxide, 40 per cent of soot and dust and 97 per cent of lead. 'Hungary's traffic pollution', *The Environmental Digest*, 67, Jan 1993, p 15. Transport contributions in London are given in Table 9.3.

13 A German study assessed the emissions from a medium-sized car, driven for 13,000 km for 10 years, and concluded that during its lifetime such a car would produce 44.3 t of carbon dioxide, 4.8 kg of sulphur dioxide, 46.8 kg of nitrogen oxides, 325 kg of carbon monoxide, 36 kg of hydrocarbons and 26.5 t of waste (including tyre and brake abrasion products such as asbestos) and lead; Whitelegg, J (1993) 'Dirty from the cradle to the grave', *The Guardian*, 30 Jul, p 18

records and death certificates. Studies may be short term (pollution episodes) and long term (ten-year or even a lifetime's duration). Special surveys may be conducted in which selected groups of people keep diaries of the incidence and severity of their illnesses. The real-world situation of epidemiological studies imposes limitations on the findings because the ambient urban atmosphere contains diverse pollutants which vary over time and from place to place. Studies have to assume that all the group under study are subjected to the same pollutant exposure, but this can vary enormously from individual to individual. Another problem of epidemiological studies is that they can conclude only that a particular health effect is associated with a particular level of pollutant: causality cannot be proved.

Given the limitations of epidemiological studies, increasing importance is being given to laboratory (controlled chamber) tests in which the response of volunteers to specific types and amounts of pollutants can be measured with precision. Naturally, to protect human volunteers the tests can only be undertaken over a narrow range of pollutant concentrations. This applies particularly to groups at risk such as people with asthma and cardiovascular diseases. Laboratory tests usually involve very small numbers of people so the results from similar studies may differ due to individual variations among each group of volunteers. In both epidemiological and toxicological studies the findings are usually suggestive rather than conclusive, so indicating the need for further research.

Redefining the Thresholds of Pollutant Effects Replicating research work undertaken several years earlier using more sensitive and accurate techniques can result in a lowering of the threshold level at which a pollutant is considered to produce a measurable adverse reaction in sensitive individuals. Some pollutants, notably carcinogenic pollutants, may have no safe threshold limit. This means the authorities must decide whether emissions of such pollutants into the environment are necessary. The rapid implementation of a ban on emissions can be extremely difficult or impossible either because it is beyond present technology to be able to do so or because it would cause unacceptable economic and social disruption. Consequently authorities may decide to reduce the emissions of known carcinogenic pollutants to as low as is practically possible with the long-term aim being to eventually ban such emissions. The WHO recognises proven or probable carcinogens as acrylonitrile, arsenic, benzene, chromium, nickel, PAHs and vinyl chloride.

WHO Air Quality Guidelines People are at risk when air pollution exceeds the guidelines advocated by the WHO to 'provide a basis for protecting public health from adverse effects of air pollution and for eliminating, or reducing to a minimum, those contaminants of air that are known or likely to be hazardous to human health and well-being'. It should be noted that the WHO definition of health is that it is a state of complete physical, mental and social well-being and not merely the absence of disease. The WHO guidelines are not mandatory standards, but instead provide a guide to national governments or groups of nations such as the European Union in setting their own standards (Tables 2.2–2.7). WHO guidelines were established for 28 air pollutants in 1987 and these guidelines are currently under review with revisions due in 1996. WHO guidelines, unlike national standards, do not consider the broader factors such as the economic and technological implications of attainment. In addition to these standards designed to protect human health and sometimes referred to as primary standards, there are secondary standards set to protect vegetation and

Table 2.2 *Examples of air quality standards and guidelines for sulphur dioxide*

Organisation and standard	Concentration (ppb)	Concentration ($\mu g/m^3$)*
WHO		
Annual mean[†‡]	19 (15–23)	50 (40–60)
24 h mean[‡]	47 (38–56)	125 (100–150)
1 h mean[‡]	130	350
10 min mean	188	500
EU limit values		
Annual mean	30 if black smoke >34	80 if black smoke >40
	45 if black smoke <34	120 if black smoke <40
Winter mean	49 if black smoke >23	130 if black smoke >60
	68 if black smoke <23	180 if black smoke <60
98th centile[§]	94 if black smoke >128	250 if black smoke >150
	132 if black smoke <128	350 if black smoke <150
EU guide values		
Annual mean	15–23	40–60
24 h average	38–56	100–150
UK		
15 min mean	100	375
US standards		
Annual average	30	80
24 h average	140	365
California		
24 h average	40	105
1 h average	250	655

* 1 $\mu g/m^3$ = 0.376 ppb.
† Annual average limit values expressed as median values; annual average guide values expressed as arithmetic means
‡ Single figure applies to Europe, the range of figures to the rest of the world.
§ Daily mean measurements in one year

Table 2.3 *Examples of air quality standards and guidelines for suspended particulate matter*

Organisation and standard	Concentration (μg/m³)
WHO	
Annual mean, black smoke	50
24 h average, black smoke	125
Annual mean, TSP*	60–90
24 h mean, TSP	120
24 h mean, thoracic particles	70
EU limit values†	
Annual mean, black smoke	80 (68)
Winter mean, black smoke	130 (111)
98th centile, black smoke	250 (213)
Annual mean, gravimetric	150
95th centile, gravimetric	300
EU guide values†	
Annual mean, black smoke	40–60 (34–51)
24 h mean, black smoke	100–150 (85–128)
UK	
24 h average, PM_{10}	50
US	
Annual arithmetic mean, PM_{10}	50
24 h average, PM_{10}	150
California	
Annual geometric mean, PM_{10}	30
24 h average, PM_{10}	50

* Total suspended particulates.
† Numbers in parentheses refer to British Standard Smoke (BS = 0.85 EU value)

aesthetic aspects of the environment such as long-range visibility and soiling of buildings.[14]

Sensitive Population Groups at Risk The WHO guidelines and national mandatory air quality standards are based on the lowest level at which a

14 A series of WHO reports assessed the health impacts of pollutants and defined health-based and environmental guidelines. For example, WHO (1979) *Sulphur Oxides and Suspended Particulate Matter*, Environmental Health Criteria 8, WHO, Geneva [other reports include oxides of nitrogen (criteria 4, 1977), lead (3, 1977 and 85, 1989), photochemical oxidants (7, 1979), carbon monoxide (13, 1979) and noise (12, 1980)]; WHO (1987) *Air Quality Guidelines for Europe*, WHO Regional Publications European Series No 23, WHO, Copenhagen. Revised WHO guidelines will be issued in late 1996.

Table 2.4 *Examples of air quality standards and guidelines for carbon monoxide*

Organisation and standard	Concentration (ppm)	Concentration (mg/m³)*
WHO		
8 h mean	9	10
1 h mean	26	30
30 min mean	52	60
15 min mean	86	100
UK		
8 h running average	10	12
US		
8 h average	9	10
1 h average	35	40
California		
8 h average	9	10
1 h average	20	23

* 1 mg/m³ = 0.859 ppm.

Table 2.5 *Examples of air quality standards and guidelines for nitrogen dioxide*

Organisation and standard	Concentration (ppb)	Concentration (μg/m³)*
WHO		
24 h mean	78	150
1 h mean‡	209 (105)	400 (200)
Monthly maximum†	99–167	190–320
EU limit value		
98th centile	105	200
EU guide value		
Annual mean (median)	26	50
98th centile (1 h)	71	135
US		
Annual average	53	100
California		
1 h average	250	478

* 1 μg/m³ = 0.523 ppb.
† Not to be exceeded more than once per month.
‡ Numbers in parentheses refer to proposed revision of the Standard in 1996.

Table 2.6 *Examples of air quality standards and guidelines for ozone*

Organisation and standard	Concentration (ppb)	Concentration (μg/m³)*
WHO		
8 h mean	50–60	100–120
1 h mean	76–100	150–200
EU limit values		
8 h mean	55	110
1 h public information	90	180
1 h public warning	180	360
UK		
8 h mean	50	100
US		
1 h average	120	240
California		
1 h average	90	180

* 1 μg/m³ = 0.500 ppb.

pollutant has been shown to produce adverse health effects or the level at which no observed health effect was demonstrated plus a margin of protection to safeguard 'sensitive groups' within the population. A safety factor of two is often adopted in calculating the standard. Sensitive groups include people with asthma, those with pre-existing heart and lung diseases (eg bronchitis, emphysema, angina, acute myocardial infarction, chronic airway obstruction), the elderly (people over 65 years of age), infants (under 2 years or even under 5 years of age) and pregnant women and their unborn babies. Such groups often represent around one-fifth of a national population

Table 2.7 *Examples of air quality standards and guidelines for lead*

Organisation and standard	Concentration (μg/m³)
WHO	
Annual mean	0.5–1.0
EU	
Annual mean	2.0
US	
Calendar quarter	1.5
California	
30 day average	1.5

in Northern countries such as the US and Britain. In some Southern countries where there may be large numbers of undernourished people the proportion of people likely to react adversely to pollution is much higher.

Elderly people are susceptible to pollutants because of their reduced lung function, which declines gradually with age. Young children are at more risk than adults for several reasons. They spend long periods outdoors playing vigorously and breathing fast and children breathe more air for their body weight than adults. Mouth breathing is common in children so the benefits of nasal scrubbing of pollutants is lost. Their airways are narrower and therefore more sensitive to inflammation. As their lungs are not fully developed, this means the potential for long-term damage in the form of developing chronic lung diseases is greater. To these groups at risk can be added people taking vigorous physical exercise (eg participants in outdoor sports and games, cyclists, joggers), outdoor workers undertaking strenuous work loads (eg road and building construction workers), people with AIDS or other diseases which have damaged the body's immune system, as well as current and ex-smokers. Athletes training or competing outdoors are at risk because of their high ventilation rates and because they switch from nose to mouth breathing, which means that the nasal filtering of pollutants is lost.

Example of an Air Quality Standard An example of an air quality standard is the WHO one-hour nitrogen dioxide guideline of 209 ppb (400 $\mu g/m^3$). This represents a maximum value not to be exceeded at any time and has been recommended on the basis that a concentration of 293 ppb (560 $\mu g/m^3$) was judged as the lowest concentration at which adverse effects were found in people with asthma and that the guideline allowed for a further margin of protection. Rather than adopt the WHO guideline value the European Union used a one-hour standard of 105 ppb (200 $\mu g/m^3$) while Japan adopted a stricter one-hour standard of 42–63 ppb (80–120 $\mu g/m^3$). However, both the European Union and Japanese standards refer to 98th centiles and not the maximum value as used by the WHO. What this means is the 98th centile of one-hour average concentrations over one year (air pollution concentrations usually follow a log-normal distribution) should not exceed 105 ppb (200 $\mu g/m^3$) for more than 2 per cent of the time, that is 175 hours. Expressed in another way the 176th highest of a series of 8760 hourly average concentrations should not exceed 105 ppb (200 $\mu g/m^3$). In other words, an urban area can conform with these mandatory standards even if hourly concentrations during some or even many hours during the year greatly exceed levels recognised to pose a health risk to some people.[15]

European Union sulphur dioxide air quality standards for daily (24-hour)

15 Elsom, D M (1995) 'Air and climate', in Morris, P and Therivel, R (eds) *Methods of Environmental Impact Assessment*, UCL Press, London, pp 120–142; the WHO recommends halving its one-hour nitrogenol dioxide guideline to 105 ppb (200 $\mu g/m^3$) in 1996

values is similarly expressed in terms of the 98th centile of all daily mean values taken throughout the year. In this case, sulphur dioxide levels can exceed the standard – with no upper level indicated – for up to seven days during the year without failing to meet the standard. As a general but not infallible guide, the 98th centile value is typically two to three times greater than the annual mean value, whereas the maximum value is typically around twice the 98th centile. The public often treat the 98th centile as a maximum value not to be exceeded and so are surprised to learn that pollution levels have exceeded this value yet no regulation has been broken because of the short duration of the exceedance. Even so, many people consider their health is at risk any time the 98th centile is exceeded.

National Variations in Air Quality Standards The strictness of air quality standards varies from country to country. Japanese air quality standards often tend to be more strict than either European Union or American standards whereas standards in most Southern countries are weaker. Standards may be amended and made more strict should new research show that a lower level of pollutant affects health than previously recognised or that medical opinion suggests the need to incorporate a greater margin of safety than previously existed. This happened in the case of carbon monoxide when the WHO in 1987 changed its earlier one-hour guideline for Europe from 35 ppm (40 mg/m^3) set in 1972 to 25 ppm (30 mg/m^3). Equally, if the results of research findings on which the setting of an air quality standard was devised are shown to be in error it may be subsequently weakened. It is not surprising that national variations in standards exist because epidemiological and toxicological studies often produce conflicting results and differing national advisers may have greater confidence in the results of some studies than others. Whereas some countries set standards to protect the most susceptible members of the population (eg the young or elderly) others set them to protect the healthy majority outside the extreme age ranges. National standards are only likely to be standardised when all countries agree to adopt, say, WHO guidelines.

In a few cases, a national government may relax a standard if in attempting to meet the standard it believes the economy, primarily the industrial production sector, is becoming less competitive in relation to foreign competition for markets. In the US the photochemical oxidant (ozone) standard was relaxed in 1979 from 80 ppb (157 µg/m^3) to 120 ppb (235 µg/m^3), much to the dismay of environmental pressure and some medical advisory groups. Even when strict air quality standards exist, as in Russia, this is no guarantee that local and central governments will try to enforce them. Standards tend to be set for individual pollutants but this fails to recognise the synergistic effects of pollutants, that is pollutants in combination may have aggregate effects on health greater than the sum of their individual effects. Only the combination of smoke and suspended particulates has been given an air quality standard by the European Union so far.

Monitoring Compliance with Standards Recognising health-based air quality standards is essential, but so too is being able to assess whether an urban area conforms to those standards. Information about the pollution levels experienced by an urban area depends on the number, location and accuracy of pollution monitors. In many urban areas there are insufficient monitors installed so there is no certainty that air quality meets air quality standards. Even when accurate pollution data are available widely throughout an urban area this does not indicate the actual amount and type of pollutants a person is breathing. Every person experiences a unique exposure to air pollutants because of the length of time they spend indoors and outdoors, their occupation and means of travelling to work, their location(s) within an urban area and their rate of breathing.

Walking for an hour in a city centre can produce very different pollution exposures depending on nearness to major roads. A comparison of measurements at streets with a high traffic density in Berlin showed a reduction of more than 50 per cent in nitrogen oxide concentrations 40–50 m from the kerbside whereas carbon monoxide decreased by 30 per cent within 4 m distance. Typically, people driving cars, cycling along a busy road in a city centre or walking along the pavement close to the kerb of a busy road experience two to five times more benzene, carbon monoxide, lead, nitrogen dioxide and suspended particulates than they would walking at a location 30–50 m away from the road. Pollution exposure in enclosed underground or multi-storey car parks and in tunnels is likely to be even greater. Drivers and passengers in cars may inhale up to 18 times as much pollution as people outside their vehicle, the worst occurring in congested slow-moving driving conditions in urban areas. Levels of benzene were found to be two to 18 times higher than ambient air and levels of carbon monoxide from two to 14 times higher. Nitrogen dioxide is also higher (1.3 to 2.5 times), especially during high-speed driving on motorways and during afternoon rush hours.[16]

Indoor Pollution In some cases, indoor exposure to emissions of nitrogen dioxide from cooking and heating appliances as well as from carbon monoxide and nitrogen dioxide from smoking tobacco adds considerably to a person's exposure to air pollution. In addition, toxics released from building materials including asbestos and formaldehyde may pose health threats, as can radioactive radon gas released from uranium-containing rocks or soil underlying some homes or from the building materials employed. The part played by indoor pollutants in causing poor health can be very important in some cases. The trend which began in the 1970s to build more energy-efficient buildings produced air-tight and poorly ventilated buildings which resulted in the 'sick building syndrome', whereby

16 Jefferiss, P, Rowell, A and Fergusson, M (1992) *The Exposure of Car Drivers and Passengers to Vehicle Emissions: Comparative Pollutant Levels Inside and Outside Vehicles*, Greenpeace, London, 10 pp

occupants report eye, nose and throat irritations, fatigue, forgetfulness, irritability and nausea. Centrally heated and airtight buildings seal in dust mites which can trigger asthma attacks.

For most pollutants the use of short-term ambient air quality standards, say of one-hour duration or even less, increasingly seem more appropriate than daily values when it is considered that most people spend 20–22 hours a day inside their home, in shops and in the workplace, about one hour a day inside a car or public transport vehicle in transit from one location to another, and perhaps as little as one hour a day outdoors. In many Southern countries indoor air pollution ranks not far behind ambient air quality as a cause of respiratory ill health. Between 400 and 700 million people in The South, mostly women and children, are exposed to high levels of indoor pollutants emitted by cooking and heating appliances.[17]

17 World Bank (1992) *World Development Report 1992: Development and the Environment*, Oxford University Press, New York, p 52

Chapter 3

Health-Threatening Pollutants

Sulphur Dioxide[1]

Characteristics and Sources Sulphur dioxide comes mainly from the combustion of sulphur-containing fossil fuels such as coal, lignite and heavy fuel oil. Coal and lignite account for about 80 per cent of the annual world-wide energy-related emissions of sulphur dioxide, with oil accounting for the rest. The relative contributions vary from country to country and in some cases sulphur dioxide emissions have fallen markedly in recent years as national energy needs are provided increasingly by low-sulphur oil (with a sulphur content of 1 per cent or less), natural gas (which emits only trace

---

1 Advisory Group on the Medical Aspects of Air Pollution Episodes (1992) *Sulphur Dioxide, Acid Aerosols and Particulates*, Second Report, HMSO, London; Bates, D V and Sizto, R (1987) 'Air pollution and hospital admissions in southern Ontario: the acid summer haze effect', *Environmental Research*, vol 43, pp 317–331; Elsom, D M (1992) *Atmospheric Pollution: a Global Problem*, Blackwell, Oxford (reviews a range of pollutants); Expert Panel on Air Quality Standards (1995) *Sulphur Dioxide*, HMSO, London; Holman, C (1991) *Air Quality and Health*, second edition, Friends of the Earth, London (reviews a range of pollutants); Parliamentary Office of Science and Technology (POST) (1994) *Breathing in Our Cities*, POST, House of Commons, London (reviews links between asthma and several pollutants); Patel, T (1994) 'Killer smog stalks the boulevards', *New Scientist*, 15 October, p 8 (summarises Paris health study); Quality of Urban Air Review Group (1993) *Urban Air Quality in the United Kingdom*, First Report, Department of the Environment, London (discusses key urban air pollutants); Read, C (1991) *Air Pollution and Child Health*, Greenpeace, London (reviews effects of a range of pollutants); Wichmann, H E, Mueller, W *et al* (1989) 'Health effects during a smog episode in West Germany in 1985', *Environmental Health Perspectives*, vol 79, pp 88–99; WHO (1987) *Air Quality Guidelines for Europe*, WHO Regional Publications, European Series No 23, WHO, Copenhagen (discusses the health effects and air quality standards for a range of pollutants); WHO (1990) *Acute Effects on Health of Smog Episodes*, WHO Regional Publications, European Series No 43, WHO, Copenhagen (discusses health effects of sulphur dioxide, suspended particulates and ozone)

amounts of sulphur dioxide) and nuclear fuels. Petrol-engined vehicles emit very little sulphur dioxide because the sulphur content of petrol is only 0.04 per cent by mass. In contrast, diesel-engined vehicles emit significant amounts of sulphur dioxide as diesel contains 0.2 per cent sulphur by mass or even more.

Today many cities in North America and western Europe have reduced domestic and industrial emissions of sulphur dioxide in urban areas so much that residents experience their greatest sulphur dioxide alongside busy roads due to diesel-engined buses, lorries and taxis as well as from an increasing number of diesel passenger cars (about 20 per cent of new vehicles currently sold in Europe). Catalytic converters fitted to petrol-engined cars can emit tiny amounts of odorous hydrogen sulphide. In cities in The South, sulphur dioxide emissions from diesel buses, trucks and taxis are a major cause of poor air quality.

Major industrial emissions of sulphur dioxide include coal- and oil-burning for electricity generation in power stations, smelting of non-ferrous ores (copper, lead, nickel and zinc), chemical processing (eg production of sulphur and sulphuric acid), production of paper from wood pulp, and waste incineration. Large coal- and oil-fired power stations, increasingly located outside urban areas, emit sulphur dioxide at such a high elevation that they normally contribute little to ground level concentrations in nearby urban areas. However, there may be a few occasions during stable weather conditions when plumes from power stations reach the ground after only limited dispersion and dilution, resulting in rapid short-term increases in sulphur dioxide concentrations. Domestic sources of sulphur dioxide include the use of coal, lignite, peat and wood for heating and cooking as well as from open burning of domestic and garden refuse.

Ambient Concentrations and Health Effects The WHO believe annual mean levels should not exceed 38 ppb (100 μg/m^3) or even less to prevent an increase in chronic respiratory illness rates. Whereas major European cities averaged concentrations annually around 38–75 ppb (100–200 μg/m^3) a decade ago, they are now mostly below 38 ppb (100 μg/m^3). London's annual mean concentration decreased from around 150 ppb (400 μg/m^3) in the early 1960s to 8–19 ppb (20–50 μg/m^3) by the 1980s. Even so, sulphur dioxide levels in some cities in western Europe, such as Belfast, Dublin, Madrid and Milan, remain relatively high. In contrast with improvements in western Europe, air quality has worsened in the past decade or two in many urban-industrial centres in eastern Europe where lignite is the dominant fuel. Serious sulphur dioxide problems also occur in the rapidly growing cities of nations in Asia, especially China, and South America where coal, lignite and high-sulphur oil are the major fuels.

Laboratory studies of people with asthma have shown consistently that sulphur dioxide, at levels only slightly higher than air quality standards, makes asthma worse. Asthma is a disorder in which a narrowing of the medium-sized air passages of the lungs causes wheezing, shortness of breath and coughing. People with asthma may wheeze at levels as low as 200 ppb (530 μg/m^3), especially if they are exercising (similar symptoms in healthy adults occur at levels of 1000 ppb or 2660 μg/m^3). This usually happens within a few minutes after the start of exercise but fortunately does not worsen with increasing exposure. Synergistic effects can occur when additional pollutants are present such that when mildly asthmatic adolescents are concurrently exposed to 120 ppb (240 μg/m^3) of ozone, their vulnerability to low concentrations of sulphur dioxide increases. Studies in France and Israel confirm that people living in areas highly polluted with sulphur dioxide experience an increased incidence of asthma compared with those in less polluted areas. Similarly, a survey of 574,000 Polish army recruits found that those who came from polluted regions were five times as likely to have asthma as those from cleaner areas. It appears that sulphur dioxide sensitises people to asthma, with the symptoms being triggered by common allergens such as pollens.

European and American research has shown that the lung function of children is temporarily impaired when daily sulphur dioxide concentrations are in the range 100 to 200 ppb (265–530 μg/m^3) and total suspended particulates between 200 and 400 μg/m^3. During such pollution episodes in the Netherlands in January 1985 and January 1987, not only did the lung function of 6–12 year old Dutch children fall by up to 5 per cent, but it remained impaired for several weeks afterwards. American studies indicate that the frequency of chronic cough, bronchitis and chest illness in pre-school children is greater in urban areas that have higher concentrations of sulphur dioxide and suspended particulates. A study of deaths and disease in Paris for the period 1987–1992 showed that when daily sulphur dioxide levels increased by 38 ppb (100 μg/m^3), deaths from heart attacks increased by 10 per cent.

Acid Aerosols High concentrations of sulphur dioxide during winter smogs are often accompanied by high concentrations of suspended particulates and acid aerosols. This makes it difficult to separate out the effects of individual pollutants or the precise nature of any synergistic effects occurring among the pollutants. Many of the early epidemiological studies of winter smogs claimed the increase in morbidity and mortality occurring during the smog was due to the combination of high concentrations of sulphur dioxide and suspended particulates. Today these claims are being re-examined with greater attention being given to the part played by acid aerosols and fine particulates. During winter fogs sulphur dioxide can be transformed by various metal impurities present in fog droplets and carbon on the surface of particulates into sulphate and sulphuric acid aerosols. The importance of winter acid aerosols in affecting health was deduced during the London smog of 1952 by veterinary surgeons at the Smithfield Club's Show. Whereas over 60 prize cattle needed treatment for acute chest symptoms, many ordinary cattle appeared unaffected. As the latter were in pens which were cleaned less frequently, it was thought the neutralising effect of ammonia in their excrement gave them some protection from the acid aerosols. One practical result of this discovery was that the authorities placed ammonia bottles with wicks in hospital wards during subsequent sulphurous smogs in an attempt to neutralise the acid aerosols. Ammonia neutralises sulphate by forming ammonium sulphate.

Sulphate aerosols are also produced during warm sunny weather when sulphur dioxide is oxidised during photochemical episodes. Research into ten years (1973–1984) of hospital admissions in southern Ontario revealed that increased admissions were linked with increased levels of sulphates and ozone. People admitted to hospital with asthmatic problems during the summer showed a clear link with sulphate levels two days earlier as well as ozone levels a day earlier. The combination of sulphates and ozone may suggest that the real cause of the health effects is sulphuric acid, which is seldom monitored directly but occurs on occasions when both sulphate and ozone levels are high. Measuring the acidity (hydrogen ion concentration or pH) of the air has yielded some success in confirming that sulphuric acid aerosols are present at times of elevated sulphate and ozone. Active children in a summer camp in Ontario were shown to experience levels exceeding 50 $\mu g/m^3$ of sulphuric acid fairly frequently and that this is close to the threshold of 70–100 $\mu g/m^3$ believed to affect the lung function of people with asthma taking part in exercise. Interestingly, as ammonia produced in the mouth appears to protect against the effects of acid air, it has been suggested that children in summer camps should avoid lemonade as it neutralises the protective ammonia.

Suspended Particulates[2]

Complexity of Suspended Particulates Particulates suspended in the air are composed of a complex mixture of organic and inorganic substances ranging from naturally generated sea salt and soil particles to combustion-

2 Brown, W (1994) 'Dying from too much dust', *New Scientist*, 12 Mar, pp 12–13; Expert Panel on Air Quality Standards (1995) *Particles*, HMSO, London; Committee on the Medical Effects of Air Pollutants (1995) *Non-Biological Particles and Health*, HMSO, London; Quality of Urban Air Review Group (1993) *Diesel Vehicle Emissions and Urban Air Quality*, Second Report, Department of the Environment, London; American studies of fine particulates include Dockery, W D, Pope, C A *et al* (1993) 'An association between air pollution and mortality in six US cities', *The New England Journal of Medicine*, vol 329, pp 1753–1759; Pope, C A, Schwartz, J and Ransom, M R (1992) 'Daily mortality and PM_{10} pollution in Utah Valley', *Archives of Environmental Health*, vol 47 (3), pp 211–217; Pope, C A, Thun, M J *et al* (1995) 'Particulate air pollution as a predictor of mortality in a prospective study of US adults', *American Journal of Respiratory and Critical Care Medicine*, vol 151, pp 669–674; Schwartz, J (1992) 'Particulate air pollution and daily mortality in Steubenville, Ohio' *American Journal of Epidemiology*, vol 135, pp 12–20; Schwartz, J and Dockery, D W (1992) 'Increased mortality in Philadelphia associated with daily air pollution concentrations', *American Review of Respiratory Disease*, vol 145, pp 600–604

created smoke particles. Particulates are released during the combustion of fossil fuels associated with power generation, home heating and cooking, motor vehicles and from a wide range of industrial processes including waste incineration. Fine particles are formed from gas to particle conversion through oxidation: sulphur dioxide to sulphuric acid and nitrogen dioxide to nitric acid. Although sulphuric acid exists in air in particle form, nitric acid is present as a vapour. Both acids react with ammonia gas, readily available in the atmosphere as a product of decomposition, to form ammonium salts. Ammonium nitrate and sulphate exist in air as solid particles at low humidities, or as solution droplets at higher humidities.

Airborne particulates are referred to as suspended particulate matter (SPM), total suspended particulate (TSP) or black smoke depending on the type of measurement technique used. To add a further complication, the British method of measuring black smoke concentrations results in its values being equivalent to 85 per cent of the values derived using the European Union standard method of measuring black smoke (refer to Table 2.3). Fine particulates may be specified by size such as PM_{10}, referring to particles less than 10 μm in diameter, or $PM_{2.5}$, referring to particles less than 2.5 μm across. Occasionally airborne particulates may be described simply as dust. This term is commonly used when discussing suspended particulates in the air of cities such as Beijing, Cairo and Mexico City where considerable amounts of soil particles or sand are blown into the city from the surrounding dry areas, adding to anthropogenic emissions of particulates. Even the Mediterranean city of Athens receives half of its suspended particulates as soil particles. Construction activities may be a significant source of dust and unsurfaced roads in and around a city can lead to the occurrence of high levels of suspended particulates during dry and windy weather conditions.

Air Quality Standards and the Significance of Particle Size It has long been considered that sulphur dioxide and suspended particulates produce similar health effects and the presence of both of these pollutants appears to lead to a worsening of health effects. Air quality guidelines and standards sometimes reflect this combined or possibly synergistic effect. The European Union recognised the synergistic effect of sulphur dioxide and suspended particulates by specifying a 98 percentile daily standard of 132 ppb (350 μg/m^3) if black smoke concentrations were less than 128 ppb (150 μg/m^3) and a lower 94 ppb (250 μg/m^3) sulphur dioxide standard if black smoke concentrations exceeded 128 ppb (150 μg/m^3).

In recent years much greater attention has been given to fine particulates, especially as improved measurement techniques have become available. The size of the particles is very relevant to discussions of the health effects of suspended particulates because size determines how deeply they penetrate into people's lungs. Large inhalable particles, 15–100 μm in diameter, are usually trapped in the nose and throat (naso-pharyngeal region) while thoracic particles 5–10 μm across reach the upper parts of the lungs (tracheal-bronchial region). In contrast, smaller respirable particles of less than 5 μm diameter reach the fine airways (respiratory bronchioles) during normal nasal breathing and even the alveolar region when breathing through the mouth, such as when exercising vigorously. Not only do the finer particles penetrate deeply into the respiratory system, but they tend to be the products of combustion so their chemical composition is usually more harmful to health than, say, clay particles derived from soils which constitute the coarser suspended particulates. The US, as did Brazil, introduced standards for fine particulates (PM_{10}) in 1986 in the form of an annual mean of 50 $\mu g/m^3$ and a 24-hour mean of 150 $\mu g/m^3$, whereas California and the UK apply more stringent standards (Table 2.2). Japan has set a 24-hour standard of 100 $\mu g/m^3$ and a one-hour standard of 200 $\mu g/m^3$. Recent epidemiological research suggests that not only is there a need for other countries to introduce air quality standards for PM_{10}, but that there may be no safe threshold for PM_{10}.

Health Effects Airborne particles may contain recondensed organic and metallic vapours making them particularly toxic. Diesel engines emit oily black fine particulates (eg soot or carbon particles) which may be impregnated with complex organic compounds such as polycyclic aromatic hydrocarbons (PAHs) which have been shown to be carcinogenic in animal studies. The PAHs are a large group of organic compounds containing two or more benzene rings with benzo(*a*)pyrene being considered the most carcinogenic. Confirming increased cancer incidence in people is extremely difficult, but surveys in Canada and the US of tens of thousands of railway workers subjected to different degrees of exposure to diesel fumes showed those exposed to diesel for at least 20 years had a significantly increased risk of lung cancer. Exposure to PAHs has been blamed for increased occupational lung cancer among coke oven and coal gas workers as well as employees in aluminium plants. Another carcinogenic pollutant is asbestos in the form of fibres being emitted into the air during the wear and tear of brakes and tyres.

Increasing recognition is being given to the part that concentrations of fine particles (PM_{10}), rather than the total amount of SPM, play in causing increased morbidity and mortality in urban areas. Even at relatively low concentrations fine particulates have been shown to cause changes in lung function and lead to increases in cardiovascular and respiratory diseases (including asthma attacks). What is most worrying is that there may be no safe limit for fine particulates. Fine particles which reach the alveoli, the deepest region of the lung, are not cleared efficiently and may be absorbed into the blood stream (as in the case of lead) or if insoluble and inhaled in sufficiently large amounts may remain in the lungs and lead to lung diseases such as emphysema.

A very detailed 15-year study of 8111 adults undertaken in six American cities indicated that people in the most polluted cities were 26 per cent more likely to die than those in the least polluted city due to fine particulates, even though all six cities met US air quality standards. The association between particle concentrations and mortality seems to be found irrespective of the different types of particles in each city. This may indicate that the role of fine particulates in causing adverse health effects is that of carrying and delivering harmful chemicals deep into the lungs. Many studies now indicate that as levels of PM_{10} increase, so do the number of deaths and hospital admissions for respiratory diseases including asthma. In general terms, the American studies suggest that when the PM_{10} concentration increases by 10 $\mu g/m^3$, the daily death rate rises by 1 per cent. Although subject to great uncertainty, this may imply that PM_{10} is responsible for 60,000 deaths in the USA and as many as 10,000 in the UK each year.

An example of a detailed American study of fine particulates was that undertaken in the Utah valley. This showed that mortality averaged 4–5 per cent higher for each 50 $\mu g/m^3$ incremental increase of concurrent day PM_{10}. On the days when concurrent day PM_{10} levels exceeded 100 $\mu g/m^3$, mortality counts averaged 11 per cent higher than on days when PM_{10} levels were less than 50 ìg/m³. As PM_{10} may be high for several consecutive days during a smog, and because PM_{10} might have a cumulative effect, five-day moving average levels were also considered. Mortality averaged 6–8 per cent higher for each 50 $\mu g/m^3$ incremental increase of five-day lagged moving average PM_{10}. During smogs when the five-day lagged moving average PM_{10} levels exceeded 100 $\mu g/m^3$, mortality counts averaged 19 per cent higher than on days when these levels were less than 50 $\mu g/m^3$. These relationships appear to be independent of other pollutants and they are observed in areas where PM_{10} concentrations are high in winter or in summer.

Fine particulates emitted by diesel-engined vehicles have been implicated in the increasing frequency of hay fever. Hay fever or seasonal allergic rhinitis, with its symptoms of itchy and watering eyes and blocked and runny noses, is caused by allergy to pollens. Apparently, hay fever in Japan was rare before 1950 but since then it has risen greatly in line with the rapid growth in numbers of diesel-powered cars. Japanese research points to diesel exhaust particles making people sensitive to hay fever triggers such as pollen by stimulating the production of antibodies active in hay fever. Vehicle pollutants were implicated as the cause of allergies in a German study of 9000 6 year olds in 1994. This showed that allergies were 1.5–2.0 times more common among children living within 50 m of a busy road than those living in the same town but further away from main roads.

Carbon Monoxide[3]

Characteristics and Sources Carbon monoxide is an odourless and colourless gas which is produced by the incomplete combustion of carbon-

3 Expert Panel on Air Quality Standards (1994) *Carbon Monoxide*, HMSO, London; WHO (1979) *Carbon Monoxide*, Environmental Health Criteria 13, WHO, Geneva

based fuels. It is formed when oxygen is scarce and fuel does not burn properly, so it is a greater problem in high-altitude cities and during cold conditions. Transport accounts for more than 90 per cent of the total emissions of carbon monoxide in most urban areas. Although many countries in The North have introduced increasingly strict emission controls for carbon monoxide, the rapid increase in numbers of vehicles and distances travelled has meant a worsening carbon monoxide problem.

Carbon monoxide concentrations depend strongly on the traffic density of streets, the distance from the kerbside, the state of the engine of the vehicle, and the weather conditions. Poorly maintained spark ignition combustion engines during idling or deceleration are a particularly important source of carbon monoxide in urban areas. In contrast with petrol engines without catalytic converters, diesel engines when adjusted properly emit little carbon monoxide. Carbon monoxide emissions are greatest when an engine is first started from cold and when the engine is idling, as at traffic lights and road junctions and during traffic jams. The busy roads of most major cities in the world experience high carbon monoxide concentrations during the morning and early evening rush hours. The highest concentrations of carbon monoxide occur near dense traffic in road intersection tunnels, underpasses and underground car parks. Exposure to carbon monoxide can be twice as high – even as much as 14 times as high has been recorded – within vehicles as it is at the roadside.

Health Effects and Air Quality Standards Carbon monoxide is a systemic poison which affects health as it interferes with the absorption of oxygen by haemoglobin, exacerbates cardiovascular disease, can affect the nerves and lead to angina pectoris. As carbon monoxide is breathed, it enters the bloodstream. Its toxicity is caused by the molecule of blood, haemoglobin, which carries oxygen around the body, having a strong affinity for carbon monoxide such that carboxyhaemoglobin (COHb) is formed occupying oxygen-binding sites. The affinity of carbon monoxide for haemoglobin is 200–240 times higher than oxygen. This reduces the oxygen-carrying capacity of the blood and has the potential to starve the brain and other tissues of oxygen. Unborn children are particularly at risk because foetal haemoglobin has an even greater affinity for carbon monoxide than adult haemoglobin such that the concentration of COHb in foetal blood can reach two to three times higher than maternal blood COHb. It also takes longer for carbon monoxide to clear from foetal blood. The foetal circulatory system cannot compensate for the reduction in oxyhaemoglobin without a sustained increase in cardiac output. Monitoring of carbon monoxide concentrations tends to emphasise eight-hour averages because of the time taken for COHb to reach equilibrium in the body. The threshold for effects is about 2 per cent COHb, which is equivalent to an eight-hour exposure at moderate activity to 15–20 ppm (17–23 mg/m^3) carbon monoxide.

Low to moderate concentrations of COHb impair thinking and perception, cause headaches, slow reflexes, reduce manual dexterity, decrease exercise capacity and cause drowsiness (though it can lead to a disturbed sleep pattern). At high concentrations, death can result, as in the case of people committing suicide by inhaling vehicle exhaust fumes. Low concentrations of COHb may cause problems for people with angina (heart disease). Studies in Boston have shown that patients with angina, exercising on treadmills, experienced chest pain much earlier if they simultaneously inhaled carbon monoxide at rates which caused COHb levels of 2 per cent – a level experienced by many smokers (tobacco smoke contains carbon monoxide) and by non-smokers exposed to traffic fumes. Bridge and tunnel workers in New York City showed a greater than expected death rate from heart disease (associated with narrowed coronary arteries) and this has been attributed to regular exposure to high levels of carbon monoxide. This raises concern that other people such as traffic policemen, traffic wardens, road sweepers and even commuters in busy cities who are exposed to high carbon monoxide levels may experience an increased incidence of heart disease.

People with congenital heart defects have low blood oxygen levels and may be at risk if the oxygen-carrying capacity of their blood is reduced even further by a small increase in COHb concentration. The people most at risk from the adverse effects of carbon monoxide include not only those with pre-existing heart illness, but also infants, pregnant women and the elderly and those with chronic bronchitis and emphysema. Pregnant women are at risk because carbon monoxide may lead to the unborn baby's mental and physical growth being retarded.

Nitrogen Oxides[4]

Species and Sources There are several nitrogen oxides, but nitrogen dioxide and nitric oxide are the most important. Nitrogen oxides are generated when combustion occurs at high temperature and naturally occurring nitrogen and oxygen in the air combine to form nitric oxide. Nitric oxide is relatively innocuous but it is normally oxidised rapidly by the ozone present in air, within minutes, to nitrogen dioxide. Combustion of fuels such as coal containing nitrogenous compounds or the combustion of nitrogen-containing chemicals release nitrogen dioxide directly, but most of the nitrogen oxides arise from the oxidation of nitrogen in air. Typically, direct emissions of nitrogen dioxide from motor vehicles – the major source of nitrogen oxides in urban areas – form only 5–10 per cent of the total nitrogen oxides released. Subsequent conversion of the 90–95 per cent nitric oxide

4 Advisory Group on the Medical Aspects of Air Pollution Episodes (1993) *Oxides of Nitrogen*, Third Report, HMSO, London; Hasselblad, V, Eddy, D M and Kotchmar, D (1992) 'Synthesis of environmental evidence: nitrogen dioxide epidemiology studies', *Journal of Air and Waste Management Association*, vol 42, pp 662–671; Photochemical Oxidants Review Group (1993) *Oxides of Nitrogen in the United Kingdom*, Second Report, Department of the Environment, London

emissions to nitrogen dioxide depends on the availability of ozone. In city centres the supply of ozone is rapidly exhausted so much of the nitric oxide remains unoxidised. Only as the nitric oxide emissions drift away from the busy roads into the suburbs, above the rooftops and over the surrounding countryside, does more ozone become available for oxidation. Consequently, nitrogen dioxide commonly constitutes around 5–40 per cent of the total nitrogen oxides at city centre roadside locations, 30–80 per cent at urban background sites and 70–100 per cent in rural areas.

Ambient Concentrations Nitrogen dioxide generally declines from the centre of the road to sites at the back of the pavement. At a busy London street with traffic flows of around 50,000 vehicles a day, levels range from 80–90 ppb (150–170 µg/m^3) in the centre of the road through 50–60 ppb (95–115 µg/m^3) at the kerb to 40–50 ppb (75–95 µg/m^3) at the back of the pavement, approximately 3 m from the kerb (though levels may vary from one side of a street to the other). Locations 10–30 m away or more experience even lower concentrations often referred to as 'urban background' concentrations. However, the rate of decrease in nitrogen dioxide concentrations from the centre of a busy road to urban background sites is less than that for pollutants such as carbon monoxide, lead and fine particulates. This arises because the atmosphere's capacity to oxidise nitric oxide to nitrogen dioxide is very limited in the vicinity of busy roads by the availability of ozone. As distance from the kerbside increases so more ozone is encountered which can oxidise nitric oxide to nitrogen dioxide. On an urban scale, rather than the microscale of considering a section across a street, nitrogen dioxide concentrations tend to be highest in city centres rather than the suburbs because of the dominance of motor vehicles as the principal source of nitrogen oxides. Peak hourly levels of nitrogen dioxide of 314 ppb (600 µg/m^3) or more have been recorded in major cities such as Amsterdam, Athens, Brussels, London, Los Angeles, Munich and Rotterdam.

Episodes of nitrogen dioxide pollution ought to occur in summer rather than winter due to the part played by photochemical oxidation of nitric oxide to nitrogen dioxide. However, winter episodes can be of similar severity, suggesting that additional means of producing nitrogen dioxide may exist, such as the rapid conversion of nitric oxide with oxygen on the surfaces of fog droplets. Additionally some episodes may be due to meteorological conditions bringing down the higher nitrogen dioxide concentrations found above the tops of buildings to the surface, a process termed fumigation.

Nitrogen dioxide, a reddish brown gas, can be oxidised to a higher oxidation state to fine nitrate and nitric acid aerosols by reactions with hydroxyl radicals, ammonia and ozone. These products are much more soluble in water and are readily removed by rain so contributing to the acid rain problem. In some parts of Europe nitrate aerosol concentrations are now double those recorded in the 1950s. Another high oxidation state produced is PAN, with a typical lifetime of six hours, which can reach high concentrations during photochemical episodes and is important for health because it is a very strong eye irritant (stronger than ozone).

Power stations, often located at the urban periphery or in rural areas, are major emitters of nitrogen oxides but are of less importance for potential adverse health effects than vehicles as their emissions take place at a great height and are normally subjected to dilution and dispersion before reaching breathing level. Power stations do not normally contribute to the episodes of high nitrogen dioxide concentrations experienced at ground level in urban areas. Their emissions are of far greater concern for their acid deposition effects on sensitive environments. Industrial sources of nitrogen oxides include waste incinerators, industrial boilers, nitric acid manufacture and chemical plants.

Health Effects Nitrogen dioxide is an oxidising agent less powerful than ozone but has similar toxic effects in humans such as injuring the smallest air passages of the lung. Acute exposure to nitrogen dioxide causes respiratory diseases such as coughs and sore throats but, together with sulphur dioxide, can aggravate bronchitis, asthma and emphysema. Young children and people with asthma are particularly at risk. Nitrogen dioxide alone probably worsens the lung function of people with chronic bronchitis and asthma at levels exceeding 300 ppb (575 $\mu g/m^3$), but not all studies confirm this. Some laboratory studies have shown that the airways of people with asthma became more sensitive after exposure to only 100 ppb (190 $\mu g/m^3$) nitrogen dioxide. This occurs because the pollutant (as do sulphur dioxide and ozone) damages the mucociliary system, consisting of fine hair-like structures on the surface of cells lining the air passages, which sweep mucus and debris towards the mouth. Typically the rate of 'beating' of the cilia to expel the impurities is reduced. In other words, nitrogen dioxide exposure can make people with asthma more susceptible to symptoms caused by other environmental factors such as pollens and housedust mites, even if it does not provoke symptoms directly, because it prevents or limits a person's ability to expel allergens. Similar effects occur among people with hay fever such that growing numbers of people are experiencing hay fever symptoms of itchy eyes and runny noses due to an increase in their sensitivity to grass and tree pollens. A few studies associate 100 ppb (190 $\mu g/m^3$) with increased hospital admissions but many others did not find this. Paris statistics for the period 1987–1992 revealed that a 52 ppb (100 $\mu g/m^3$) daily rise in nitrogen dioxide was associated with a 63 per cent rise in the number of people calling their doctors with asthma attacks and a 17 per cent rise in people going to hospital for the same reason.

Laboratory studies have shown that nitrogen dioxide concentrations of 400 ppb (765 $\mu g/m^3$), levels experienced occasionally in urban areas, increase susceptibility to infection. A study of 1225 pre-school children in four regions in Switzerland attempted to examine the relationship between nitrogen dioxide concentrations and daily respiratory symptoms such as cough, sore throat, fever, running nose and earache for a period of six weeks in 1985 and 1986. Nitrogen dioxide levels were measured outside the children's homes as well as by using personal exposure samplers attached to each child. The frequency of respiratory symptoms per child per day was shown to increase with increasing levels of outdoor nitrogen dioxide.

Volatile Organic Compounds[5]

Characteristics and Sources Volatile organic compounds (VOCs) refer to a wide range of organic compounds including hydrocarbons (alkanes, alkenes, aromatics), oxygenates (alcohols, aldehydes, ketones, acids, ethers) and halogen-containing species (eg methyl chloroform, trichloroethylene). They are all organic compounds of carbon and are sufficiently volatile (meaning they readily evaporate) to exist as vapour in the air. For example, benzene is a clear colourless liquid with a boiling point of only 80°C. Emissions of VOCs result from incomplete fuel combustion or from evaporated unburned petrol from vehicle fuel tanks and carburettors as well as from leakage during the transport, storage and distribution of fuel to service stations. Leakage from the natural gas distribution network also adds VOCs such as ethane. Domestic sources include paints and solvents, consumer products, adhesives and fuel combustion. Methane is the most abundant VOC on the global scale, produced mainly by natural processes such as the decomposition of organic matter in rice paddies and natural woodlands, but its relatively low reactivity means it is of limited importance in pollution–health considerations except indirectly – that is, it is an important greenhouse gas and contributes to global warming. It is common for researchers examining health effects of VOCs to restrict their studies to non-methane VOCs.

An important part played by VOCs in air pollution problems is that they contribute to the formation of photochemical oxidants such as ozone. The potential of VOCs to create ozone varies with each compound. It has been quantified as the photochemical ozone creation potential (POCP). Values vary from the relative inactive 0.7 for methane, 4.0 for ethane, 18.9 for benzene, 41.4 for *n*-butane, 56.3 for toluene and 100.0 for ethylene. The VOCs with the greatest photochemical reactivity usually contain unsaturated double bonds such as in ethane, propane (alkanes), butadiene (an alkene) or toluene, xylene and trimethylbenzene (aromatics).

5 Expert Panel on Air Quality Standards (1994) *Benzene*, HMSO, London; Expert Panel on Air Quality Standards (1994) *1,3-Butadiene*, HMSO, London; Jefferiss, P, Rowell, A and Fergusson, M (1992) *The Exposure of Car Drivers and Passengers to Vehicle Emissions*, Greenpeace, London; Read, R and Read, C (1991) 'Breathing can be hazardous to your health', *New Scientist*, 23 Feb, pp 34–37 (refers to US studies of benzene and other pollutants)

Health Effects Some VOCs cause eye and skin irritation, drowsiness, coughing and sneezing, whereas others such as benzene and 1,3-butadiene emitted by petrol exhausts are also carcinogenics, causing leukaemia. Benzene, like benzo(*a*)pyrene, is classified as a genotoxic carcinogen, which means it directly affects the genetic material of the cell (the DNA) and as such no absolutely safe level of exposure can be defined. This aromatic hydrocarbon occurs naturally in crude oil and forms during the upgrading of fuel oil. The dominant emissions of benzene in urban atmospheres are from petrol exhausts (being one of many unburnt hydrocarbons), petrol during refuelling and by evaporation from fuel tanks. In unleaded fuel, aromatic hydrocarbons (as well as olefines) replace lead as the means of raising the octane level. This results in higher exhaust emissions of benzene (and butadiene from olefines) from vehicles using unleaded petrol in a vehicle not fitted with a catalytic converter. In the European Union the benzene content is limited to 5 per cent by volume, although typically fuels contain about 2–4 per cent in most European countries. Diesel accounts for only a relatively small proportion of emissions of benzene (about 9 per cent in the UK in 1991).

A study of 748 workers in the rubber industry exposed to benzene over ten years showed that this group of people were 5.6 times more likely to have low white blood cell counts and develop leukaemia than the general population. According to the WHO and US EPA, 0.3 ppb (1 $\mu g/m^3$) produces an estimated lifetime risk of leukaemia of 4–8 per million, with the risk being proportional to the concentration. Estimates of the number of people who may develop leukaemia in the Los Angeles basin as a result of exposure to benzene are put at 100–780 per million people exposed. People inside vehicles in a slow-moving stream of traffic may be exposed to two to three times higher concentrations of benzene than those walking alongside the road due to leaks into the interior from the exhaust system and due to emissions from car exhausts in front. A few researchers have suggested that the higher rates of leukaemia among children in the suburbs and commuter villages could be linked to benzene exposure during prolonged car journeys.

Air Quality Standards and Ambient Concentrations Only a few countries have set benzene air quality standards, perhaps reflecting that according to the WHO there is no known safe threshold. The Netherlands adopted an annual standard of 3 ppb (10 $\mu g/m^3$) in 1993 (and also Germany from 1998), whereas an advisory group to the UK Government suggested setting a running annual average of 5 ppb (16 $\mu g/m^3$), but qualified this by concluding that as benzene is a genotoxic carcinogen and as, in principle, exposure to such substances should be kept as low as practicable, the government should set a deadline for reducing this to 1 ppb (3 $\mu g/m^3$). Current benzene levels in UK cities indicate that some locations experience annual levels close to 5 ppb (16 $\mu g/m^3$) and that all locations currently exceed 1 ppb (3 $\mu g/m^3$). The growing concern about the adverse health effects of benzene has resulted in greater attention being given to reducing the benzene content of petrol, reducing the volatility of petrol, which will reduce evaporative emissions (providing the aromatic hydrocarbon content is not increased at the same time), installing vapour recovery systems at petrol pumps and in vehicles, and fitting catalytic converters which reduce benzene emissions.

Ozone[6]

Characteristics and Formation Photochemical reactions between nitrogen oxides and VOCs (and involving carbon monoxide) in sunlight create oxidants such as ozone, a triatomic oxygen molecule. In other words, ozone is a secondary pollutant. The main sources of the precursor emissions which lead to ozone formation are motor vehicles and power stations for nitrogen oxides and motor vehicles and evaporation losses from organic solvents and the petrochemical industries for most of the VOCs. Ozone, a faintly bluish gas, is the dominant oxidant formed during photochemical reactions and comprises about 90 per cent of the total. Other oxidants created include PAN, peroxybenzol nitrate, hydrogen peroxide and nitric acid, whereas the photochemical reactions also create fine particulates which give photochemical smogs a hazy appearance.

Tropospheric and Stratospheric Ozone Concern for increasing concentrations of ozone in the lower atmosphere (troposphere) should not be confused with the problem of the depletion of naturally occurring ozone in the upper atmosphere (stratosphere). Stratospheric ozone is formed at altitudes between 12 and 40 km, known as the ozone layer, by sunlight splitting oxygen molecules into oxygen atoms which then combine to form ozone. Stratospheric ozone is being depleted by chlorine-containing compounds such as CFCs, carbon tetrachloride and methyl chloroform. The depletion is accentuated at the cold poles, especially in Antarctica during springtime where it has created what is popularly referred to as the 'ozone hole'. Stratospheric ozone plays a vital part in protecting people, plants and animals by absorbing harmful ultraviolet radiation from the sun which would otherwise increase skin cancer, cause cataracts, damage crops and kill phytoplankton. Another benefit of the ozone layer is that it is warmed during the process of absorption of ultraviolet radiation and forms a thermal lid to the atmosphere. This lid traps virtually all atmospheric moisture below

6 Advisory Group on the Medical Aspects of Air Pollution Episodes (1991) *Ozone*, First Report, HMSO, London; Edwards, R (1995) 'Ozone alert follows cancer warning', *New Scientist*, 27 May, p 4; Expert Panel on Air Quality Standards (1994) *Ozone*, HMSO, London; Lippmann, M (1991) 'Health effects of tropospheric ozone', *Environmental Science and Technology*, vol 25, pp 1954–1962; Office of Technology Assessment (1989) *Catching Our Breath: Next Steps for Reducing Urban Ozone*, US Congress, Washington DC; Photochemical Oxidants Review Group (1993) *Ozone in the United Kingdom 1993*, Third Report, Department of the Environment, London

it, so enabling cloud and precipitation processes to operate, which in turn sustain life on our planet.

Some stratospheric ozone does diffuse down into the lower atmosphere producing a naturally occurring background concentration of ozone of about 10–15 per cent of the tropospheric total. Occasionally brief intrusions of stratospheric air, rich in ozone, can plunge towards the surface, temporarily increasing surface concentrations. This usually happens during disturbed weather conditions such as those associated with the passing of a cold front when urban-generated levels of ozone are not particularly high anyway. One link between the tropospheric and stratospheric ozone problems is that the depletion of ozone levels in the upper atmosphere will allow increased levels of ultraviolet radiation to reach the lower atmosphere. This increase in ultraviolet radiation will speed up the rate of photochemical reactions which produce ozone in the lower atmosphere and so worsen urban air quality.

Ambient Concentrations Ozone is as much a pollutant of rural as urban areas. Indeed, rural areas often experience higher ozone concentrations than urban areas, especially the traffic-congested city centres. This arises for two main reasons. Firstly, city centres record lower ozone levels than suburban or rural areas because some pollutants remove ozone from the air. Nitric oxide emitted from motor vehicles is one such ozone-scavenging pollutant, as are unsaturated hydrocarbons such as alkenes. Secondly, VOCs vary in their degree of reactivity such that photochemical reactions that lead to ozone formation may take an hour or several hours to operate. During the time taken to create ozone the urban plume of precursor pollutants may have drifted many tens of kilometres downwind of cities, increasing rural ozone concentrations there by as much as 70 ppb (140 $\mu g/m^3$). Ozone may continue to be created many hundreds of kilometres downwind of major cities during daylight hours.

During stable weather conditions associated with an anticyclone, vast quantities of precursor emissions from many urban–industrial areas often become trapped above a low-level temperature inversion and drift a thousand kilometres or more across state and national boundaries. There is sufficient time for even the least-reactive VOCs to contribute to ozone formation during this spell of sunny warm weather conditions. This rich plume of ozone remains undiminished because it is isolated from having contact with the ground and from the scavenging effects of fresh nitric oxide emissions released by urban areas. This reservoir of ozone may be brought down to the ground in areas very distant from the original source of the precursor emissions when the temperature inversion breaks down under the thermal turbulence produced by strong afternoon solar heating. In contrast, any ozone lying close to the ground after sunset is depleted by contact with the surface (the process of dry deposition) and by chemical reactions with nitric oxide. Hence ozone levels close to the ground may approach zero and remain so until next morning when sunlight begins to trigger ozone formation from the fresh precursor emissions and/or when the night-time stable or inversion layer of the atmosphere breaks down, bringing down ozone that had been stored aloft. If for some reason an inversion breaks down during the night it is possible that ozone trapped aloft is transported downwards, producing an unexpected but short-lived rise in ozone concentrations at night.

The annual mean ozone concentration in Europe appears to be increasing at a rate of about 1–2 per cent, mainly in response to increasing emissions of nitrogen oxides and VOCs from traffic. Whereas summer background levels in 'clean' areas were about 10–20 ppb (20–40 $\mu g/m^3$) a century ago, they are today in the range 20–40 ppb (40–80 $\mu g/m^3$). However, trends at individual sites vary greatly. At most UK rural sites the trend is upward, but in southern England ozone concentrations have declined recently at sites where nitrogen oxide levels are high and where they are increasing. This occurs because of the increased scavenging of ozone by emissions of nitric oxides. Consequently, pollution control legislation which reduces nitrogen oxide emissions could lead initially to a short-term increase in ozone levels.

Not surprisingly, because of the role of photochemical reactions in ozone formation, ozone concentrations are greatest during daylight hours and during periods of warm, sunny and stable weather conditions. Air temperatures exceeding 20°C are generally needed as this speeds up the rate of chemical reactions and also increases the evaporative emissions of VOCs. In recent years, peak hourly concentrations of around 150 ppb (300 $\mu g/m^3$) have occurred in southern Britain, Belgium and the Netherlands compared with peaks of 275–300 ppb (550–600 $\mu g/m^3$) measured in the Athens basin and in northern Italy. In the Los Angeles basin peak values have shown a decline in recent decades from peak hourly values of over 600 ppb (1200 $\mu g/m^3$) in the 1950s to 200–300 ppb (400–600 $\mu g/m^3$) during the 1990s. In contrast, Mexico City has gained a worsening reputation for ozone in recent years with peak hourly values typically reaching 400–600 ppb (800–1200 $\mu g/m^3$).

Air Quality Standards Ozone concentrations are usually measured as hourly concentrations, with the maximum hourly concentration during a day being used as a guide to the severity of ozone pollution to which people are exposed. Although peak hourly concentrations of ozone are held responsible for causing the most severe health effects, some researchers suggest that ozone levels measured over a longer period may be more important to health. Many locations today reveal a diurnal ozone cycle which incorporates both a locally generated midday sharp peak and a regionally transported, less pronounced plateau in the late afternoon. The local and regional contributions can merge together to give six to eight hours of sustained high ozone concentrations. Broad but less pronounced ozone peaks appear to have become more commonplace in Europe and the US than 20–30 years ago as the atmosphere has become more widely contaminated by precursor pollutants. The WHO specify an eight-hour guideline of 50–60 ppb (100–120 µg/m^3) and it is likely that nations will increasingly adopt this or a similar standard in addition to their mandatory one-hour ozone standard. In 1994, the advisory group to the UK Government recommended adopting an ozone air quality standard in the form of a running eight-hour average of 50 ppb (100 µg/m^3).

Short-term Health Effects Ozone is extremely reactive, being one of the strongest oxidising agents (oxidants) known. It can react with almost any type of biological substance. It can crack stretched rubber and ladder nylon stockings at very low levels and cause paint and fabrics to fade. Therefore it is not surprising that it can harm delicate lung tissues as well as impair the body's defences against bacteria and viruses. Ozone causes damage at the point of contact: the respiratory tract. Owing to its low solubility in water it is absorbed to a much lesser degree in the naso-pharyngeal region than, say, sulphur dioxide. Consequently, it penetrates much deeper into the peripheral regions of the lung, into the tiniest air passages. The low solubility of ozone in water is also probably the reason for its weak eye-irritating properties compared with other compounds present in photochemical smogs such as PAN. Whichever oxidant is to blame, photochemical smogs usually cause eye irritation, which often leads to eye fatigue and blurred vision.

High ozone levels make patients with asthma worse, impair lung function, and increase both respiratory tract infections and hospital admissions. When daily ozone levels increase by 50 ppb (100 µg/m^3) in Paris, admissions of elderly people with chronic breathing problems rise by 20 per cent and lower respiratory tract infections in children by 24 per cent. Like sulphur dioxide and nitrogen dioxide, ozone sensitises people with asthma to common allergens such as pollen by damaging the ability of the cells which line the respiratory tract to sweep out invading pollen and bacteria. Laboratory tests have shown that people with asthma breathing air with 120 ppb (240 µg/m^3) of ozone for an hour reacted to half the dose of ragweed pollen compared with their reaction when breathing clean air. Ozone can worsen other chronic respiratory diseases such as bronchitis by reducing resistance to respiratory infections and so increasing the frequency of colds or more serious diseases such as pneumonia.

Ozone affects the health of the population at low levels when physical exercise is combined with several hours' exposure to low-level concentrations – that is, the tissue dose is enhanced by an increased respiratory rate. The duration and intensity of exposure are of prime importance: several hours of exposure to levels above a threshold may be more important than the maximum concentration to which a population is exposed. Physical exercise during the afternoon, a time of the day when ozone levels are highest, exposes many people to high doses of ozone. Even low levels of ozone can cause symptoms such as coughing, choking, shortness of breath, excess sputum, throat tickle, raspy throat, nausea and impaired lung function when exercising. Such effects mean that top-class competitive athletes can seldom perform at their best even when levels of ozone are relatively low – as some athletes discovered when the Olympics were held in Los Angeles in 1984.

The role of physical exercise in determining exposure to ozone highlights that those individuals whose health is most at risk from ozone are not the people with asthma or chronic bronchitis – the population group most sensitive to pollutants such as sulphur dioxide – but those people engaged in prolonged, strenuous physical activity such as adults engaged in sport and children participating in school games or at play. During light, intermittent exercise, lasting only an hour or two, an ozone concentration of 300 ppb (600 $\mu g/m^3$) causes irritation. Studies at a New Jersey summer camp found that when children were exposed to an eight-hour average ozone level of around 100 ppb (200 $\mu g/m^3$) they experienced a temporary impairment of lung function. Healthy exercising men exposed to ozone levels of 120 ppb (240 $\mu g/m^3$) for seven hours found their lung function decreased by 12 per cent and experienced breathing difficulties, especially an inability to take deep breaths. Studies suggest that although children are as sensitive as adults to ozone causing lung function changes, they appear less aware of any accompanying respiratory irritation than adults. Given that the background level of ozone is relatively close to the threshold concentration of ozone which causes adverse health effects it is possible that, if annual trends continue, all sunny days may pose a threat to people exercising in terms of causing eye, nose and throat irritation, coughs, fatigue, headaches and chest discomfort.

Long-term Health Effects Long-term exposure of laboratory rats to ozone has shown that irreversible functional and morphological changes to their lungs occur that imply premature ageing of the lung. Epidemiological studies in Los Angeles suggest that its residents experience a decrease in lung function and an increase in chronic obstructive pulmonary disease – that is, emphysema and chronic bronchitis – compared with residents from less polluted regions. However, ozone may be only one contributing pollutant to chronic obstructive pulmonary disease as levels of suspended particulates were also high in the study area. Research in Los Angeles involving post-mortems of the lungs of healthy young non-smokers killed in accidents revealed inflammation of the bronchioles – bronchiolitis – which may be due to long-term exposure to the high ozone levels of the Los Angeles basin. Such effects are similar to that evident in cigarette smokers.

With ozone levels currently exceeding federal health standards of 120 ppb (240 $\mu g/m^3$) in parts of the Los Angeles basin for three months of the year – but for far longer periods in the past – it is not surprising that some researchers claim that children born and brought up there will grow up with 10–15 per cent less lung capacity than children elsewhere. Children are more likely than adults to develop ozone-related lung damage because, for their body size, children inhale several times more air than adults and they breathe faster (through their mouths), particularly during strenuous physical activity. In addition, they spend more time outdoors than any other population group.

Lead and Other Toxic Metals[7]

Trace Metals Trace metals, usually occurring in particulate form, are released from ferrous and non-ferrous metal smelting and finishing, battery manufacturing, waste incinerators, motor vehicles, cement and fertiliser production and during the combustion of fossil fuels. Metal forms of arsenic, chromium and nickel are known to be carcinogenic. Metals can damage the cardiovascular and pulmonary systems, cause skin disease and affect the central nervous system. Specifically, arsenic can produce lung cancer and dermatological disorders; beryllium can result in dermatitis and ulcers; cadmium is harmful to the kidneys; chromium can cause lung and gastrointestinal cancers; nickel can trigger respiratory illnesses, birth defects, and nasal and lung cancers; and lead can cause liver and kidney damage as well as neurological effects. Whereas concentrations of many metals pose a health risk in 'hot-spots', often surrounding a specific point source such as an industrial plant, lead is a much more widespread pollutant.

Airborne Lead The main source of lead in the urban atmosphere is from the combustion of leaded petrol in which lead has been added as an anti-knock agent and as a lubricant for valve seats in the form of tetraethyl and tetramethyl lead. Lead prevents knocking – the distinctive 'pinking' noise which occurs when there is a spontaneous ignition of the petrol and air mixture in the corner of the cylinder furthest from the spark plug (the end-gas zone). Adding lead to petrol is equivalent in engine combustion of using petrol with a higher octane number (the percentage of very high knock-resistant types of hydrocarbons), but it is a cheaper method of boosting the octane quality of petrol than undertaking intensive refining. This practice was begun in the 1930s, although by the mid-1970s countries such as the US and Japan had begun to reduce the lead content of petrol, followed by the European Union in the late 1970s. After combustion the lead is released

7 Harrison, R M (1993) 'A perspective on lead pollution and health 1972–1992', *Journal of the Royal Society of Health*, Jun, pp 142–148; Royal Commission on Environmental Pollution (1993) *Lead in the Environment*, Ninth Report, HMSO, London; WHO (1991) *Impact on Human Health of Air Pollution in Europe*, WHO Regional Office for Europe, Copenhagen (briefly reviews health effects of arsenic, cadmium, mercury and lead as well as summer-type and winter-type pollution episodes); Wishart, A (1992) 'Lead campaigner cleared of fraud', *New Scientist*, 30 May, p 7 (refers to the controversy concerning the validity of the earliest study, by Herbert Needleman in 1979, which had claimed that even at low doses lead affected children's behaviour); Wright, B (1992) 'High lead levels may permanently lower IQ', *New Scientist*, 29 Feb, p 13 (Australian study results)

through exhaust emissions into the air in the form of fine inorganic particles which can be inhaled.

American research suggests that a blood lead level of 0.15 μg/ml is associated with an atmospheric concentration of 1.5 $\mu g/m^3$. The concentration of lead in blood is used as an indicator of recent exposure to lead, both from inhaled airborne lead and from the ingestion of lead in food and drinks. Adverse health effects increase in severity with increasing blood lead levels. As lead is not readily excreted, it affects the kidneys, liver, nervous system and blood-forming organs. The effects of lead range from increased blood pressure (increasing the risk of a heart attack in middle-aged men) and disturbed kidney and reproductive functions to irreversible brain damage. In Australia it was estimated that if the elimination of lead in petrol could reduce blood lead levels by half it would reduce average blood pressure levels by 1–2 points in 35–64 year olds, thereby resulting in 12,000 fewer people annually in this age range needing treatment for hypertension. In addition, there would be 6000–12,000 fewer heart attacks and up to 2655 lives would be saved.

Children appear to be most at risk and it is claimed that high levels of lead in the blood affect their neurobehaviour, with such children experiencing behavioural problems, lower intelligence quotients (IQs) and difficulty in concentrating. However, claims for lead affecting behaviour and IQ remain controversial. Suggestions as to why lead may be affecting IQ levels include lead interfering with the role of calcium in brain cell development. Perinatal exposure to low levels of lead may affect the length of gestation and infant mental and physical development (eg resulting in a lower birth weight and subsequent impaired physical growth).

Ambient Levels of Airborne Lead Many cities in The North such as London, Los Angeles, New York and Tokyo have largely overcome previous lead pollution problems as the lead content in petrol has been successively reduced and as unleaded petrol has come to dominate petrol sales. Typically lead concentrations in US and UK cities have dropped by more than 90 per cent since the early 1980s. California banned the sale of leaded petrol in 1992 and the US, as a whole, banned sales in 1995. Unleaded petrol was introduced not only because of concern about the effects of lead on health, but because vehicles fitted with catalytic converters which reduce emissions of carbon monoxide, nitrogen dioxide and hydrocarbons only work effectively with unleaded petrol (lead 'poisons' the catalyst).

Relatively low traffic densities in Beijing and Moscow have helped to ensure airborne lead is not a problem in these cities at the present time, but such a problem may develop as the number of motor vehicles increases. The use of ethanol or gasohol (a blend of ethanol and petrol) as the dominant fuel for motor vehicles in the Brazilian cities of Rio de Janeiro and São Paulo has minimised airborne lead concentrations. In contrast, large cities such as Bangkok, Cairo, Jakarta, Karachi, Manila and Mexico City still face serious airborne lead problems. In Bangkok, excessive exposure to lead is estimated to cause 200,000 to 500,000 cases of hypertension, resulting in up to 400 deaths a year. In addition, it is claimed that children have lost four or more IQ points on average by the age of 7 years because of exposure to elevated lead levels. In Mexico City it is estimated that seven out of ten children have had their development stunted by lead poisoning (although other pollutants may also have played a part).

Conclusions: Responding to the Pollution Threat

Sulphur dioxide, acid aerosols, suspended particulates, fine particulates, carbon monoxide, nitrogen dioxide, VOCs, ozone and lead all pose potential threats to the health and well-being of the inhabitants of an urban area. To be able to assess the seriousness of those threats and then to take effective actions that will deal with the pollution problems, the city authorities need to set up an appropriate framework that will eventually enable them to achieve and sustain healthy urban air quality. The next two chapters outline what is needed to produce an effective urban air quality management system.

Chapter 4

Developing an Effective Framework for Urban Air Quality Management

Framework for Urban Air Quality Management

If urban air quality fails to meet mandatory or advisory health-based air quality standards then sensitive members of the community or even most of the community may be subject to unacceptable health risks. In such a situation the city authorities and national government need to establish a framework which enables them to take actions which will ensure that air quality is improved and that eventually air quality standards or guidelines are reached and maintained. This may involve applying short and long term pollution control (emission-reduction) policies and measures. For example, temporary traffic restrictions or industrial production cutbacks may be imposed during a smog to prevent further short-term air quality deterioration while the authorities pursue a long-term strategy involving changes to the entire city's land use, energy and transport policies.

Before costly emission-reduction actions are taken the authorities will want to know the likely air quality effectiveness of alternative pollution control policies and measures. This is especially important when there is a range of emission-reduction measures that could be employed, each of which differ in cost and difficulty of implementation. This chapter is concerned with how the authorities should go about establishing and operating an air quality management system for managing air quality in both the short and long term. Many questions need to be answered and many factors considered when setting up an effective urban air quality management system. An obvious starting point is to establish whether an urban area even has an air pollution problem or whether it may have one in the near future. This requires monitoring and modelling the ambient levels of a wide range of pollutants over different time-scales and locations to assess whether health-based air quality standards are being met once such standards have been agreed. For some urban areas this requires establishing a network of pollutant monitors but for most this means improving and expanding an existing network. If air quality fails to meet the standards, as is the case in far too many of the world's cities, then pollution control policies and measures need to be introduced.

Even if air quality is acceptable at present there is a need to continue monitoring to be assured it will remain so. Monitoring needs to be combined with the means to predict air quality levels in, say, ten years time taking into account likely changes in land use, energy and transport policies as well as trends in population and the number and use of motor vehicles. To be able to predict future air quality levels requires a knowledge of current and planned emission rates from different sources and locations within the urban area and, in some cases, a measure of the pollution imported from other urban areas. Prediction involves using numerical models (differing pollutants and scales of investigation may require different models) to estimate how the spatial pattern of emission rates is transformed by the atmospheric processes of dilution, dispersion and chemical reactions into ground level pollution concentrations. The model is first applied to the existing situation so that pollution monitors can assess the accuracy of the model. If it is of acceptable accuracy it can then be applied with confidence to future conditions based on various scenarios of changes to the urban pattern of emission rates. The model results can provide the authorities with essential insights into the likely air quality impact of specific land use, energy and transport policies.

The components of an urban air quality management system include an air quality monitoring network, emission inventories, numerical prediction models, air quality standards and public information bands, and a range of cost-effective pollution control policies and measures, together with the resources and powers to impose them.[1] This chapter discusses each

1 Archer, G (1995) 'Use of air quality standards and local air quality management in the European Union and other countries', *Clean Air*, vol 25, pp 16–27; Elsom, D M (1994) 'The development of urban air quality management systems in the United Kingdom', in Baldasano, J M, Brebbia, C A, Power, H and Zanetti, P (eds) *Air Pollution*, vol 2, Pollution Control and Monitoring, Computational Mechanics, Southampton, pp 545–552; Elsom, D M and Crabbe, H (1995) 'Developing effective urban air quality management systems in the United Kingdom: case studies', *Proceedings of the 10th World Clean Air Congress, Espoo, Finland*, vol 3, Finnish Air Pollution Prevention Society, Helsinki, paper 508; Elsom, D M and Crabbe, H (1995) 'Practical issues involved in developing effective local air quality management in the United Kingdom', in Power, H *et al* (eds) *Air Pollution*, Computational Mechanics, Southampton, pp 483–492; Longhurst, J W S, Lindley, S J and Conlan, D E (1994) 'Towards local air quality management in the United Kingdom', in Baldasano, J M, Brebbia, C A, Power, H and Zanetti, P (eds) *Air Pollution*, vol 2, Pollution Control and Monitoring, Computational Mechanics, pp 525–532; Longhurst, J W S, Lindley, S J and Conlan, D E (1995) 'Advances in local air quality management in the United Kingdom' in Power, H (op cit)

component separately, but it should be borne in mind that they all form part of an integrated system (Figure 4.1). If inadequate attention is given by the authorities to one component it is likely to result in limitations in the effectiveness of the entire system. Many cities in the world have developed some form of urban air quality management system, although many have not reached the sophistication and completeness ultimately needed by urban air quality managers.

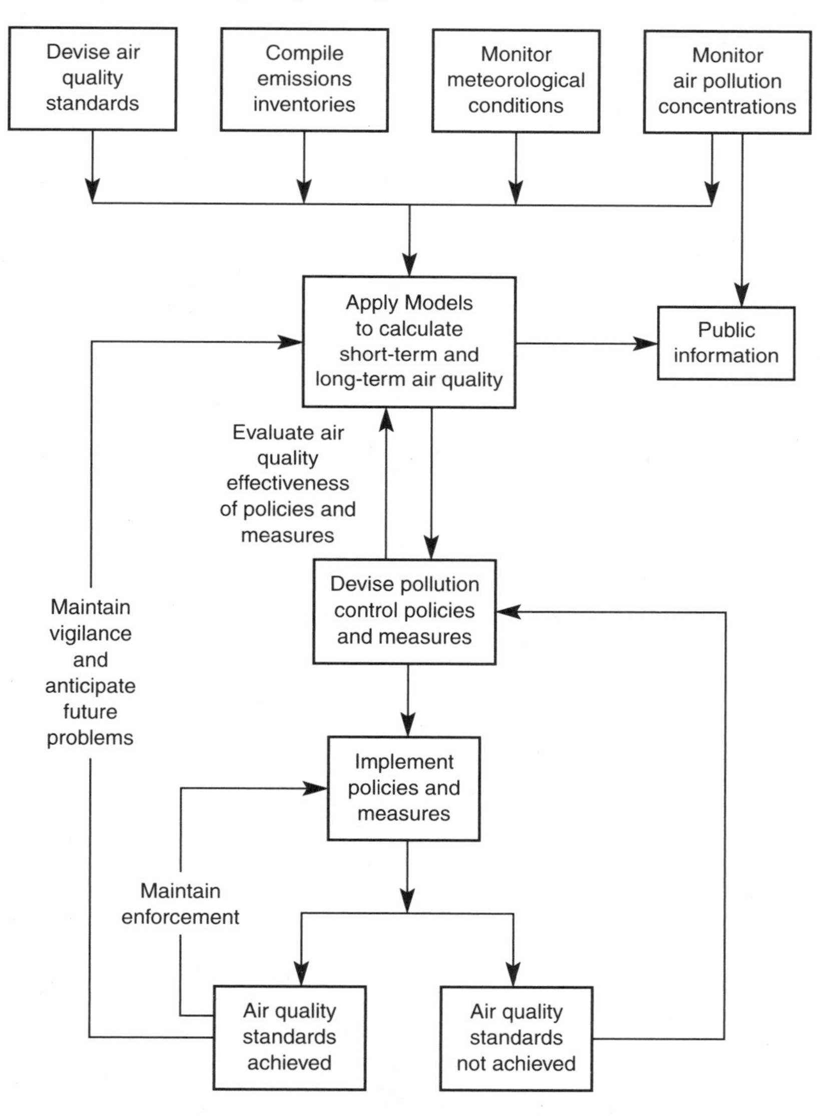

Figure 4.1 *Framework for air quality management*

Air Quality Monitoring Networks

Objectives of Monitoring In the context of air quality management, pollution monitoring networks are employed with several objectives in mind:

- to assess whether or not air quality meets health-based standards or guidelines to assess the degree of health risk posed to the population by different pollutants in various parts of the city (ie to identify pollution hot-spots);
- to identify short-term periods during which health-based standards are exceeded so that the public can receive warnings and be offered advice about how they can minimise risks to their health and the authorities can justify the introduction of temporary emission-reduction measures (a smog alert system);
- to measure changes in pollution concentrations to assess the effectiveness of short-term (eg temporary traffic bans) and/or long-term pollution control policies and measures (eg transport policies, alternative fuels, more stringent vehicle emission standards);
- to establish long-term trends in pollution concentrations with a view to assessing why those changes are occurring (eg changing activity patterns, growth in vehicle emissions);
- to validate numerical prediction models and provide confidence in the accuracy of their results on which authorities will base their short-term and/or long-term pollution control actions;
- to check that licensed premises (eg industrial plants) comply with pollution regulations (eg emission limits);
- to provide data for the preparation of an environmental impact statement for a proposed large project (eg monitoring before and after development);
- to provide information to improve our understanding of the atmospheric processes transforming emissions to concentrations.

What Pollutants Should be Monitored? Knowledge of ground level concentrations of a wide range of pollutants throughout the urban area are desired. In practice, sulphur dioxide, suspended particulates (including PM_{10}), carbon monoxide, nitrogen dioxide, VOCs (eg benzene), ozone and airborne lead pose the most common threats to the health of the community and it is these pollutants that are the focus of attention of most urban-wide pollution monitoring networks. Toxic chemicals (eg ammonia, fluoride) or toxic metals other than lead (eg cadmium) can cause localised health problems around individual industrial sources such as chemical industries, waste incinerators and metal-processing plants and require small-scale monitoring networks to be established around the point source in question.

Pollutants pose differing health risks so the monitoring network density should reflect this situation by concentrating on the pollutants posing the greatest threat to health. Currently in many Northern countries the health effects of nitrogen dioxide, PM_{10} and benzene are causing concern, whereas concentrations of sulphur dioxide and airborne lead have fallen so low in recent years that these pollutants no longer pose a health problem except near some industrial sources. Such a situation allows the monitoring network for sulphur dioxide and airborne lead to be reduced to a minimum (eg restricted to sites monitoring the long-term trend and any remaining pollution hot-spots such as industrial plants) while expanding the nitrogen dioxide, PM_{10} and benzene monitoring network. Clearly an air quality monitoring network should reflect changing situations and concerns as well as new research results. Additional pollutants may have to be monitored or a network that was once assumed to have a satisfactory number of monitors may have to be expanded. For example, only in recent years have some countries recognised the health threat posed by PM_{10} and benzene. In the case of ozone, recent research suggests that although concentrations in urban areas are generally lower than the surrounding rural areas there may be localised areas where ozone levels are similar to rural areas. This uncertainty needs investigating by expanding the ozone monitoring urban network.

Selecting Monitoring Sites and Network Density A dense automated network measuring all major pollutants and providing continuous up to the minute data to a central control – where visual displays provide the urban-wide air quality situation – is the ideal monitoring network for air quality management, but the high cost of this computerised system often precludes its realisation in practice. Instead a compromise has to be reached between cost and the type of data needed.[2] If the number of monitoring sites has to be restricted then authorities need to focus on pollution hot-spots such as traffic-congested city centres and industrial sites as well as a few 'urban background' sites which can provide a guideline to the typical pollution levels to which large numbers of the urban community are exposed. Representative urban sites may be located in densely-populated areas, shopping centres, railway stations, etc. The validity of a single fixed site to provide an indication of community exposure can be questioned so it is appropriate to use other monitors for short-term periods at various urban locations to assess the degree to which the one site is indeed representative. Such a strategy establishes which parts of the urban area are not represented by the single site and so may need monitoring. The use of a mobile monitor enabling short-term urban traverses to be undertaken may

2 Barrowcliffe, R (1992) 'Air quality monitoring', *Environmental Policy and Practice*, vol 1(4), pp 3–26; Calori, G, Finzi, G and Tonezzer, C (1994) 'A decision support system for air quality network design', *Environmental Monitoring and Assessment*, vol 33, pp 101–114; Department of the Environment (1994) *Improving Air Quality: a Discussion Paper on Air Quality Standards and Management*, Department of the Environment, London; Munn, R E (1981) *The Design of Air Quality Monitoring Networks*, Macmillan, London

be another way of verifying representation, as may the use of a large number of cheap passive monitors such as diffusion tubes. The use of different types of monitoring equipment highlights the question as to whether measurements obtained from different types of equipment are compatible. Compatibility can be tested by operating the different equipment side by side at the same location for a trial period.

When finance is available to establish a larger network of monitoring sites various network designs may be used. One option is to place a monitor as near as possible to a regular grid network as this provides the most convenient type of data for input into numerical prediction models. Berlin uses 31 continuously operating sulphur dioxide monitors arranged in a grid network of 4 by 4 km across the city (an additional 16 short-term monitors were placed within one of the larger squares to form a 1 by 1 km network for a test period in 1984–1985).[3] Another option, more commonly applied as it is less costly, is to locate monitors in differing land use and urban activity areas such as the city centre, residential, commercial and industrial areas in an attempt to obtain pollution values representative of that type of urban zone. Either type of design may include additional monitors or sub-networks to measure the effect of traffic emissions on air quality in potential pollution hot-spots such as congested city centre streets. Public pressure may play a part in deciding whether other pollution hot-spots are monitored such as around specific industrial plants. A traffic-centred network may involve monitors being placed in the middle of a busy road, at the kerbside, at the back of the pavement and at a short distance away from the road. Information collected from this network enables relationships to be established concerning the rate of change of air quality with distance from the road. Urban monitoring networks for a variety of pollutants may be established for many different purposes, with the result that urban areas contain a diverse collection of monitors. Finally, it may be appropriate to locate monitors at the urban periphery to assess the amount of pollution being imported to and exported from the city.

Site selection for the monitors can involve other factors such as the need for security to protect against vandalism (this usually means the air intake is located 2.5 m or more above the ground), the need for a power supply, 24-hour access to the site, whether planning permission will be given for the installation of a large cabin of multi-pollutant monitoring equipment, and the possible influence from indoor and localised sources which may make the data unrepresentative of the wider area. As pollution concentrations are strongly influenced by atmospheric conditions and because weather data are needed as input into short-term prediction models, pollution monitoring stations may include equipment to measure wind speed and direction, temperature, precipitation, relative humidity and air pressure.

3 Lahmann, E (1990) *Winter Smog in Germany*, Air Hygiene Report No 3, WHO Collaborating Centre for Air Quality Management and Air Pollution Control, Berlin, p 49

Although an automated network of sites providing real-time information transmitted to a central point is essential for the management of short-term air pollution episodes or smogs, it is of less importance for some aspects of long-term air quality management such as ensuring that annual mean concentrations meet air quality standards. However, air quality management needs to include both short- and long-term management and so the transmission of real-time data by means of telephone lines is important. Pollution concentrations are needed not only for averaging times of daily (24-hour) periods, but also for hourly and even 15-minute periods as short-term peaks can cause acute health effects (Figure 4.2). Some high-resolution equipment can monitor concentrations continuously every few minutes or even less but such detailed information is seldom needed except to check instrument performance. If relationships between pollution concentrations such as annual means and 98th centile concentrations can be established it is possible to use relatively simple equipment to monitor the annual mean concentrations from which higher resolution concentrations can be estimated.

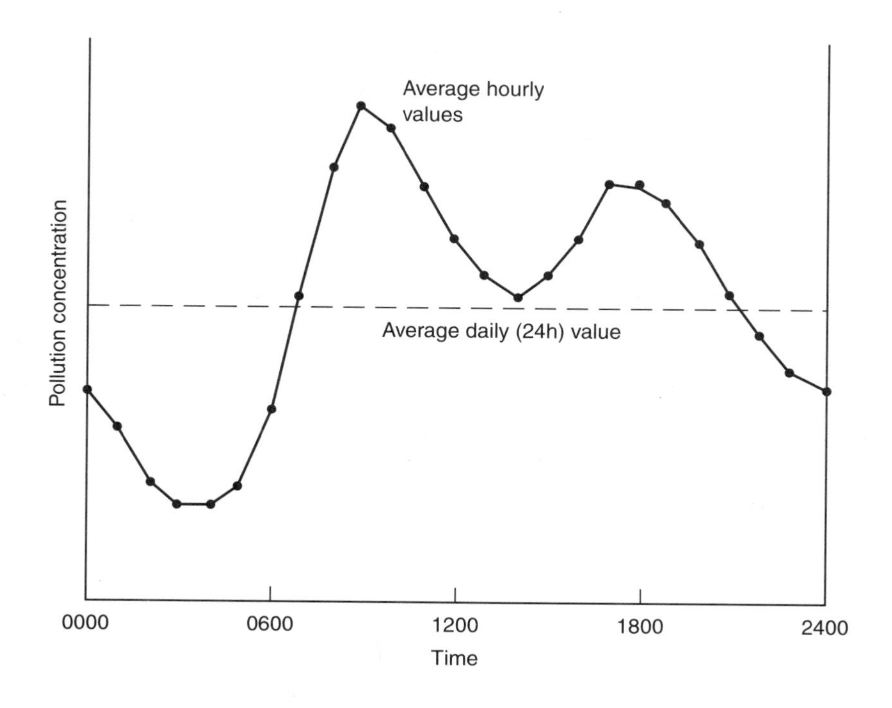

Figure 4.2 *How daily (24 h) averaging values may conceal hourly peaks of pollution concentrations that may pose serious health risks. The diurnal pollution cycle depicted is typical of that produced by traffic emissions such as carbon monoxide and nitrogen oxides*

Methods of Measuring Pollutants

The methods chosen to measure air pollution concentrations depend on several factors including the intended use of the data, the budget available to purchase and operate the equipment, the expertise of technicians to operate and service the equipment, access to advanced technology and whether particular methods are specified in air quality legislation, as is often the case. Installing, operating and maintaining monitoring equipment is a skilful technical task as monitors need regular servicing, testing, cross-checking and recalibrating to ensure accurate data are being collected. For some monitoring methods, laboratory analyses of the collected samples may also be needed.

Methods of measuring pollutants tend to be either continuous automated systems or discontinuous, manual systems. Automated analysers are costly but can monitor pollutant concentrations more or less continuously and can record short-term peaks (hourly or even a few minutes) as well as daily, monthly and annual averages. Their results can be transmitted rapidly to a central control so that air quality managers have the opportunity to decide whether, say, short-term emission-reduction measures need to be introduced. Manual systems involve laboratory analyses of samples of the air collected over a period of time (seldom less than a day and sometimes weekly). For some pollutants there may be several sophisticated or simple measuring methods available. Unfortunately, the results from each method may not be directly comparable, which leads to problems when trying to compare air pollutant levels in one location with another or when assessing the long-term trends of a pollutant where the monitoring method has changed over the years. Of course, as new measuring techniques are developed or existing techniques improved, so monitors need to be replaced. However, it is important in understanding long-term air quality trends that one or more sites in an urban area either continue operating the same method or that there is a period during which the new and old monitors are run side by side to assess comparability of the measurements. The most common methods used for measuring particulate and gaseous pollutants are explained in the following sections.[4]

---

4 Butterwick, L, Harrison, R and Merritt, Q (1991) *Handbook for Urban Air Improvement*, Commission of the European Communities, Brussels; Harrison, R M and Perry, R (1986) *Handbook of Air Pollution Analysis* (second edition) Chapman and Hall, London; Mucke, H-G, Manns, H, Turowski, E and Nitz, G (1995) *European Intercomparison Workshops on Air Quality Monitoring: Measuring of Sulphur Dioxide, Nitric Oxide and Nitrogen Dioxide*, Air Hygiene Report No 7, vol 1, WHO Collaborating Centre for Air Quality Management and Air Pollution Control, Berlin; Quality of Urban Air Review Group (1993) *Urban Air Quality in the United Kingdom*, First Report, Department of the Environment, London; Rice, J and Beevers, S (1995) *The London Air Quality Manual*, South East Institute of Public Health, Tunbridge Wells

Sulphur Dioxide The simplest method is the net acidity 'bubbler' method. Filtered air is bubbled through a dilute oxidising solution of hydrogen peroxide adjusted to pH 4.5. Any sulphur dioxide present forms sulphuric acid which is titrated against standard alkali. Daily samples provide a measure of the amount of sulphur dioxide in the air, although the method assumes that any other acid or alkali such as ammonia in the air is negligible (which may not always be the case). The spectrophotometric pararosaniline method (or West Gaeke method) involves bubbling air through a dipotassium tetrachloromercurate solution, which causes a red/purple colour change whose intensity, measured at a wavelength of 560 nm, is proportional to the amount of sulphur dioxide in the air.

A more advanced and real-time method which enables ten-minute or hourly concentrations of sulphur dioxide to be measured is the continuous ultraviolet fluorescence analyser technique. This uses the principle that sulphur dioxide will fluoresce (around the wavelength of 340 nm) – that is, it will give off energy in the form of light – after being irradiated with ultraviolet radiation (with a wavelength of 214 nm). The intensity of the light is directly proportional to the concentration of sulphur dioxide in the air being sampled. An alternative method is to use differential optical absorption spectrometry (DOAS), which can provide measurements averaged over five minutes if needed. This technique is used in the Swedish OPSIS monitoring system. It uses the principle that a gas absorbs wavelengths which are unique to itself. A xenon lamp transmits a beam of light with a known spectrum across a known distance (usually several hundred metres) to a receptor where the spectrum is then reanalysed. By comparing the intensity of light at the wavelength absorbed uniquely by a specific gas with the intensity of light at a wavelength which is not absorbed by any gas, the concentration of gas can be inferred.

Suspended Particulate Matter There are various methods of monitoring SPM with concentrations being expressed as mass per volume (eg $\mu g/m^3$). One traditional simple method, the smoke shade reflectance method, measures concentrations of 'black smoke' (typically particles up to 10–15 µm in diameter). Air is drawn through a white filter paper on which particles form a black stain which is measured using a portable reflectometer. The darkness of the stain is converted into mass per volume using a standard calibration graph. The calibration graph may vary nationally (eg the UK version produces black smoke concentrations equivalent to 85 per cent of European Union standard values). This smoke stain method measures fine respirable black material, mainly originating from incomplete combustion, but is influenced strongly by the colour of the particulates. The gravimetric method for TSP uses the weight of the particulates collected on a filter paper through which air has passed. Since 1987 the high-volume gravimetric sampler used in the US has had a 10 µm particle size selective inlet to provide measurements of PM_{10}.

The greater importance of small particles, the thoracic and respirable particle size ranges (approximately less than 10 and 2.5 μm, respectively), has meant that monitoring increasingly focuses on fine particulates. Unlike the previous methods which require analysis of the material collected on the filters, the tapered element oscillating microbalance (TEOM) uses filter-based sampling but with real-time mass measurement capability. The microbalance consists of a sophisticated electronics system built around a tapered element. A hollow tube is attached to a platform at its wide end and has an exchangeable filter cartridge mounted on its tip. The filter cartridge is usually that for PM_{10} but filters for $PM_{2.5}$ or even $PM_{1.6}$ may be used (but not at the same time).

The tapered element is vibrated at its natural frequency. The heated particulate-laden sample stream is drawn through a heated inlet to a cartridge containing a Teflon-coated glass fibre filter, where the particulate collects. As the particulate mass gathers on the filter cartridge, the tube's natural frequency of oscillation decreases. Based on the direct relationship between mass and frequency, the instrument's microprocessor computes the total mass accumulation on the filter, as well as the mass rate and mass concentration, in real time with this information being transmitted to a control centre. The TEOM gravimetric method is widely used, although Germany is promoting in preference a laser-based method which measures particle numbers.

A recent important development for monitoring fine particulates is the vibrating tube impactor which, unlike the TEOM, can determine the total mass of different size fractions simultaneously. It consists of four glass U-tubes connected in series. Each successive tube has a smaller bore so that the intake air accelerates as it passes from tube to tube. The tubes are arranged to have successively more acute bends. When air enters the first tube, the larger heavier particles have too much momentum to negotiate the bend and so they collide with the tube wall and stick there. Progressively smaller particles are similarly deposited in each tube. The increased velocity, and therefore momentum, of the particles as they pass from tube to tube makes it more likely that they will be deposited. The tubes are vibrated at a fixed frequency and the heavier each tube becomes, as it collects particles, the greater the energy needed to maintain the vibration. This can then be related to the total mass and mass rate of the particles.

There is no simple relationship between the concentrations measured by all these various techniques and this makes the comparison of health risks in countries throughout the world very difficult, if not almost impossible.

Carbon Monoxide Carbon monoxide can be measured using the principle of infra-red radiation absorption by this gas. Many molecules absorb radiation but all have characteristic spectra and for carbon monoxide the amount absorbed at a wavelength of around 4.67 μm is proportional to the concentration. Carbon dioxide and water vapour molecules can interfere with the transmission of infra-red radiation around this wavelength but the instrument overcomes this problem by also measuring absorbences at wavelengths not absorbed by carbon monoxide and making appropriate corrections in the perceived concentration of carbon monoxide.

Nitrogen Oxides The chemiluminescent dry gas analyser provides continuous monitoring of nitric oxide, nitrogen dioxide and total nitrogen oxides. It operates using the principle of chemiluminescence, a process where light is emitted by an excited molecule at a temperature at which light rays would not normally be expected following a chemical reaction. The principle has parallels with the fluorescence method but in this case the excitation of the molecules is achieved through chemical reaction with ozone (produced by the instrument) rather than a physical stimulus. The amount of light emitted is proportional to the concentration of the nitric oxide present in the sample. The analyser splits the sampled air into two streams for analysis. The first measures the nitric oxide present and the second stream measures total nitrogen oxides. In this second sample, nitrogen dioxide is reduced to nitric oxide by passing a sample of the air through a catalytic molybdenum converter and then all the nitric oxide present is subjected to the chemical reaction with ozone. Subtracting the results of the first sample from the second gives the concentration of nitrogen dioxide. Nitrogen dioxide can also be measured using the DOAS system described previously.

Volatile Organic Compounds Gas chromatography can be used to provide accurate measurements of species-specific VOCs such as benzene. Air is drawn through an adsorption tube for a pre-set time and fixed flow-rate. The tube is then heated and the compounds adsorbed onto the tube packing are driven onto a concentrator. When the transfer is complete, the concentrator is heated and the compounds are carried on to a capillary column in a flow of helium gas. These are then measured by a flame ionisation or electron capture detector. By 1996, the UK Automatic Hydrocarbon Network was comprised of 12 urban monitoring sites which automatically collect and measure 26 hydrocarbon species for each hour of the day. The DOAS system can provide hourly measurements of some hydrocarbons including benzene and toluene using their absorption bands in the range 250–300 nm.

Ozone Ozone can be measured continuously (every minute) and automatically using the principle that ozone molecules absorb ultraviolet radiation at 253.7 nm. The ultraviolet photometric instrument compares the amount of ultraviolet radiation at this wavelength which is transmitted by the ozone-free air supplied by the instrument and the sampled air. The instrument contains an in-built ozone generator (ozone being produced by irradiating oxygen with ultraviolet radiation at a wavelength of 185 nm) which is used for calibration. Ozone can also be measured using the chemiluminescence method, whereby sampled air is mixed with ethylene. The two gases react to produce light emissions in the 350–600 nm ranges, with the concentration of ozone being proportional to the intensity of emissions. The DOAS system can also measure ozone.

Trace Metals Lead particles and other metals such as cadmium are collected on filters and subsequently determined by various means in the laboratory to obtain, say, weekly concentrations. Common practice is to digest the filter in nitric acid and to determine the metal ions in solution using atomic absorption spectrometry. Alternatively, samples are collected by drawing air through a filter which is then analysed using an X-ray spectrometer. When irradiated with X-rays, metal pollutants absorb energy and then re-emit the energy at wavelengths characteristic of each metal present. Concentrations are determined from the intensity of secondary X-rays emitted at these characteristic wavelengths.

Passive Samplers: Diffusion Tubes Many of the techniques provide continuous real-time measurements, but in some situations useful air quality information can be gained using simple equipment such as diffusion tubes. These inexpensive passive samplers absorb the pollutant onto two stainless-steel gauze discs placed at the bottom of a short cylinder open to the atmosphere at the other end (exposed in a downward direction to prevent rain or dust entering the tube). After exposure the tubes are sent for laboratory analyses. For example, nitrogen dioxide is absorbed and converted to nitrite by triethanolamine coating the metal gauze after diffusion along the transparent acrylic tube (71 mm long by 11 mm internal diameter). The nitrogen dioxide concentration is then determined spectrophotometrically after the nitrite has been reacted with a colour-forming reagent, the colour intensity being dependent on the initial concentration of nitrogen dioxide gas absorbed.

Diffusion tubes have been developed for ammonia, benzene, carbon monoxide, hydrogen sulphide, nitrogen dioxide, ozone and sulphur dioxide. In areas of high pollution concentrations they can produce results for daily or even three-hourly exposures, although in areas of low concentrations they are usually exposed for a week, several weeks or even a month at a time. A national network of more than 400 diffusion tubes enabled nitrogen dioxide concentrations in the UK to be mapped in 1986 and 1991, followed up in 1993 with a third national survey using 1200 diffusion tubes. Many urban areas have used these inexpensive tubes to map the spatial patterns of various pollutants. Diffusion tube data must be treated with caution as the variation between readings from tube to tube and site to site can be significant. They are particularly subject to the influence of wind, which can cause turbulence at the tube inlet, effectively reducing the diffusion length and causing a more rapid uptake of the pollutant. Comparison of nitrogen dioxide concentrations from diffusion tubes with more accurate chemiluminescence monitor data has shown that the tubes produce higher readings. Even so, the weekly exposure of diffusion tubes has been used to infer daily averages, whereas monthly mean concentrations for, say, nitrogen dioxide are commonly used to estimate the annual mean and even 98th centile concentrations.[5]

Urban Pollutant Emission Inventories

Understanding the nature and strength of sources of air pollutants is a first step towards eventually controlling those emissions and securing a healthy atmosphere. This requires the compilation of an urban emissions inventory which is a list of the location and type of pollutant sources in an urban area together with the amount of each pollutant discharged in a specified period.[6]

Once an emission inventory has been compiled it needs regular updating as new industrial sources are added or when new controls on emissions are introduced. Most countries have compiled national emission inventories, but there is a need for more city inventories. Information in an inventory should include emission rates from individual point sources such as industrial plants and power stations (often with elevated stacks), from area sources such as housing estates (low-level sources) and from line sources such as motor vehicles along a road and trains on a railway track. Emission sources may be grouped according to fuel type (eg coal and smokeless fuels, light and heavy fuel oil, petrol and diesel, gas and solid waste).

Some pollutants pose enormous problems when compiling their emission inventories as there is limited information readily available, as for VOCs. In

---

5 Bower, J S, Lampert, J S, Stevenson, K J *et al* (1991) 'A diffusion tube survey of nitrogen dioxide concentrations in urban areas in the UK', *Atmospheric Environment*, vol 25B, pp 255–265; Campbell, G W, Stedman, J R and Stevenson, K J (1994) 'A survey of nitrogen dioxide concentrations in the UK using diffusion tubes, July–December 1991', *Atmospheric Environment*, vol 28, pp 477–486; Gair, G A et al (1991) 'Development of a simple passive technique for the determination of nitrogen dioxide in a remote continental location', *Atmospheric Environment*, vol 25A, pp 1927–1939; Grosjean, D and Hisham, M W M (1992) 'A passive sampler for atmospheric ozone', *Journal of Air and Management Waste Association*, vol 42, pp 169–173; Palmes, E D, Gunnison, A F, Dimattio, J and Tomczyk, C (1976) 'Personal sampler for nitrogen dioxide', *American Industrial Hygiene Association Journal*, vol 37, pp 570–577

6 Chell, M and Hutchinson, D (1993) *London Energy Study*, London Research Centre, London; Hutchinson, D (1994) *Emission Inventories in Practice – London and the West Midlands*, paper presented at the National Society for Clean Air and Environmental Protection (NSCA) Local Air Quality Management Workshop, Abingdon, April 1994, NSCA, Brighton; Longhurst, J W S, Lindley, S J, Conlan, D E and Watson, A F R (1994) 'Emissions of air pollutants in the north west region of England', in Baldasano, J M, Brebbia, C A, Power, H and Zanetti, P (eds) *Air Pollution*, vol 2, Pollution Control and Monitoring, Computational Mechanics, Southampton, pp 99–106; Timmis, R J and Walker, C A (1988) *Dispersion Modelling of Air-quality Changes due to Smoke Control: a Case Study for Leek*, Report 638 (AP), Warren Spring Laboratory, Stevenage; US Environmental Protection Agency (1994) *Encyclopedia of Emission Inventory Methods*, Report EPA-600/X-94-026a, USEPA, Research Triangle Park, NC

other cases difficulties arise because pollutants such as ozone and to a lesser extent nitrogen dioxide are not emitted directly into the atmosphere but are secondary pollutants formed chemically from other pollutants. Inventories for secondary pollutants require sophisticated models incorporating the chemical reactions which transform primary pollutants into secondary pollutants.

Industrial plants, because they usually have to demonstrate that they are complying with legislated emission limits, keep detailed records of stack emissions of the major pollutants which can be used as input to an urban emission inventory. Sulphur dioxide emissions from large individual premises heated by fuel oil can be readily estimated if records of the amount of fuel consumed are kept and the sulphur content of the fuel is known. Allowance needs to be made when some of the sulphur is not released into the atmosphere as sulphur dioxide but is retained in the ash. For coal the retention of sulphur in the ash depends critically on the temperature of the combustion processes and this temperature has increased as technology has improved, typically being about 10 per cent. Emissions of sulphur dioxide can be determined by multiplying the mass of fuel consumed (eg tonnes per year), its fractional sulphur content and the fraction of sulphur retained in the ash (zero in the case of liquid fuels).

Estimating emissions of sulphur dioxide is a relatively simple task, mainly because emissions depend primarily on the sulphur content of the fuels. This is not the case for other pollutants. Emissions of nitrogen oxides depend mainly on the conditions of combustion (especially temperature) and to a lesser extent the fuel properties, whereas carbon monoxide is emitted by a variety of sources, each of which is characterised by differing emission factors. Additional complications occur for estimating emissions of VOCs as natural emissions make up a large proportion of the total emissions, for example about 40 per cent in Europe, mainly from terpenes and isoprene hydrocarbons from forests.

Residential (domestic) emissions are usually estimated as an area emission over, say, 1 km grid squares. Emissions are determined from records of the number and type of heating systems within the area weighted by emission factors for each type of equipment and records of household fuel consumption and fuel deliveries, or even enquiries to individual households. Within any residential area shops, offices and garages may be located which may require additional enquiries and questionnaires. If residential area emissions are needed for shorter periods (eg daily) than supplied by fuel consumption figures (eg monthly, three-monthly), then assumptions need to be made about the use of heating systems. This usually involves the concept of 'degree-days' which assumes that when the outdoor temperature falls below a critical value of, say, 15°C, domestic heating systems will be operated. In other words, emissions from domestic heating systems can be estimated from average daily or even hourly temperature values.

Emission factors are used to obtain emission rates for a wide range of pollutants from many types of sources. Vehicle emissions at a particular location or length of road are calculated using traffic census data weighted according to emission factors determined by laboratory measurements of exhaust emissions from a sample of vehicles. Emissions from motor vehicles are usually expressed as a weight of pollutants per standard distance (eg grams per kilometre, pounds per mile). The emissions from vehicles are influenced by many considerations such as the type of fuel used, the type of engine design, the presence of pollution controls (eg catalytic converters, carbon canisters), the vehicle's age, its state of maintenance, driver behaviour, traffic conditions and the vehicle's speed.

Estimates of emissions from motor vehicles are usually made for a particular location or stretch of road or, say, a one kilometre grid square over a specified time period. This requires traffic census data on the number and different classes of vehicles (eg cars, light goods vehicles, medium goods vehicles, heavy goods vehicles, taxis, buses and motorcycles) as well as the percentages of diesel- and petrol-engined vehicles. Obviously it is impossible for traffic census data to assess all these factors affecting emission rates, so generalisations and assumptions have to be made about the vehicle stock and driver behaviour, which are incorporated into the emission factors used. Emissions from motor vehicles are calculated by considering the emission factor per vehicle type and vehicle speed (eg grams per kilometre), traffic activity (eg vehicle kilometres) for vehicle type and vehicle speed, and the percentage of vehicle type fuelled by a specific fuel (eg leaded petrol). Given the complexity and time-consuming nature of determining vehicle emissions in this way, it is not unusual for a more simplistic approach to be adopted such as using one emission factor weighted by the known number of vehicles travelling during a specified time period at an assumed mean speed. Detailed emission factors may not be available in some countries, but factors from other countries may be used and modified for, say, fuel sulphur content.

Emission inventories are a vital part of air quality management systems in that decisions on implementing emission-reduction measures need to be based on a clear understanding of how much each emission source – power stations, industry, home heating, traffic – contributes to any air pollution problem in the city, otherwise costly decisions could be made that are unnecessary or ineffective.

Predicting Pollution Concentrations

A numerical pollution model is used to predict how spatial patterns of emission rates from sources at differing heights are transformed into the near-ground level pollution concentrations to which people are exposed. The model simplifies the behaviour of the atmosphere by applying certain assumptions about how pollutant emissions are diluted, dispersed and, in some cases, altered chemically or photochemically.[7] It is important that the model is validated as confidence in the prediction will be greater if it can be shown that it can predict current pollution levels from existing emission rates. Most models used today are emission inventory–diffusion models which need the use of a computer. Occasionally, in urban areas with complex topography, a physical scale model may be constructed in a wind tunnel in an attempt to predict the behaviour of emissions, with the results being used to improve a numerical model which then takes over from the physical model.

Numerical dispersion (emission inventory–diffusion) models are used to predict pollution concentrations hours or days ahead in the case of smogs and years or even decades ahead for long-term air quality management. In the case of short-term prediction, the earlier a smog can be forecast, the greater the number of options available to tackle the smog. Numerical prediction models incorporate detailed information on the source strength of point (eg large industrial plants), area (eg aggregate emissions from residential districts) and line (eg cars, railways) emission sources in the urban area (emission inventory) using a spatial resolution of a 1 by 1 km grid. Emission rates will be specified over different time-scales depending on whether the model is used for short- or long-term prediction. Short-term models need to allow for the pattern of emission rates to vary diurnally and weekly (eg weekend versus weekday) in accordance with the weather conditions (eg degree-days) and seasonal differences (eg home heating during the colder months).

---

7 Barrowcliffe, R (1993) *The Practical Use of Dispersion Models to Predict Air Quality Impacts*, Environmental Resources Management, London; Benarie, M M (1987) 'The limits of air pollution modelling', *Atmospheric Environment*, vol 21, pp 1–5; Carruthers, D J, Holroyd, R J, Hunt, J C R, Weng, W S, Robins, A G, Apsley, D D, Thomson, D J and Smith, F B (1994) 'UK-ADMS: a new approach to modelling dispersion in the Earths's atmospheric boundary layer', *Journal of Wind Engineering and Industrial Aerodynamics*, vol 52, pp 139–153; Department of Transport (1994) *Design Manual for Roads and Bridges*, vol 11, Environmental Assessment, Section 3, HMSO, London; Eerens, H C, Sliggers, C J and van Hout, K D (1993) 'The CAR model: the Dutch method to determine city street air quality', *Atmospheric Environment*, vol 27B, pp 389–399; Elsom, D M (1995) 'Air and climate', in Morris, P and Therivel, R (eds) *Methods of Environmental Impact Assessment*, UCL Press, London; Hackman, M P and Stedman, J R (1992) *A Revised Short-period Model for Air Pollution*, Report LR 874 (AP), Warren Spring Laboratory, Stevenage; Hunt, J C R, Holroyd, R J, Carruthers, D J, Robins, A G, Apsley, D D, Smith, F B, Thomson, D J (1991) 'Developments in modelling air pollution for regulatory uses', in van Dop, H and Steyn, D G (eds), *Air Pollution Modelling and its Application VIII*, Plenum Press, New York; Royal Meteorological Society (1995) *Atmospheric Dispersion Modelling: Guidelines on the Justification of Choice and Use of Models, and the Communication and Reporting of Results*, RMS, Reading; Simms, K (1991) 'Modelling traffic pollution', *Clean Air*, vol 21, pp 191–196; Williams, M L (1982) *Air Pollution Dispersion in Street Canyons – Comparisons of a Simple Model with Measured Data*, Report LR 423 (AP), Warren Spring Laboratory, Stevenage; Zannetti, P (1990) *Air Pollution Modeling*, Computational Mechanics, Southampton

A numerical dispersion model has the advantage that it can predict local variations in pollution levels within the city, identifying pollution hot-spots. It can fill in the gaps between monitoring stations by predicting current pollution concentrations in those areas. More important is the fact that it is used to predict the concentrations arising from changing emission sources and rates. For primary pollutants most models incorporate only the physical aspects of atmospheric influences on emissions, including wind speed and vertical stability. The most commonly used dispersion model is the Gaussian model. This assumes the pollution spreads outwards in a cone-shaped plume aligned to the wind direction in such a way that the distribution of pollution concentration decreases away from the plume axis in horizontal and vertical planes according to a specific mathematical 'Gaussian' equation.

The axis of the plume does not normally coincide with the height of the stack as the density and momentum of the emissions quickly carries the plume to a higher elevation, known as the effective stack height. Density and momentum are related to the temperature of the pollutants discharged and the exit velocity of the emissions, respectively. Generally, the higher the effective stack height and the stronger the winds, the greater is the dilution of the pollutants and the lower the pollution concentrations experienced at ground level. The maximum ground level concentration experienced from a pollution plume is where the plume first reaches the ground. The rate of dispersion of the plume, and consequently the pollution concentrations experienced at any location at the surface, are a function of wind speed and direction and atmospheric stability. Gaussian models are frequently used to predict pollution concentrations from a single source such as an industrial stack and there are various modifications that can be made to the model such as incorporating the effects of nearby buildings, plume meander and dry deposition.

Gaussian models are also used for area sources (eg construction sites, car parks, urban areas, regions) and line sources (eg roads). They are more complex to apply to urban areas than to a single emission source and usually rely on dividing the area into a series of boxes and allowing for the transfer of pollutants between boxes in a downwind direction. The US Environmental Protection Agency offers a range of well-established models. Gaussian models form the basis of various commercially available urban models (eg the Indic Airviro system developed in Sweden). A new generation of models is becoming available such as the UK atmospheric dispersion modelling system, which will eventually replace the Gaussian models first developed in the late 1950s and 1960s. Gaussian models assume a Gaussian dispersion process and rely on meteorological measurements made near the ground which were assumed to be an adequate representation of the state of the whole boundary layer. However, this is an oversimplification even though the models give reasonable results. Advances in the understanding of both the structure of the atmospheric boundary layer and dispersion have meant that better models can now be produced. The new generation models take into account the common atmospheric situation when turbulence and diffusion characteristics vary significantly with height in the boundary layer. This and other improved assumptions used in the new models should give rise to more accurate predictions of pollution concentrations over a wide range of atmospheric conditions.

Given the rapid fall-off of traffic-related pollutants with distance from roads several dispersion models have been developed specifically to predict pollution concentrations at various distances from roads using known traffic flow (mean vehicle speed, flow-rate) and meteorological conditions (eg wind speed and direction). Examples include the CALINE models of the Californian Department of Transportation and the CAR model (calculation of air pollution from road traffic) used in the Netherlands. The latter calculates the total emission from the traffic in a street by the daily traffic volume, the fraction of passenger cars, the mean velocity and the emissions from the vehicles. Dispersion is related to the type of street (streets being divided into types according to the buildings nearby), the distance from the middle of the street and a regional wind speed factor. Simple graphical models are available such as the UK Department of Transport graphical screening model. As with all pollution prediction models it is important to assess the accuracy of traffic pollution models by comparing predictions of current pollution levels with monitored data where they are available.

Non-chemical dispersion models are of little use for photochemical models which must include details of the chemical and/or photochemical processes involved in their formation and destruction. Secondary pollutants such as ozone involve regional transport and even urban models need to consider the import of ozone or its precursor pollutants. Trajectory models over long-range transport scales may be needed. For nitrogen oxides it is usual to model the composite pollutant, which is the sum of nitric oxide and nitrogen dioxide as this composite pollutant is approximately conserved within the urban area, even though the proportions of nitric oxide and nitrogen dioxide may vary. For modelling, it is convenient to express nitrogen oxides as nitrogen dioxide in mass terms.

In some cases imported pollution can contribute considerably to urban pollution, especially in the case of smogs, and it is necessary to incorporate this background concentration. Background pollutants may be derived from the rest of the country or from across national boundaries and seas. This may require nesting the urban model within a model using a coarser grid. It may vary within the urban area, being greater in one part than another. Another problem in forecasting pollution levels from day to day is that pollution carryover can occur when pollutants are lifted aloft and trapped above or between inversions overnight before being brought back to the surface the next morning. This pollution carryover from the previous day can cause errors when forecasts are based only on the pertaining meteorological and emission conditions and it can obscure expected differences in pollution levels between weekdays and weekends.

Meteorological data will be needed as input data for numerical prediction models such as wind speed and direction, air temperature, atmospheric stability and boundary layer depth (and surface heat flux for the new generation models). Information on winds and temperature as well as relative humidity is usually available from one or more urban meteorological stations, sometimes rooftop sites. Atmospheric stability and mixing depth can be derived from radiosonde ascents undertaken at a nearby urban–peripheral airport. However, such a location does not provide a good indication of the nature of the urban boundary atmosphere, which may be unstable due to the urban heat island and turbulence. Normally some modification is applied to rural-derived values to make them more representative of the urban situation. An acoustic radar located in the urban area is a better but much more expensive source of information on atmospheric stability, including the heights of temperature inversions. Finally, broad estimates of atmospheric stability for the Gaussian models (eg Pasquill–Smith categories which correspond to mixing layer depth) can be obtained using a nomogram involving solar radiation, cloud cover and mean wind speed.

In general, predictive modelling poses serious difficulties for effective air quality management because it is usually complex and requires specialist staff to undertake the modelling work, there is a limited number of appropriate models available and they are inevitably of limited accuracy. However, the evaluation of policy options necessitates their incorporation into air quality management. When models are used it is important not to treat them as a 'black box', but rather to be aware of the assumptions used and their limitations. Models are normally more useful when comparing the air quality improvement of different emission-reduction measures – that is, relative concentrations are more important than absolute concentrations.

Air Quality Standards and Public Information Bands

Short-term (eg hourly, daily) and long-term (eg annual) health-based air quality standards, whose exceedance should result in action being taken to improve air quality, are a key component of an effective air quality management framework (refer to Chapters 2 and 3). Smog alert or alarm levels for pollution episodes also need specifying (explored further in Chapter 5). It is useful if air quality standards and smog alert thresholds are incorporated into public information bands which enable the public to be aware of the relative safety or threat posed by the air quality they are experiencing. If the public have confidence in the authorities then it is not necessary to provide absolute levels of each pollutant, which to many of the public are confusing or meaningless anyway. Rather it is more appropriate to use an index which groups the concentrations of a pollutant or preferably several pollutants into broad bands described variously as indicating good, moderate, poor and hazardous air quality (or alternative descriptive terms). When the air quality is described as, say, very poor or hazardous it would imply to the public that their health is at risk and actions may be expected of them. Actions may involve not using their cars and using public transport instead or turning down their central heating system. They would also need to be advised about ways to reduce their exposure to the unhealthy air quality.

Public air quality information, both current and forecast, needs to be readily available to the public via the news media (eg radio, television, daily newspapers) and telephone. It needs to be displayed prominently alongside roads or in shopping centres using electronic display boards and screens. The information needs to be current (or forecast) air quality information for that locality, which means that nearby real-time automatic monitors are needed to provide regularly updated hourly information. Currently there are too many city authorities who are monitoring air quality but then failing to disseminate that information to the public in a meaningful way.[8]

Some of the most useful pollution indices that are used specify bandings such that if air quality reaches the health-based air quality standard for a pollutant it is given a number of 100. If air quality is worse than the health-based standard the number rises above 100, whereas if it is better than the standard it lies below 100 (the total range of the index may be from zero to, say, 500). This process can be applied to all pollutants measured within an urban area to produce sub-indices. Then the highest sub-index determines the air quality index and the banding notified to the public. In other words, what is important to the public is to be informed whether their health is at risk from air pollution and not specifically which pollutant.

However, in some cases it may be necessary to inform the public which pollutant has determined the banding issued because specific actions may be needed which target emissions of that pollutant or if there are particular groups of people particularly at risk from one type of pollutant. One of the most widely used pollution indicators is the US Pollutant Standards Index, developed in the mid-1970s and adopted in modified forms by other countries (eg Canada, Taiwan) and cities (eg Helsinki, Hong Kong) around the world. The number 100 corresponds to the health-based air quality standard for a range of pollutants (Table 4.1). The Helsinki air quality index was developed in 1993 and the level of 100 for each pollutant is either based on national or WHO air quality guidelines (Table 4.2). The index is linear above 100. The level of 50 is half the air quality guidelines and a background level of 10 is designated. Some countries use alternative numerical ranges such as the national public information bands introduced in the UK in 1990. Hourly concentrations for three pollutants are grouped into four bands to which a descriptor is applied (Table 4.3). The bands have not been adopted by all urban areas as several cities either use alternative descriptors

---

8 Crabbe, H and Elsom, D M (1995) 'Local air quality management in the UK survey', *Clean Air*, vol 25, pp 95–107; Hedges, A (1994) *Involving the Public: Communicating Air Quality Data and Individual Responses*, paper presented at the National Society for Clean Air and Environmental Protection (NSCA) Air Quality Management Workshop, Abingdon, April 1994, NSCA, Brighton

Table 4.1 *Comparison of the US Pollutants Standards Index (PSI) values with pollutant concentrations, health descriptions and PSI colours*

Index	Air quality level	PM_{10} 24 h (μg/m³)	SO_2 24 h (μg/m³)	CO 8 h (ppm)	O_3 1 h (ppm)	NO_2 1 h (ppm)	Health effect descriptor	PSI colour
500	Significant harm	600	2620	50	0.6	2.0	300–400 = hazardous	Red
400	Emergency	500	2100	40	0.5	1.6		
300	Warning	420	1600	30	0.4	1.2	200–300 = very unhealthful	Orange
200	Alert	350	800	15	0.2	0.6	100–200 = unhealthful	Yellow
100	National standards	150	365	9	0.12	*	50–100 = moderate	Green
50	Half of standard	50	80†	4.5	0.06	*	0–50 = good	Blue
0		0	0	0	0	*		

* No index value reported at concentration levels below those specified by 'alert level' criteria.

† Annual primary national ambient air quality standard.

(replacing good by moderate or fair and replacing very good by good) or they have defined their own stricter bands.[9]

Conclusions: Difficult, but Vital

Setting up pollution monitoring networks, compiling emission inventories and defining air quality standards can be costly, time consuming and difficult, but it is necessary if the goal of healthy air quality is to be attained and sustained. Once these components of the air quality management framework exist, modelling work can be undertaken to assess the

9 Aarnio, P, Hamekoski, K, Koskentalo, T and Virtanen, T (1995)'Air quality, monitoring and air quality index in the Helsinki metropolitan area, Finland', *Proceedings of the 10th World Clean Air Congress, Espoo, Finland*, vol 2, Finnish Air Pollution Prevention Society, Helsinki, paper 201; Lee, F Y P and Gervat, G P (1995) 'The air pollution index system in Hong Kong', *Proceedings of the 10th World Clean Air Congress, Espoo, Finland*, vol 3, Finnish Air Pollution Prevention Society, Helsinki, paper 524

Table 4.2 *Helsinki air quality index*

Index	CO 1 h (mg/m³)	CO 8 h (mg/m³)	NO_2 1 h (μg/m³)	NO_2 24 h (μg/m³)	SO_2 1 h (μg/m³)	SO_2 24 h (μg/m³)	O_3 1 h (μg/m³)	PM_{10} 24 h (μg/m³)
50	4	4	35	35	40	40	75	35
100	20	8	150	70	250	80	150	70
200	40	16	300	140	500	160	300	140

Index	Description	Health effects
≤50	Good	No effects
51–100	Fair	Adverse effects probable
101–150	Passable	Adverse effects possible on sensitive individuals
≥150	Poor	Adverse effects possible on sensitive subpopulation

effectiveness of various pollution control policies and measures and the interactions between them considered to ensure that one policy does not undermine the benefits of another. Given that the implementation of land use, transport and energy policies involves many different groups within a city and that some of the resources and legislative powers may reside with the national government, there is clearly a need for co-ordination, although one group should be charged with overseeing the whole package.

Table 4.3 *UK public information air quality bands and descriptors (ppb)*

Pollutant	Very good	Good	Poor	Very poor
Ozone	0–49	50–89	90–179	>180
Sulphur dioxide	0–59	60–124	125–399	>400
Nitrogen dioxide	0–49	50–99	100–299	>300

Chapter 5

Developing Smog Alert Systems

Short-term Pollution Episodes and the Need for a Smog Alert System

There are occasions, short-term episodes (smogs) lasting a few hours or days, when air pollution concentrations reach health-threatening or dangerous levels well above air quality standards. Smogs occur when urban emissions are relatively high and stagnant meteorological conditions fail to dilute and disperse the pollutants sufficiently. Concern over the adverse health effects of smogs has led to many city and national authorities introducing schemes to warn of, as well as forecast, the occurrence of smogs. The authorities can then advise the community of the potential health threats of the poor air quality and the actions the public can take to minimise their exposure to high pollution levels. The authorities can encourage voluntary actions or require mandatory short-term measures to reduce pollutant emissions during the smog.

Measures aimed at preventing a worsening of air quality include restricting the number and type of vehicles permitted to enter the problem area, reducing energy consumption in residential and public buildings (eg reduce the heating during winter or air conditioning during summer smogs) and requiring industry to cut emissions. It is unlikely that emission-reduction measures can prevent a smog occurring but they can reduce the severity, duration and even the spatial extent of the smog (Figure 5.1). The earlier a smog alert can be issued, the greater its effectiveness as it allows the community more time to make plans to reduce emissions (eg delaying shopping trips, sharing cars, opting for public transport) and for sensitive groups to ensure they do not expose themselves unnecessarily to poor air quality.

Smog alerts comprise two or, more commonly, three stages (Figure 5.2). The first stage triggers the issuing of a health advisory warning together

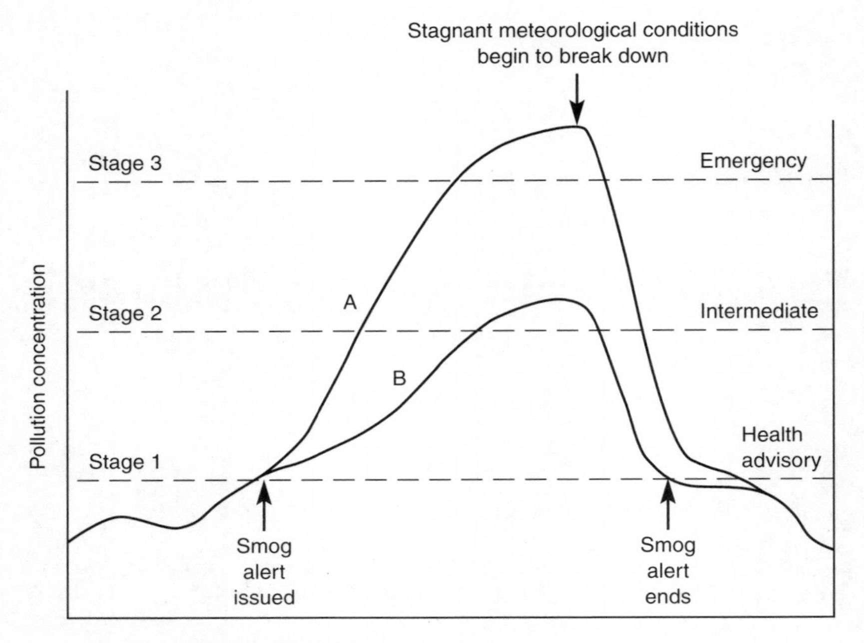

Figure 5.1 *Implementing voluntary and mandatory actions to reduce emissions at the start of a smog (or earlier) can reduce the severity and duration of the smog. In this way, an emergency stage 3 smog alert can be prevented even though people's health still remains at risk during the smog at the lower alert stages*

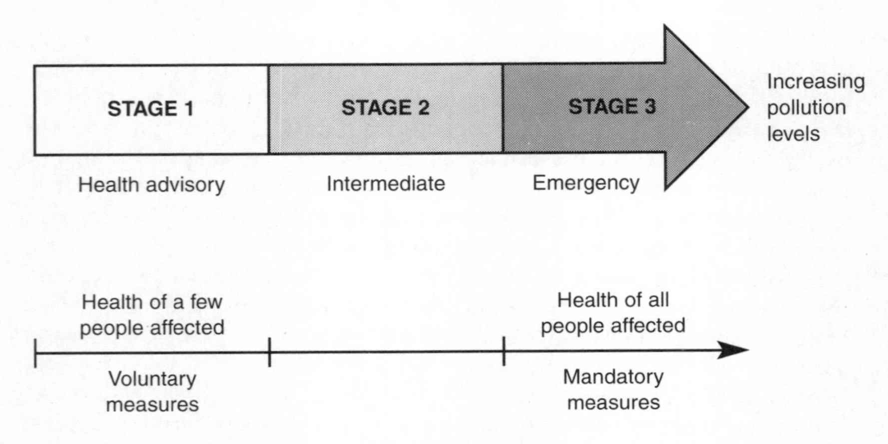

Figure 5.2 *Stages of smog alert schemes*

with requests for voluntary action to reduce emissions (eg asking the public not to make inessential car journeys). The second stage introduces mandatory pollution control measures (eg requiring certain industrial plants to reduce emissions by 30%), while the third stage requires more stringent measures (eg traffic bans and closure of industrial plants). Many cities around the world operate smog alert systems. One of the first smog alert schemes was devised for London when an emergency hospital alert plan was set up following the infamous 1952 sulphurous smog. However, the subsequent decline of smoke and sulphur dioxide levels meant that the alert was never brought into operation. The first public smog alert is credited to Los Angeles, when in 1969 it was agreed that schoolchildren should not be required to undertake games when oxidant (ozone) levels reached 350 ppb (700 $\mu g/m^3$) because vigorous outdoor exercise increased the pollution dose they received. Unfortunately, since then the issuing of smog alerts has become necessary in many of the world's cities.

An effective smog alert scheme requires co-ordination between city and central government departments and groups (eg environmental health, transport, planning, police, hospitals, meteorological service). This may be best achieved through the creation of a new agency that has the executive powers and resources to take overall charge during a smog. However, whatever the structure adopted for issuing and acting on the smog alert, the success of the scheme is dependent on the co-operation of the whole urban community and its willingness to accept restrictions on various activities. This highlights the need for widespread consultation and public awareness campaigns before a smog alert scheme is initiated.

Forecasting the Smog Alert

A smog occurs because of a combination of a short-term increase in emissions (eg increased traffic emissions, increase in heating of homes during a cold spell) and unfavourable stagnant meteorological conditions. During winter smogs, sub-freezing temperatures, a strong surface or low-level temperature inversion (ie a low atmospheric mixing depth) and light winds or calm conditions are all important factors influencing the build-up of pollution levels. Sub-freezing temperatures create a high energy demand for heating of homes and offices which increases emissions from fuels burned either in the buildings or at power stations. Cold weather results in increased emissions from vehicles as the engines (and catalytic converters) take longer to reach their optimum efficiency. High temperatures increase the evaporation of ozone-forming VOCs from vehicle fuel as well as from products such as oil-based paints, glues, varnishes and wood preservatives. Light winds and a low atmospheric mixing height produce a reduced volume of air into which the pollutants are dispersed and diluted. When a snow cover is present it creates a smooth surface which is less conducive to pollutants being removed from the air by impaction and absorption. Low temperatures may enhance some atmospheric chemical reactions when mist and fog droplets or even particulates are present (eg oxidation of nitric oxide to nitrogen dioxide). The presence of fog, especially in winter, can make the smog worse as it reduces the amount of sunlight reaching the ground, which would heat the surface and generate turbulence that may help to mix and dilute the ground-level pollutants. In addition, solar radiation absorbed at the top of the fog may increase the temperature at that height, so strengthening the surface-based temperature inversion that is usually present and so limiting dilution of the pollutants.

City centres usually experience higher air temperatures than the surrounding rural areas due to time-lag differences in the heating and cooling rates of urban buildings and roads compared with rural fields. This heat-island effect may affect the spatial distribution of pollution levels. When the heat-island intensity reaches 2–3°C, this urban–rural temperature difference produces a small air pressure difference which induces a light breeze flowing radially into the urban centre from the surrounding countryside. This cool breeze, blowing at only 2–3 m/s, brings cleaner rural air to the urban fringe, but transfers suburban pollutants towards the city centre, so increasing pollution levels there. The effects of such breezes on pollution levels are not well documented but during a smog in Manchester, UK in December 1962 the urban-induced country breeze redistributed smoke concentrations within the conurbation, increasing peak 24-hour levels from 4564 to 5575 $\mu g/m^3$ near the city centre. This 25 per cent increase in the inner city concentration was accompanied by a compensatory decrease in the outer suburbs and urban fringe.

The location of an urban area can increase its susceptibility to smogs by accentuating unfavourable meteorological conditions locally. When a city lies in a basin or valley, the slopes act like the sides of a box and a temperature inversion may form the box lid, so trapping the pollutants. Under anticyclonic conditions, cold air drains down the valley sides, cooling the valley bottom and strengthening the inversion (measured as the temperature difference between the top and bottom of the valley). Pollutants are unable to disperse from the valley or basin and the air quality deteriorates considerably.

Land and sea breeze circulations can play a part in aggravating coastal city smog problems. During the night an offshore land breeze sweeps the pollutants out to sea, but then an onshore sea breeze brings them back the next day. Land and sea breeze circulations seldom extend to more than a few hundred metres depth, but that may be sufficient to trap pollutant emissions from most sources, even tall stacks. Such circulations may trap a power station plume towards the top of its circulation and eventually bring it down to ground level. In the case of photochemical pollution, the precursor emissions which lead to ozone formation may be transported by the land breeze out over the sea at night. The next day, after photochemical reactions have converted the precursor emissions into ozone over the sea (where fresh emissions of ozone-scavenging pollutants such as nitric oxide and alkenes are absent), the ozone may be brought onshore.

In Greater Athens, land and sea breeze circulations are responsible in part for the coastal locations of Thessaloniki and Nea Karvali experiencing higher ozone levels than Athens during July and August. During these months, night-time land breezes transport precursor emissions from the Athens basin out to sea where photochemical reactions form ozone in the following morning's daylight. Sea breezes then bring the pollution onshore but they fail to reach inland as far as Athens because they are opposed by northerly Etesian winds flowing over the city. Sea breezes are not always associated with a worsening of air quality. The leading edge of a cool sea breeze (sea breeze front) may push air pollutants ahead of it as it advances inland such that it is followed by clean marine air. Such a situation occurred during the infamous smog of 25 July 1973 in the Los Angeles basin, when ozone concentrations ahead of the front during the late afternoon exceeded 500 ppb (100 μg/m^3), while levels fell to 150 ppb (300 μg/m^3) or less behind the front. Athens, Melbourne and Los Angeles are among a number of major cities whose pollution levels can be influenced strongly by land and sea breeze circulations.[1]

Another problem in forecasting pollution levels from day to day is that pollution carryover can occur as, for example, in the case of photochemical smogs when the precursor pollutants have been lifted aloft and become trapped above or between inversions. Such a pollution layer is cut off from fresh emissions of ozone-scavenging compounds and from dry deposition to the ground. Not only does this prolong the lifetime of the ozone, but it allows photochemical reactions to proceed until all the precursors have been used up to produce an ozone-rich layer. In contrast, the layer below it in contact with the ground becomes depleted of ozone by ground deposition and by reaction with nitric oxide. When morning arrives, the polluted layer from the previous day may become entrained in the deepening atmospheric mixing layer during the morning, such that surface ozone levels increase abruptly to high values. Not surprisingly, such pollution carryover effects can cause problems when attempting to forecast air quality. Pollution carryover may also be responsible for lessening the differences in pollution levels that might be expected to occur between weekdays and weekends.

All the above factors play a part in determining the pollution levels that result from a given amount of emissions. This understanding of the processes involved is used by state meteorological offices or pollution control agencies to forecast daily and hourly air quality levels which are communicated to the public as well as providing the basis for smog alerts. Forecast schemes vary in complexity, ranging from simple empirically based schemes to more complex numerical dispersion models incorporating detailed local emission inventories. The latter have the advantage that they can predict spatial variations in pollution levels across the city (ie identifying

---

1 Blumenthal, D L, White, W H and Smith, T B (1978) 'Anatomy of a Los Angeles smog episode: pollutant transport in the daytime sea breeze regime', *Atmospheric Environment*, vol 12, pp 893–907

pollution hot-spots) and they are necessary for predicting the likely effects of any planned emission-reduction measures. One complication facing all forecast schemes is that pollution from sources outside the immediate area may be contributing to the smog – that is, pollutants from neighbouring urban–industrial complexes or even from sources in other countries. Long-distance transfer of pollutants is a particular problem when attempting to forecast ozone concentrations.

Setting the Threshold Levels for Smog Alert Stages

The threshold pollution levels for each smog alert stage vary from country to country (and sometimes within a country) as for air quality standards and guidelines (Table 5.1). If short-term air quality standards for individual or combinations of pollutants exist, then these provide an appropriate value for the smog alert stage 1 threshold. However, some cities may exceed the air quality standard every day for several months of the year. In such situations, the authorities may set a higher pollution concentration to define smogs – that is, short-term pollution episodes – believing that if smog alerts are issued too frequently few people will heed the health warning and

Table 5.1 *Selected national smog alert levels for various pollutants*

Country and pollutant	Stage 1: health advisory	Stage 2: intermediate	Stage 3: emergency
Carbon monoxide (ppm)			
Germany	26 (3 h)	39 (3 h)	52 (3 h)
Greece	13 (8 h)	21 (8 h)	30 (8 h)
Hungary	17 (3 h)	26 (3 h)	34 (3 h)
US	15 (8 h)	30 (8 h)	40 (8 h)
Nitrogen dioxide (ppb)			
Germany	313 (3 h)	523 (3 h)	732 (3 h)
Greece	105 (1 h)	262 (1 h)	366 (1 h)
Hungary	183 (3 h)	314 (3 h)	418 (3 h)
US	590 (1 h)	1182 (1 h)	1569 (1 h)
Ozone (ppb)			
Greece	100 (1 h)	150 (1 h)	250 (1 h)
Hungary	100 (3 h)	150 (3 h)	200 (3 h)
US	200 (1 h)	400 (1 h)	500 (1 h)
US (Los Angeles)	200 (1 h)	350 (1 h)	500 (1 h)
Sulphur dioxide (ppb)			
Germany	225 (3 h)	450 (3 h)	675 (3 h)
Greece	75 (24 h)	150 (24 h)	188 (24 h)
Hungary	150 (3 h)	225 (3 h)	300 (3 h)
US	300 (24 h)	600 (24 h)	790 (24 h)

requests for voluntary emission reductions. On the other hand, setting the smog alert threshold too high means that some of the population will be exposed to harmful pollution levels without realising this.

In some countries smog alerts are simply the higher values in an index used regularly to inform the public about daily and hourly air quality levels. This approach has the advantage that the public are already familiar with what an index means. For example, the US aims to make the smog alerts for a range of pollutants readily understandable to the public through the use of the Pollutant Standards Index (PSI). The PSI levels for the three smog alert stages are 200 (stage 1), 300 (stage 2) and 400 (stage 3, or emergency). The situation PSI values are reported by newspapers, radio and television regularly in all US urban areas with populations exceeding 200,000. The adoption of this index across the country ensures that people are readily aware of air quality in whatever city they are visiting. California adopts a slight variation when reporting PSI levels. In September 1991 it introduced a health advisory level at 138 or higher (corresponding to 150 ppb ozone), advising athletes and children to avoid strenuous outdoor activities. It also issues its stage 2 alert at 275 rather than 300.

Informing the Public

Smog alerts are announced via newspapers, radio and television. Electronic display signs may be switched on along main roads and in public places. In some situations, the police may issue warnings over tannoys and even helicopters have been used to broadcast alerts. Simply issuing smog alerts can cause health problems for some members of the community as they may equate a smog warning with the threat of danger and this in itself promotes anxiety. Given this situation it is vital that smog alerts are issued in such a way that they do not cause panic and confusion. In some individuals, research projects in Germany and the US have shown that a smog alert generates such a fear of exposure to pollution that it may suffice to trigger anxiety-induced symptoms that mimic the expected adverse health effects (even when a pollution risk is not present).

Although great efforts are needed to ensure the public are alerted to smogs, smog alerts are more likely to be effective if they are seen as a natural extension of the public realising that it is in their interests to be kept informed about air quality on a regular basis. This highlights the need for a campaign of public awareness and education about the reasons why the city experiences smogs and the health implications of poor air quality, together with ways to tackle the pollution problems not only during smogs, but also in the long term. Campaigns can take many forms such as distributing information leaflets, talks in schools and at local community meetings, articles in newspapers and magazines, and programmes on the radio and television. Many of the public, unless living near a pollution hot-spot, are often unaware of the health threats posed by poor air quality as well as the large economic losses due to lost hours at work by workers with pollution-related illnesses and the increased burden that they pose on the health services. The short-term (and long-term) voluntary emission-reduction measures needed during a smog are more likely to be undertaken if the public understand the need for these measures and are willing to accept the inconvenience and additional costs that these measures may cause. Effective urban air quality management relies on support from the community. Indeed, one of the most effective times to gather public support for introducing long-term pollution control programmes is during and after smogs. Just as the 1952 smog in London galvanised public and media opinion to press the government for national Clean Air legislation, so smogs in Athens, Mexico City and cities in many other parts of the world have triggered a demand for remedial action.

It is clear from this discussion that the public need to be fully involved when the authorities attempt to manage urban air quality. Three areas of involvement can be identified.

- A public awareness and education campaign is needed to explain the causes of poor air quality and the potential health risks posed by poor

Table 5.2 *Educational campaign leaflet, 'Ten Ways to Clear the Air', produced by the San Diego Air Pollution Control District, California*

1	Reduce your driving. Whenever possible, combine errands, car-pool, use public transportation, ride a bicycle or walk. Telecommute (work from home) or work longer hours fewer days a week
2	Keep your car in good running condition and the tyres properly inflated. Also, use less-polluting cleaner-burning gasoline or drive a clean-fuel vehicle
3	Don't top off your gas tank. Gasoline spillage evaporates and contributes to smog. It also contains toxic pollutants
4	Support the Smog Check programme. Removing emission control equipment does not improve engine performance
5	Report 'smoking' vehicles. Call 1-800-28-SMOKE to report vehicles with excessive tailpipe emissions
6	Around the home, avoid the use of aerosol spray products. Most aerosol propellants contribute to smog
7	Use water-based paints and solvents. Oil-based paints contain three to five times more toxic solvents than water-based, latex paints. Also, keep lids closed when not in use and paint with brushes or rollers rather than sprayers
8	When you fire up the barbecue, use an electric probe, a chimney that uses newspapers or new lighter fluid that produces less emissions than traditional charcoal lighter
9	Use energy-efficient lighting wherever possible. Make sure lights and appliances are turned off when not in use. In addition, raise the temperature level on your air conditioner a few degrees in summer and turn down the heat a few degrees in winter
10	Install solar energy. Water and space heating account for more than 50 per cent of household energy use

air quality, together with what can be done to tackle the pollution problem in the short and long term (Table 5.2).

- A public information system is needed to inform the public regularly about the state of air quality. Up to date air quality levels (and forecasts) need to be communicated to the public in a readily understandable form.
- Smog alerts (two or three stages) need to be issued giving clear advice to the public or sensitive groups about what actions they can take to minimise risks to their health during episodes of poor air quality. In addition, the voluntary and mandatory measures needed to reduce emissions need to be specified (Table 5.3). After the smog, information on the effectiveness of the measures should be issued to the public.

Table 5.3 *Leaflet giving advice on what to do during a smog episode distributed by the San Joaquin Valley Unified Air Pollution Control District, California*

The following protective measures are recommended to be taken by:
sensitive persons, persons with chronic lung disease or asthma, the elderly, the chronically ill, exercising adults and children, and healthy individuals who feel the effects at any level

1 Avoid strenuous outdoor physical activity (athletic activities, jogging, etc) during an episode. Avoid exertion or excitement which increases your breathing rate. Plan other diverting indoor activity for children and adolescents. At stage 1 and 2 smog alerts, outdoor activities should be increasingly more restrictive. Children should be kept indoors
2 Remain indoors until the episode is terminated. Keep doors and windows closed if possible. (Indoor concentrations of ozone are about one-half that of the outdoor levels.) Use your air conditioner to recirculate indoor air and keep cool. High temperatures may add stress to the pollutant effects
3 Do not smoke (and avoid places where others are smoking). Pollutants from smoking may aggravate the effects of ozone
4 Avoid aerosols, dusts, fumes and other irritants. Reduce activities such as cooking, hobbies or cleaning that produce irritants to the nose, eyes and lungs
5 Avoid traffic-congested areas where pollutants are being generated if you must be outside
6 Avoid contact with persons suffering from respiratory infections
7 Plan your activities. During air pollution seasons, listen to media forecasts or call 1-800-SMOG-INFO for daily update. Postpone unnecessary activities on predicted episode days. Use cool morning hours for exercise and outdoor activities
8 Expect onset or increasing severity of symptoms with increasing ozone levels (coughing, wheezing, phlegm, shortness of breath, headaches, chest discomfort and pain)

Consult your physician if symptoms persist. Know what medications to use for specific symptoms. Maintain ample fluid intake. Know the location of your nearest emergency treatment facility

Health Warnings

An announcement of a smog alert needs to be accompanied by clear advice on what actions people can take to minimise their exposure to the high pollution concentrations. It is important that this advice reaches those people particularly at risk such as people with asthma, those with respiratory disease, infants, the elderly and pregnant women as well as healthy people participating in vigorous exercise (eg athletes, cyclists, schoolchildren). They need to be advised to stay indoors and close windows (pollution levels are usually much lower indoors), to delay or postpone unnecessary journeys (lessening their own outdoor exposure as well as reducing vehicle emissions) and avoid strenuous outdoor activities (which lead to a greater intake of pollutants). The simple message 'don't jog in the smog' makes very good sense because vigorous exercise increases the pollution dose received as more pollution is breathed in and is taken deep into the lungs. Breathing through the mouth when exercising also means the pollution-scrubbing effects of nasal hairs when breathing normally through the nose do not apply. Schools need to be advised that outdoor games should be cancelled and children kept indoors during their lunch break as well as being told not to play outdoors when they reach home. During some smogs in Mexico City, schools are closed not only to lessen the exposure of the pupils to smog on their way to and from school, but also to reduce the amount of traffic on the roads.

Staff at hospitals and health clinics need to be warned to expect increased admissions. Appointments for outpatients may have to be cancelled and routine operations postponed if staff and facilities are needed to deal with the smog victims. In some extreme cases, very sick people, and those with asthma, bronchitis and heart disease, may be taken to hospital or health centres as a precaution if it is thought that their illness is likely to worsen. In the Czech Republic, extra vitamins are given out in hospitals and health centres to increase people's resistance to the adverse health effects of the smog, especially as pollutants lower a person's resistance to infections. Some people evacuate themselves from the city if they feel their health will be seriously threatened. Many people in Prague try to send their children away during the school holidays because of the threat of winter smogs.

It is not uncommon for cyclists, traffic wardens and traffic police to wear masks during smogs. In December 1990, authorities in the city of Most, again in the Czech Republic, 80 km north of Prague, distributed 20,000 smog masks to children to reduce their exposure to frequent winter smogs. Some masks reduce the intake of airborne particulates but not pollution gases unless an activated carbon filter is incorporated. Remaining indoors during smogs is a sensible precaution, especially for sensitive groups in the population, as pollution levels indoors may be 20–80 per cent lower depending on the building's ventilation. However, it should be remembered that there are some situations when indoor concentrations are unhealthy due to levels of high nitrogen dioxide emitted from inefficient gas heating systems or cooking stoves.

Emission-reduction Measures

Both voluntary and mandatory emission-reduction measures may be introduced during smogs, with more stringent measures introduced as the air quality deteriorates.[2] To reduce traffic emissions the public are urged not to make inessential journeys, not to leave engines idling unnecessarily, to share vehicles, to reduce speed, to use public transport instead of cars and to stagger working hours. Use of the metro, park and ride and rail may be encouraged during smogs by offering reduced fares or waiving them altogether. Traffic congestion may be eased by requesting companies to stagger working hours. Government offices may be closed to reduce commuting by their staff (eg first undertaken by Los Angeles authorities in July 1973 during a stage 3 episode but now adopted in Mexico City). Older poorly maintained vehicles usually emit disproportionately more pollutants than newer vehicles, so discouraging their use is desirable. Some cities make telephone lines available for the public to report polluting vehicles and so heightened awareness of such a facility during smogs may discourage use of the worst pollution offenders (Los Angeles introduced the 1-800-CUT-SMOG line in 1988). Voluntary requests to the public not to use cars unless essential may meet with limited success. During the UK ozone episode on 15 July 1994, fewer than one in ten motorists responded to requests to leave their cars at home even though six out of ten had heard the smog alert warnings.[3] During the ozone episodes of summer 1995 the situation had improved slightly with 18 per cent of drivers surveyed having decided against using their car at least once during periods of poor air quality.

If voluntary measures fail to reduce traffic sufficiently, enforced measures may be needed. Private traffic may be banned from pollution hot-spots, often the city centre. Only zero-emission (eg electric) or low-emission vehicles (eg those running on cleaner fuels such as methanol, those fitted with catalytic converters) may be allowed. Such a procedure requires pre-smog planning in that clean vehicles need to display an exemption permit. In Berlin, since the late 1980s, only cars fitted with catalytic converters have been permitted access to the city during a smog alert and this is enforced using a windscreen sticker system. Motorists not displaying stickers are stopped by the police, fined and ordered to leave their vehicle at that point. Not only did this measure reduce emissions but it encouraged many more motorists to buy cars vehicles fitted with catalytic converters well before

2 Elsom, D M (1992) *Atmospheric Pollution: a Global Problem*, second edition, Blackwell, Oxford, pp 182–192, especially table 7.5

3 Department of the Environment (1994) *Report of a Telephone Omnibus Survey*, prepared by BMRB International, London, 55 pp; Hamer, M (1994) 'Drivers ignore smog alert', *New Scientist*, 30 Jul, 12

European Union legislation required all new vehicles from 1993 to have them fitted. Since August 1995, cars without catalytic converters and high-emission diesel vehicles can be banned from the roads in Germany during ozone alerts. The ban may be difficult to implement, and of limited effectiveness, because there are so many exempted vehicles (eg tourists, public-service vehicles, taxis). Ride-sharing may be encouraged by allowing access to pollution hot-spots only to vehicles with two or more occupants. When this scheme was tried in Indonesia it started a new business with young boys hiring themselves as extra passengers on the edges of the cities. Banning cars until mid-morning during winter smogs is sometimes tried (eg the Ruhr) on the basis that by mid-morning heating by the sun has had time to increase thermal turbulence such that the resultant mixing increases dispersion of the emissions.

Parking fees can be increased, free parking zones withdrawn and higher fines for illegal parking introduced. If a road pricing system is in operation within the city, the charges could be increased during the smog. However, it is essential that public transport alternatives are available for those people priced off the road. Traffic that is moving is less polluting than engine-idling stationary traffic, so temporarily banning parking along major routes as in Madrid may help to make traffic flow more easily and reduce vehicle emissions overall. Conversely, lowering speed limits reduces emissions (especially nitrogen oxides) and can ease congestion along busy motorways.

Traffic may be reduced temporarily (as well as permanently) by arbitrary means such as allowing only odd-numbered registration vehicles to enter the inner city on odd dates and even numbers on even dates. Permanent schemes that require cars not to be used on one day a week can be extended to two days as in Mexico City during smogs. Fines are imposed on anyone breaking such regulations. However, in practice, it seems that such schemes fail to make much difference to traffic flows. In the case of odd and even licence plates many families ensure they own two cars, one with an odd- and one with an even-numbered registration. Often the second car bought especially to overcome this ban is an older and more polluting vehicle.

Emissions from residential areas can be reduced by urging people to reduce home heating, switch off air conditioning and reduce energy consumption in general. Home heating fuels which are particularly polluting such as coal and lignite could be banned, although such a measure is more appropriate as a long-term pollution control strategy (eg designation of smoke control areas in which only authorised smokeless fuels may be used). Reminders to the public of such fuel restrictions may ensure there are fewer people who ignore this regulation during the smog. Garden incinerators, bonfires and barbecues may be discouraged as well as the use of certain household and decorating products (eg solvent-based paints, varnishes, glues, cleaning agents, aerosols) which release VOCs contributing to photochemical smogs.

Industry may be required to reduce emissions by 30, 40 or 50 per cent or even cease production completely. Exceptions usually apply to those industrial activities providing essential community services. These may include power stations unless a national grid system of electricity generation allows local stations to close. Even so, in northern Bohemia, the Czech Republic, the lignite-burning power stations are closed down when there is a smog alert. In other countries, reductions in industrial emissions are achieved by switching to, say, low-sulphur fuels which have been stocked in readiness for such an occasion. One of the problems faced by the authorities is ensuring that industry complies with this demand. Large fines for failure to comply provide an incentive, but city authorities need increased staff and resources to monitor compliance. During a photochemical smog, closure of businesses emitting large amounts of VOCs could be considered because of their contribution to ozone formation. This may include paint-spraying shops, dry cleaning stores and even petrol stations which do not have vapour recovery systems installed at the pumps. Allowing petrol stations only to sell reformulated or oxygenated fuel during a smog is another measure that could be applied (although the practicalities of introducing such a measure mean that this restriction is usually applied to an entire smog season).

As high stacks contribute lower amounts to local pollution than low stacks, some industrial plants may be asked to switch temporarily their emissions through tall stacks. If that is not possible, industrial plants with low stacks may be told to cut or stop production, whereas those plants with high stacks are unaffected. During the second stage smog alert in the Rijnmond–Rotterdam area of the Netherlands, industrial emissions from stacks below 40 m are prohibited.[4] Of course, although stacks taller than 150 or even 100 m (in which emissions are released at high velocities and high temperature so increasing their buoyancy) may contribute little to local emissions during smogs, they may add to the pollution burden in distant cities as the pollutants drift with the stronger winds that are usually found above a shallow temperature inversion.

Are Short-term Emission-reduction Measures Effective?

The choice of emission-reduction measures to implement during a smog needs to be based on a detailed understanding of the contribution that each emission source makes to the smog. The availability of detailed emission inventories, real-time air quality information from a dense network of pollution monitors and numerical dispersion models may be vital to select the most appropriate pollution control measures. The public will need convincing that traffic restrictions in the city centre are likely to result in significant urban air quality benefits overall rather than simply shifting the

---

4 Tellagen, E (1988) 'The Kingdom of the Netherlands', in Rhode, B (ed) *Air Pollution in Europe*, vol 1, Western Europe, Occasional Paper No 4, European Coordination Centre for Research and Documentation in the Social Sciences, Vienna, pp 145–163

pollution to suburban or peripheral locations due to the resulting increased traffic volume and congestion in those localities. After a smog the public will expect confirmation that the emission-reduction measures introduced were indeed justified. Many cities do not yet possess the air quality management system to offer this reassurance except in general terms.

Photochemistry complicates the relationship between pollutant emissions and the resulting pollution concentrations of secondary pollutants such as ozone and nitrogen dioxide. Ozone is produced from nitrogen oxides and VOCs, but decreases in ozone levels are less than proportional to the reduction in these precursor pollutants. Substantial VOC and/or nitrogen oxides in the range of more than 50 per cent may be necessary to decrease ozone levels significantly during smogs. Moreover, research suggests that although reducing VOC emissions alone may cause a zero or beneficial effect, reductions in nitrogen oxides alone may cause counter-productive effects (Figure 5.3).[5] For example, a substantial decrease in fresh emissions of nitric oxide in city centres due to traffic restrictions can actually cause ozone levels to increase in those areas because the nitric oxide formerly acted as a local ozone scavenger.

The oxidising capacity of the atmosphere is important when considering the poor air quality that nitrogen oxides give rise to. For example, air quality managers need to know whether a 50 per cent reduction in emissions of nitrogen oxides will result in a 50 per cent decrease in nitrogen dioxide levels. Hourly data from a London kerbside site provide two different answers to this question (Figure 5.4). At low nitrogen dioxide concentrations, nitrogen dioxide concentrations seem relatively unaffected by changes in emissions of nitrogen oxides, highlighting the limited oxidising capacity of the urban atmosphere. However, at the higher nitrogen dioxide concentrations typical of smogs, nitrogen dioxide concentrations decrease rapidly with reductions in emissions of nitrogen oxides. In other words, there is every reason to believe that nitrogen dioxide levels during smogs can be

5 Wolff, G T and Korsog, P E (1992) 'Ozone control strategies based on the ratio of volatile organic compounds to nitrogen oxides', *Journal of Air and Waste Management Association*, vol 42, pp 1173–1177; Zierock, K-H (1988) *Environment and Quality of Life, Photochemical Oxidants: Summary of Studies Relevant to an Abatement Policy*, Commission of the European Communities, Brussels. In Los Angeles it appears that reducing peak ozone levels can be achieved more effectively by reducing VOCs alone compared with nitrogen oxide reductions, or even equal reductions of both precursor pollutants. In fact, reducing VOCs and nitrogen oxides simultaneously requires larger percentage reductions for both than the reduction required when VOCs alone are reduced. However, the VOC reduction strategy is only the most efficient on average and the optimum strategy varies according to temporal and spatial variations in the VOC/NO_x ratio and in temperature; Kelly, N A and Gunst, R F (1990) 'Response of ozone to changes in hydrocarbon and nitrogen oxide concentrations in outdoor smog chambers filled with Los Angeles air', *Atmospheric Environment*, vol 24A, pp 2999–3005

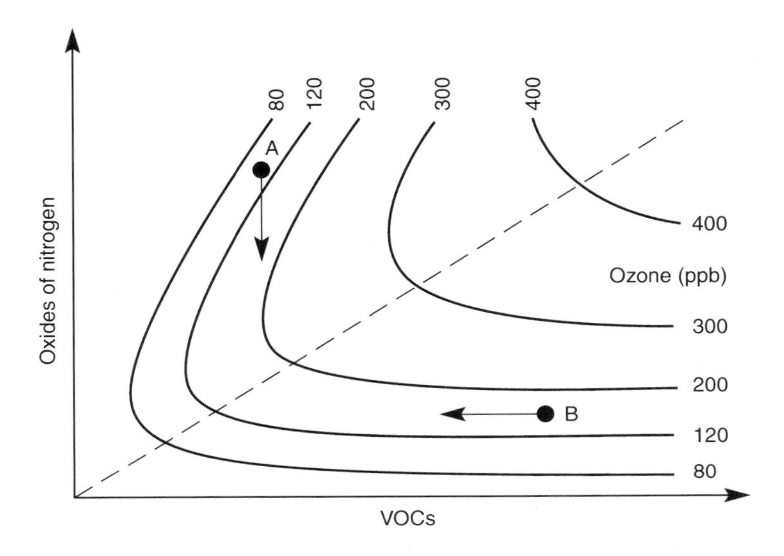

Figure 5.3 *Peak ozone levels as a function of levels of VOCs and nitrogen oxides. Changes in ozone levels as a result of reductions in VOCs and/or nitrogen oxides depend on the relative position of a city's VOC/nitrogen oxides ratio on the graph. In the worst scenario (A), reducing nitrogen oxides alone may cause ozone levels to increase, whereas in (B) reducing VOCs may cause no change in ozone levels. Ozone can be reduced most effectively when reductions in VOCs and nitrogen oxides occur in the 'knee' region of the graph (broken line)*

reduced to acceptable levels if low-level emissions, primarily from traffic, are reduced sufficiently.[6]

There are relatively few detailed assessments of the air quality effectiveness of short-term pollution control (emission-reduction) measures. Los Angeles authorities point out that no stage 3 episode has been declared in the basin since July 1973 and they credit this, in part, to the emission-reduction measures taken during stages 1 and 2 of a smog. During a five-day winter smog in January 1985 in the Ruhr, Germany, it was estimated that emission-reduction measures had reduced overall emissions by about 30 per cent, including 14 per cent sulphur dioxide from power plants, 40–50 per cent nitric oxide from traffic, 20 per cent carbon monoxide from traffic and 20 per cent sulphur dioxide from traffic. During a four-day smog in west Berlin in February 1987, traffic bans and industrial restrictions

6 Derwent, R G and Middleton, D R (1995) 'Analysis and interpretation of air quality data from an urban roadside location in central London over the period from July 1991 to July 1992', *Atmospheric Environment*, vol 29, pp 923–946; Quality of Urban Air Review Group (1993) *Diesel Vehicle Emissions and Urban Air Quality*, Second Report, HMSO, London, pp 62–63

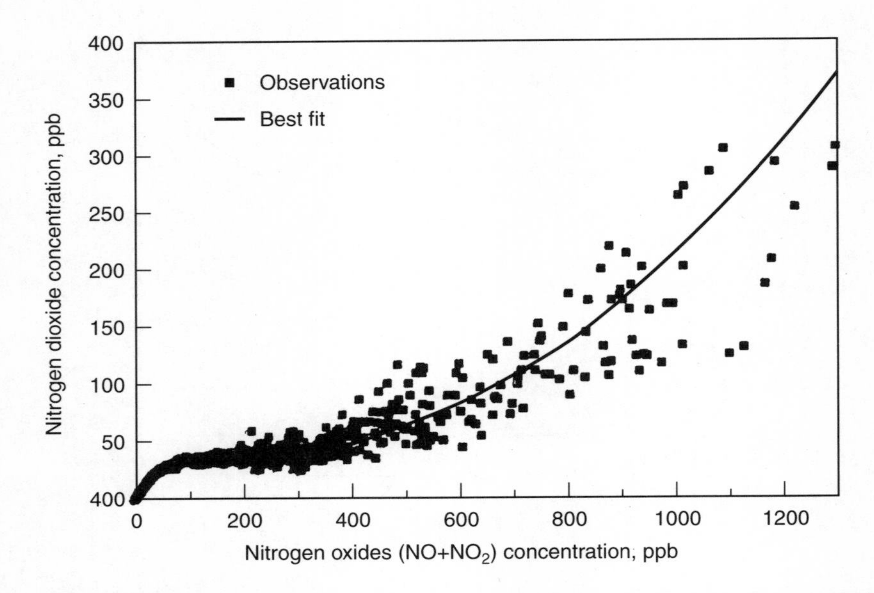

Figure 5.4 *Relationship between hourly mean concentrations of nitrogen dioxide and nitrogen oxides at a London roadside location*

Source: Quality of Urban Air Review Group (1993) *Diesel Vehicle Emissions and Urban Air Quality*, Second Report, Department of the Environment, London, p 63

prevented 500 t of carbon monoxide, 40 t of oxides of nitrogen, 5 t of soot and 0.6 t of sulphur dioxide from being added to the city's air. Around 800 companies reduced their emissions by 40 per cent and 400,000 people switched from cars to public transport. During the smog, when daily concentrations of suspended particulate matter and sulphur dioxide reached 500 $\mu g/m^3$ and 338 ppb (900 $\mu g/m^3$), respectively, the authorities suggested that if diesel engines had not been classed as low-polluting engines and exempt from the traffic ban they could have prevented a further 2 t of soot from being added to the air as well as some sulphur dioxide.[7]

In an attempt to determine the effectiveness of various control measures an experiment was undertaken in the town of Heilbronn/Neckarsulm, north of Stuttgart, Germany. For four days in June 1994 this town was closed to

7 Lubkert, B (1989) 'Characteristics of the mid-January 1985 sulphur dioxide smog episode in central Europe: report from an international workshop', *Atmospheric Environment*, vol 23, pp 611–623; MacKenzie, D (1987) 'Smog brings Germany to a standstill', *New Scientist*, 12 February, p 22; Weir, F (1993) 'A critique of UK air quality', *Environmental Health*, Nov, pp 351–355; WHO (1990) *Acute Effects on Health of Smog Episodes*, WHO Regional Publications, European Series, No 43, WHO, Copenhagen

all cars except those fitted with three-way catalytic converters and all but the lowest emission diesel-engined lorries to measure the air quality impact. The result was a 40 per cent reduction in road traffic and 50 per cent increase in public transport use, producing a 40 per cent fall in nitrogen dioxide concentrations and a halving of benzene concentrations from 4 to 2 $\mu g/m^3$. At the same time, a speed limit of 60 kph (37 mph) was imposed on a nearby autobahn to examine the effects of traffic speed on pollution levels. Measurements near the autobahn were inconclusive.[8]

Banning certain types of vehicles from city centres during smogs may not always reduce traffic emissions as much as desired. Allowing only cars fitted with catalytic converters assumes that these vehicles are low polluters. However, current catalytic converters (ie those without pre-warming capabilities) take several minutes – perhaps as many as eight minutes – to reach their operating temperature, during which time exhaust emissions are uncontrolled. As such cars operate on a richer mixture than cars not fitted with catalytic converters they actually emit more pollution than non-catalytic cars. This problem becomes significant when it is realised that in the UK 26 per cent of car journeys are less than 3 km (2 miles) and 60 per cent of car journeys are less than 8 km (5 miles).[9] The greater demand for public transport during a traffic ban results in increased numbers of diesel buses and taxis in the city centre but not all may be low polluters. In some cases bus companies bring out every available bus to cope with demand, including those needing servicing and even the oldest most fuel-inefficient vehicles. In some traffic bans the number of vehicles deemed exempt from the ban can be considerable. For example, traffic was banned in Rome centre for five hours during a smog in November 1994. Exceptions to the ban included politicians, the disabled, taxis, newspaper, medicine and food delivery vehicles, diplomats, motorists from the Vatican, emergency services vehicles, and funeral processions. The ban was brought to an end an hour earlier than planned when it was realised that the Italian national football team was due to play an important match and that civil unrest might erupt unless fans could get home to watch the match on television.[10]

The authorities need to be careful that some emission-reduction measures do not increase the population's exposure to pollutants. For example, a ban on private cars may reduce vehicular emissions but may increase an individual's length of exposure to poor air quality by causing them to walk, cycle or wait for public transport. It is important for city authorities to ensure that there is sufficient public transport available to cope with a large increase in the number of passengers and that passengers are not left

8 Edwards, R (1994) 'German banger cuts pollution', *New Scientist*, 20 Aug, p 9; 'German experiment reduces carcinogens', *The Environmental Digest*, 83/84, May/Jun 1994, p 16

9 Holman, C, Wade, J and Fergusson, M (1993) *Future Emissions from Cars 1990 to 2025: the Importance of the Cold Start Emissions Penalty*, World Wide Fund for Nature UK, Godalming, p 15

10 'Rome traffic banned', *The Environmental Digest*, 89/90, Nov/Dec 1994, p 13

waiting for lengthy periods at bus stops while breathing polluted kerbside air. Asking the public to reduce the heating in their homes during winter smogs may cause the elderly to suffer hypothermia, while urging people to turn off their air conditioning during summer smogs may increase the number of cases of hyperthermia.

When emission-reduction measures are applied during a smog they need to be justified in terms of their effectiveness in reducing emissions, pollution concentrations and public exposure to unhealthy air quality. Introducing needless short-term measures can be worse than useless because they may cause economic disruption, induce stress and anxiety among the public, increase some people's exposure to poor air quality, and may undermine public support for long-term measures needed to produce a long-lasting improvement in air quality.[11]

Neutralising the Smog

There have been many suggestions but few attempts to neutralise smogs – that is, remove the pollution or nullify the harmful effects of the pollutants present. At a very small-scale, some success was achieved during the 1952 London smog when ammonia bottles with wicks were placed in hospital wards in an attempt to neutralise the acid aerosols. A parliamentary enquiry into the smog received various suggestions about how to tackle the problem, including using very high frequency sound waves to cause the smog particles to coagulate and fall out.

As smogs are basically polluted fogs, it could be judged that there have been many successful attempts at clearing smogs, or at least small areas within a smog. Fog removal along airport runways has long been practised and has been shown to be successful when the fog is seeded with dry ice or silver iodide. Alternatively, it can be evaporated by heat such as produced by an array of jet engines in the case of the French airport system. The gap in the fog usually lasts only for a short time unless the seeding or heating is continued. Very few attempts have been made to disperse smog on an urban scale but in June 1988 the authorities in Santiago, Chile, resorted to using aircraft to spray the smog with water and detergent to encourage the removal of the fine airborne particulates present. In 1981, it was suggested that spraying a photochemical smog with diethylhydroxylamine would neutralise the ozone present. It is claimed this would pose no threat to health but it has not been attempted.[12]

Technofix solutions to smogs have long been desired by many people because it would simply mean they could carry on with their polluting activities regardless. It is not surprising that many technical solutions were

---

11 'Experience with smog alert systems in Europe', *WHO Collaborating Centre for Air Quality Management and Air Pollution Control Newsletter*, 6, Jun 1990, WHO, Langen, Germany, pp 8–10

12 Elsom (1992) op cit, p 188

suggested in Los Angeles in the 1950s when photochemical smogs were worsening in frequency and severity and the car-loving public were unwilling to accept that smogs could only be curbed through vehicle restrictions. Some people suggested that as sunlight was an essential ingredient for photochemical smog, aircraft could create a high-altitude white smokescreen umbrella to shield the city from sunlight. Others suggested digging huge tunnels through the mountains encircling the Los Angeles basin and installing gigantic fans to remove the smog. Even helicopters were suggested as a means of increasing turbulence and so encouraging the dispersal of the smog. One recent approach suggested to reduce Los Angeles smog levels is for cars to be fitted with fans which suck in polluted air (even when parked) which then reacts with a coating of catalytic paint. The ozone and carbon monoxide in the air would react with the warmed catalytic coating to produce oxygen and carbon dioxide, respectively.[13]

The technofix approach continues today based on the recognition that pollutants from tall industrial stacks, emitted at high temperatures and velocities, can penetrate a temperature inversion and so do not contribute to local pollution levels. Researchers in Mexico City have proposed using 100 giant industrial fans to suck in polluted air, heat it up and then blow it upwards in the form of vortices which would punch through the temperature inversion. Currently, this proposal is limited to mathematical modelling experiments.[14]

Short-term Versus Long-term Solutions to the Smog Problem

Smogs are episodes of poor air quality which pose a serious risk to the public's health lasting for a few hours or days. They occur when urban emissions are relatively high and stagnant meteorological conditions fail to sufficiently dilute and disperse the pollutants. If the health threat posed by poor air quality can be lessened by short-term reductions in emissions, then it is right to attempt to do so. However, it is important that efforts to tackle smogs do not undermine the commitment of the public or the government to long-term measures to improve air quality. Smog alert systems consume considerable resources which could be diverted to reducing pollution emissions in the long term. It is important that the public do not accept smog alert systems as a substitute for introducing more costly and lifestyle-changing measures that tackle the root of the air pollution problem. On the other hand, a severe smog which results in widespread illness and premature deaths among the elderly or sick can provide the stimulus for the public, the media and environmental pressure groups to campaign for

---

13 Goddard, A (1995) 'Banish smog with a lick of paint', *New Scientist*, 20 May, p 20

14 Rodriguez Valdes, A, Palacio Perez, A, Navarro Gonzalez, I and Sanchez Bribiesca, J L (1993) 'Feasibility of mechanical means for air pollution mitigation in Mexico City', in Zanetti, P, Brebbia, C A, Garcia Gardea, J E and Ayala Milian, G (eds) *Air Pollution*, Computational Mechanics, Southampton, pp 719–726; 'Mexico City pollution reaches new high', *The Environmental Digest*, 57, Mar 1992, p 11

the implementation of stringent long-term pollution control measures. The 1952 smog in London was one of the earliest examples of providing a trigger that eventually resulted in strong anti-pollution legislation despite some government reluctance to take action.

Conclusions: Reducing Baseline Emissions in the Long Term

Ultimately, the solution to the smog problem is to reduce emissions throughout an urban area to a low level and, in the case of pollution imported from outside the city boundaries, to reduce emissions similarly on a regional, national and international scale. The international dimension of smogs has been highlighted during several recent winters when sulphur dioxide and suspended particulates from eastern Europe and the Ruhr district of Germany have drifted westwards to create smog problems for the Netherlands and Belgium. In addition, many photochemical smogs have their origin in emissions of nitrogen oxides and VOCs from neighbouring countries. It seems unlikely that temporary measures would be adopted in one country to prevent a smog occurring a day or even several days later in another. In such cases the solution lies in international agreements for long-term emission reductions.

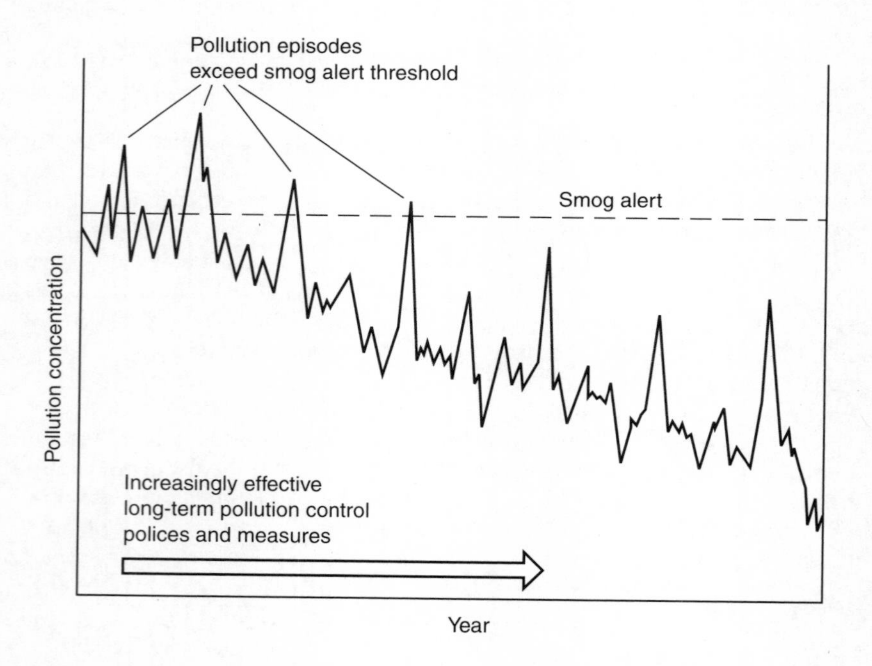

Figure 5.5 *Reducing baseline emissions over several years will eventually reduce the frequency of occasions when smog alert levels are exceeded, although variability in weather conditions from year to year may obscure this trend for a while*

Reducing emissions to a low level (and eventually to a minimal level) will eliminate smogs as there is a limit to which atmospheric conditions can concentrate and/or convert emissions to produce high pollution concentrations. As the baseline or average pollution level in an urban area declines, so the severity and frequency of smogs will decrease. This trend may be unclear initially, being obscured by random occurrences of stagnant meteorological conditions, but in the long term the beneficial effects of reducing baseline emissions become clear (Figure 5.5). In some cases, changes in the climate characteristics of a region (eg changing frequency of anticyclones bringing stagnant meteorological conditions, rising temperatures due to global warming) may delay the improvements but, eventually, as emissions continue to fall, the threat of smogs will diminish.

Chapter 6

Cleaner Fuels and Cleaner Cars

Introduction

Smog alert systems can alleviate the worst excesses of the pollution problem but cannot prevent smogs from re-occurring during stagnant weather conditions. The solution to the problem of urban populations experiencing poor air quality is a long-term commitment to reduce pollutant emissions to achieve healthy air quality. Reducing the emissions per motor vehicle can be achieved through the introduction of more fuel-efficient engines, the use of cleaner fuels and improved technology. Where private cars remain the principal means of travel within an urban area, a technological approach to pollution control would be to replace existing diesel- and petrol-engined cars with zero-emission vehicles. The speed with which cleaner fuels and cleaner vehicles are introduced will be influenced greatly by the commitment of city and national governments to improving air quality as they can set stringent technology-forcing emission and fuel efficiency standards as well as using economic instruments to influence adoption (eg tax incentives to encourage vehicle owners to use less polluting fuels and buy zero-emission vehicles).

Exhaust Emission Standards

Emission standards for vehicles can be tightened as improved engine technologies, pollution control equipment and fuels become available. Alternatively, emission standards may be set to force the automobile and oil industries to develop improvements at a faster pace than they would have otherwise. The US and Japan have been leaders in successive tightening of emission standards but the European Union is beginning to catch up. Vehicle emission standards in the European Union were tightened significantly with new cars from 1993 (stage 1), requiring the fitting of catalytic converters (Table 6.1). From 1996 a further reduction (stage 2)

Table 6.1 *European Union (EU) emission standards for cars*

Type	CO	HC + NO_x	Particulates
EU stage 1 (1993)			
Petrol and diesel	3.16	1.13	0.18
EU stage 2 (1997)			
Petrol	2.20	0.50	—
Diesel, indirect injection	1.00	0.70	0.08
Diesel, direct injection	1.00	0.90	0.10
EU stage 3 (2000) as proposed by the European Parliament			
Petrol	1.00	0.10 (HC) 0.10 (NO_x)	
Diesel	0.50	0.10 (HC) 0.30 (NO_x)	0.03

takes place in petrol-engined vehicle emission limits of 30 per cent for carbon monoxide and 56 per cent for hydrocarbons plus nitrogen oxides over the 1993 levels. This European Union directive applies to new vehicle types from 1996 and to all new vehicles from 1997 and brings the European Union broadly in line with 1994 US federal standards. The European Union plans to promote further reductions in emissions by the year 2000 (stage 3) with a joint auto-oil research programme examining the potential improvements of cleaner engine technologies and fuels to produce ultra-low emitting vehicles. Stage 3 emission standards will equate approximately with California's ultra-low emission vehicle standards.[1]

Catalytic Converters

To meet new emission standards for cars, catalytic converters have been required to be fitted in cars in the US and Japan since the 1970s, in the European Union since 1993 and in four southeast Asian countries (Malaysia, Singapore, Taiwan and Thailand) also since 1993. Catalytic converters are of two basic types. The simplest is an oxidation catalyst which consists of a canister fitted with a porous ceramic element, coated with a thin layer of platinum or other noble metal of the platinum group (the catalyst), in which air and the exhaust gases are mixed to convert carbon monoxide and hydrocarbons to carbon dioxide and water vapour. Its disadvantage is that

1 Royal Commission on Environmental Pollution (1994) *Eighteenth Report: Transport and the Environment*, HMSO, London, pp 120–124. Comparison between, say, European Union and US emission standards is difficult because each use different test cycles. As well as setting standards for hydrocarbons (HC) + NO_x the US sets standards for NO_x, total HC and non-methane HC

it does not reduce nitrogen oxides. Oxidation catalysts are appropriate for diesel engines but function better if the fuel contains as little sulphur as possible.

The three-way catalyst is the type usually fitted to petrol-engined vehicles. It is a similar canister but with a different mixture of platinum metals: platinum catalyses reactions to remove hydrocarbons and carbon monoxide whereas rhodium removes nitrogen oxides. It needs careful control of the fuel/air ratio. Too little air (oxygen) and the engine produces more carbon monoxide and hydrocarbons. Too much air and the engine emits more nitrogen oxides. For optimum efficiency it must operate around an air to fuel ratio of 14.7:1, known at the stoichiometric ratio. To regulate the ratio, a device called a Lambda sensor is fitted to the exhaust system. It measures the oxygen content of the exhaust gases and feeds information electronically to the fuel injection control or carburettor to keep the air/fuel mixture at the optimum level. The three-way catalyst converts carbon monoxide, hydrocarbons and nitrogen oxides to carbon dioxide, water vapour and nitrogen (Figure 6.1).

The use of catalytic converters requires unleaded petrol as lead poisons the catalyst, preventing it from functioning correctly. Regular vehicle inspections are needed to ensure the catalyst is working correctly as it can be tampered with, removed, poisoned by lead or damaged in some way. The catalyst system plus Lambda sensor is referred as a regulated, controlled or closed-loop system. Whereas the controlled three-way catalyst can achieve emission reductions of 80–95 per cent in test conditions or 75–80 per cent in all driving conditions (ie taking into account its initial poor performance from cold starts), the uncontrolled three-way catalyst reduces emissions at best by 50–70 per cent. One of the disadvantages of three-way catalysts is that as the engines are constrained to operate very near the stoichiometric ratio, the additional fuel savings offered by lean-burn engines cannot be used. According to UK research a car fitted with a catalytic converter has a fuel consumption 3–9 per cent higher than one without, and carbon dioxide emissions can be 9–23 per cent greater.[2]

One problem with catalytic converters is that they take several minutes to warm up to their operational 'light-off' temperature of around 300–400°C during which emissions go unchecked. The length of many urban journeys may be only a few kilometres (miles) so this can be a serious limitation of such pollution control equipment. Additionally, a catalyst can 'go out' when the engine is idling in congested traffic as it falls below the temperature at which it operates effectively. Conversely, at high driving speeds, if temperatures exceed 800°C, a catalyst can fail. Engine misfiring or 'bump starting' can also cause failures as can malfunction of the Lambda sensor used to determine the air to fuel ratio. Perhaps 5 per cent of all catalytic converters may fail and have to be replaced in the first three years. In

---

2 'Catalytic converters study published', *The Environmental Digest*, 56, Feb 1992, pp 13–14

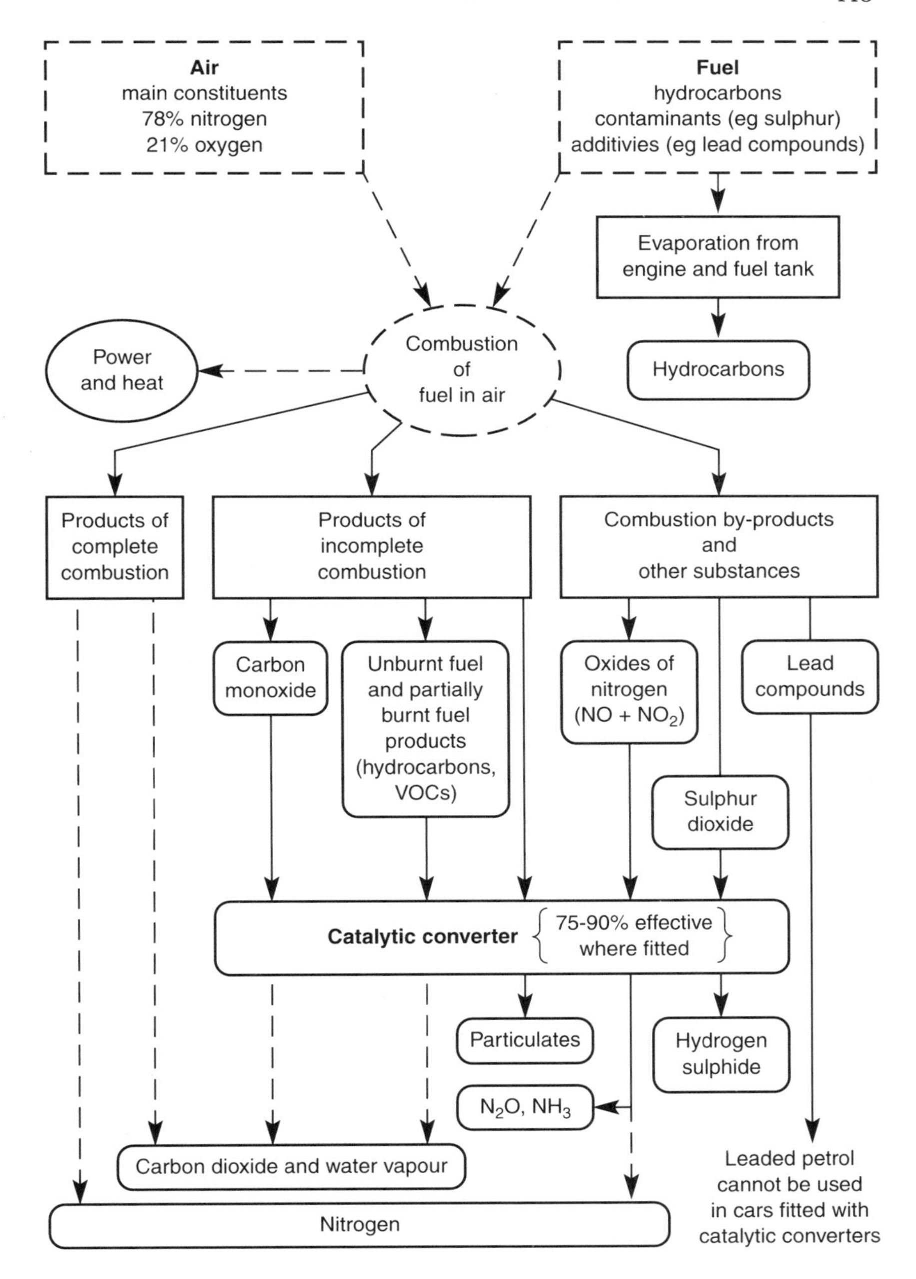

Figure 6.1 *Pollutants emitted by petrol-engined vehicles*

Source: Royal Commission on Environmental Pollution (1994) *Eighteenth Report, Transport and the Environment*, HMSO, London, p 22

Sweden, which has had catalytic converters fitted in cars since 1989, the failure rate after five years was found to be up to 15 per cent in some makes of cars. Consequently, especially on cold days of calm and stable weather conditions, carbon monoxide will remain a significant problem, especially along busy streets, at road junctions, in tunnels and at traffic lights until the motor industry tackles the problems of 'cold start' emissions by speeding up the time taken for the catalyst to begin operating.[3]

Technology improvements should soon lead to pre-warmed or quick 'light up' catalysts becoming standard (with a dashboard light to indicate when it is functioning correctly). By 1995 there was a growing number of car manufacturers offering some method of quickly warming the catalysts to their operating temperature. However, existing cars will still give rise to excessive cold start emissions (Figure 6.2). Emission performance

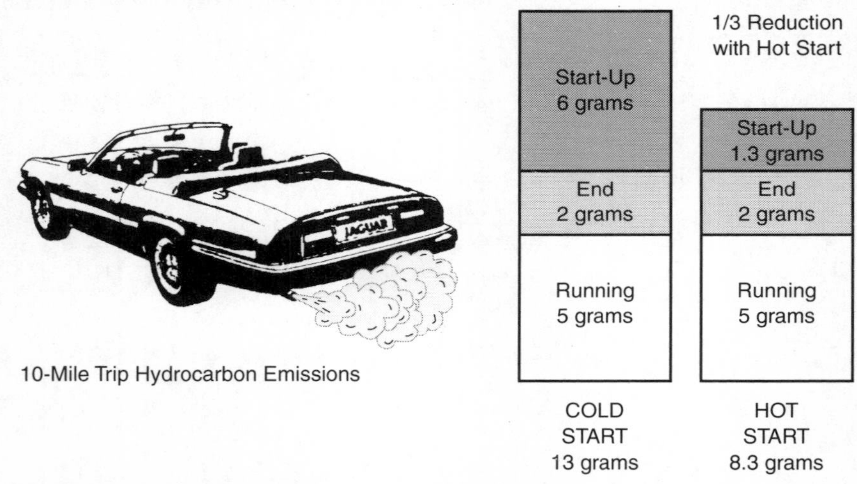

Figure 6.2 *Comparison of the amount of hydrocarbons emitted from a petrol-engined car fitted with a catalytic converter during a cold start and a hot start. Around half of the hydrocarbons emitted during a short trip happen during the cold start*

Source: Data based on an assessment by the Californian Air Resources Board

deterioration of cars fitted with catalytic converters is another issue that manufacturers need to address. European research suggests that on average cars fitted with catalysts deteriorate such that carbon monoxide emissions increase from 1 g/km at new to 3 g/km at 80,000 km (50,000 miles) and hydrocarbons plus nitrogen oxides from around 0.4 g/km at new to 1.0 g/km after 80,000 km. California has required improved warranties on catalytic converters from 1990 cars onwards, extending the seven year and 110,000

3 Holman, C, Wade, J and Fergusson, M (1993) *Future Emissions from Cars 1990 to 2025: the Importance of the Cold Start Emissions Penalty*, World Wide Fund for Nature UK, Godalming

km (70,000 miles) warranty to 10 years and 160,000 km (100,000 miles). This will improve the reliance of the systems and ensure that repairs are undertaken instead of being waived as too costly as has been permitted under the 'smog check' (emissions testing) programme. Since 1994 California has required new cars to be fitted with computerised systems with dashboard warning lights to indicate any malfunction in the pollution control equipment which needs repair. It is possible that the technology may eventually become available to measure the total amount of pollutant emissions a vehicle produces in a year, which could then be the basis for applying the polluter pays principle, taxing vehicle owners according to their pollution impact. It would certainly encourage car owners to keep their vehicles better maintained.

Vehicle Emissions Testing and the Identification of Gross Polluters

Periodic vehicle exhaust emissions testing is intended to identify vehicles that fail to meet mandatory emission standards and so require repair (or scrapping if repair is not possible). For example, one badly maintained car can produce as much pollution as up to 40 cleaner vehicles. Emissions tests are usually part of a larger vehicle inspection/maintenance (I/M) programme which examines whether a vehicle is safe and roadworthy. Checks can be made to assess whether a vehicle's pollution control equipment is functioning correctly and has not been tampered with or, in the case of older vehicles, whether engine maintenance has been adequate to meet the less stringent emission standards applied to older vehicles. The 'smog check' has been implemented in the US for many years and has been introduced more recently in Europe. From September 1995, the amount of carbon monoxide emitted by petrol-engined cars in the UK must not exceed 4.5 per cent for 1973–1986 vehicles and 3.5 per cent for post-1986 vehicles. For diesel-engined vehicles the level of smoke opacity must not exceed 2.5/m for non-turbo-charged engines and 3.0/m for turbo-charged engines. However, these emission standards need extending to include other exhaust pollutants. The European Union is proposing to standardise vehicle inspection tests, starting when a vehicle is four years old and then continuing at two year intervals. This compares with Germany's annual test beginning when a car is one year old, France's two year interval test not beginning until the car's seventh year, and the UK's test which is compulsory every year from the car's third birthday.[4]

Inspection and maintenance programmes usually measure exhaust emissions while the vehicle is stationary, with its engine at idle for several minutes. The US Clean Air Amendments of 1990 require states with serious or worse ozone or carbon monoxide non-attainment areas to implement an enhanced I/M programme. This requires vehicles to be tested under load

4 Royal Commission on Environmental Pollution (1994) op cit, p 141

conditions over a simulated urban driving cycle using a treadmill device termed a dynamometer. It also requires inspection of the small carbon canisters fitted to vehicles, intended to control evaporative emissions of hydrocarbons, to ensure that these have not been disconnected or are not malfunctioning. Inspection station networks can be either centralised (high volume test facilities with no repair facilities) or decentralised (licensed vehicle repair facilities which can perform repairs as well as inspect the vehicle). California's enhanced I/M inspection programme intends to assign vehicles to test-only centralised stations where there is a likelihood that they are a high polluter. The I/M programmes have been claimed to be very successful in reducing vehicle emissions. For example, the I/M programme for cars together with fleet renewal in New York reduced emissions of nitrogen oxides by 38 per cent and carbon monoxide by 34 per cent between 1980 and 1987. California's smog check introduced in 1984 was aimed at reducing vehicle emissions by 25 per cent by 1994.[5]

Given that newer vehicles tend to be much less polluting than older vehicles, the average age of the vehicle fleet and the rate at which it is renewed can contribute significantly in lowering total vehicle emissions in an urban area. The average age of vehicles in many countries may be around ten years. In the US the average age of cars on the road is eight years but 25 years ago it was only five years. This trend is thought to be due to the relatively higher prices of new vehicles and increased durability of older cars. Governments can speed up fleet renewal by introducing vehicle scrapping schemes whereby older vehicles are scrapped in exchange for a government grant towards the cost of purchasing a new (and cleaner) car. In 1990, California offered $700 for pre-1971 models and eventually retired over 8000 vehicles. The Spanish government's offer of $750 to owners who scrapped their old cars produced a 19 per cent rise in sales of new vehicles in 1994. In 1993, Budapest city council offered the 120,000 owners of grossly polluting two-stroke vehicles grants and loans for four-stroke vehicles or public transport passes. If owners chose the free public transport passes they received a two-year pass for giving up a Trabant and a three-year pass for a Wartburg.[6]

Emissions testing using remote sensing of vehicles as they are being driven along roads (rather than using laboratory analysers in pre-arranged static tests) is gaining increased attention from governments. This is because it is cheaper and quicker, being able to test thousands of vehicles

---

5 Klausmeier, R and Kishan, S (1995) 'World-wide developments in motor vehicle inspection/maintenance (I/M) programs', *Proceedings of the 10th World Clean Air Congress, Espoo, Finland*, vol 3, Finnish Air Pollution Prevention Society, Helsinki, paper 546; Lawson, D R (1993) 'Passing the test – human behaviour and California's smog check programme', *Air and Waste*, vol 43, pp 1567–1575

6 Centre for Exploitation of Science and Technology (1993) *The UK Environmental Foresight Project, vol 2, Road Transport and the Environment*, HMSO, London, p 97; 'American cars older than ever', *The Environmental Digest*, 86, Aug 1994, p 15; 'DDR cars: getting them off the streets', *Acid News*, 5, Dec 1993, p 5

in a relatively short time. One of the remote sensing devices most widely used is the system called the Fuel Efficiency Automobile Test (FEAT) developed by Donald Stedman at the University of Denver in 1987. It uses infra-red spectrometry to provide an analysis of carbon monoxide and hydrocarbon emissions from a vehicle as it passes through an infra-red beam directed across a road. An ultraviolet-based system has now been added to measure nitrogen oxides and opacity (smoke).[7]

If remote sensing replaced periodic static testing of all vehicles it would have to be located in several places across an urban area to ensure that few vehicles escaped detection. However, the accuracy of remote sensing is not as good as the static tests, especially for hydrocarbons and nitrogen oxides. This has prompted many governments to use remote sensing as an excellent measure to support rather than replace existing periodic I/M inspections as it can identify gross polluters between the periodic tests. This will enable the enforcement agencies to discover vehicles whose owners have tampered with pollution control equipment (ie reset controls) after having passed an emissions test, those who possess fraudulent emission test certificates, and those vehicles whose poor maintenance has allowed the efficiency of the vehicle engine to deteriorate since the test. Whether remote sensing leads to on the spot fines for polluting vehicles or simply a requirement that the owner takes the vehicle for a full inspection test within a set time period may be determined by how accurate remote sensing devices are considered to be compared with testing at I/M stations.

Remote sensing has been particularly useful in recent years in highlighting the fact that some vehicles are responsible for excessive emissions such that one 'gross polluter' can produce as much as 40–50 times the exhaust emissions of a 'clean' car. Tests in four cities in the UK highlight this situation (Table 6.2). The highest emitting 10 per cent of the vehicles contributed 40–59 per cent of total vehicle emissions for carbon monoxide and 52–67 per cent of total vehicle emissions of hydrocarbons. In contrast, the cleanest 70 per cent of the vehicles contributed only 8–23 per cent of total carbon monoxide emissions and 7–21 per cent of total hydrocarbon emissions. The four cities produced a range of values because the vehicles sampled were

---

7 When a vehicle breaks the FEAT infra-red beam a measurement is taken of the absorption in front of the vehicle and as the vehicle exits the beam. The detector converts the incident infra-red radiation to a voltage signal, thus allowing the carbon monoxide to carbon dioxide and hydrocarbon to carbon dioxide ratios to be calculated from the measured voltage changes both in front and behind the vehicle. The carbon monoxide/carbon dioxide and hydrocarbon/carbon dioxide ratios are the only valid measurements that can be made because the instrument cannot distinguish the intensity or position of the exhaust plume. However, using appropriate known relationships, values can be derived for the effective air/fuel ratio, the emissions of carbon monoxide or hydrocarbons in grams per gallon (or litre) of fuel, the emissions of carbon monoxide or hydrocarbons per mile (km) and the percentage carbon monoxide or hydrocarbons. The system is calibrated daily with a certified gas mixture. A video camera can be focused on the rear of the vehicles as they pass so that their licence plates can be recorded.

Table 6.2 *Contribution of exhaust emissions from the dirtiest 10 per cent and cleanest 70 per cent of vehicles to total emissions of carbon monoxide and hydrocarbons in four UK cities measured using remote sensing techniques*

City	Percentage of total CO emissions contributed by dirtiest 10 per cent of vehicles	Percentage of total HC emissions contributed by dirtiest 10 per cent of vehicles	Percentage of total CO emissions contributed by cleanest 70 per cent of vehicles	Percentage of total HC emissions contributed by cleanest 70 per cent of vehicles
London	57	66	11	10
Edinburgh	41	52	23	21
Leicester	40	53	22	20
Middlesborough	59	67	8	7

Source: Muncaster (1994)[8].

characterised by differing proportions of cold-starting vehicles (with their higher emission levels), differing speeds and driving conditions (low or high speed, cruising or decelerating), and differing vehicle age distributions and compositions (petrol and diesel, catalysts and non-catalysts).[8] These remote sensing surveys clearly indicate the enormous air quality benefits that could be gained by using legislation and enforcement measures to clean up the gross polluters. Targeting gross polluters offers a simple and cost-effective measure. In general, legislative and economic measures which encourage proper maintenance of vehicles should improve air quality significantly.

Some diesel-powered vehicles produce excessive emissions of particulates, especially fine particulates (PM_{10}), which can be a serious threat to health. The worst polluters are the poorly maintained vehicles, those using poor quality fuels and those whose emission controls have been tampered with. Periodic vehicle testing programmes may not always be effective in identifying these gross polluters. Many of the mechanical problems that cause excessive smoke emissions are very expensive to repair. This leads to vehicle owners taking temporary measures to disguise high smoke emissions when the vehicle is tested. Actions include using higher grade diesel fuel during the test or adding a smoke-suppressant additive to the fuel. In Chile, it is reported that owners have reduced smoke opacity by adding a handful of gravel or some water to the vertical exhaust pipe to

8 Muncaster, G (1994) 'Experience with remote sensing', *paper presented at the National Society for Clean Air and Environmental Protection (NSCA) Seminar of Targeting Traffic Pollution – Options for Local Air Quality Management, 8 December 1994*, NSCA, Brighton

suppress the smoke temporarily. Such problems point to the need for random roadside inspections to catch the gross polluters in addition to periodic opacity testing. In some countries, the public are encouraged to play a part in identifying 'dirty diesels' by passing on details of smoky lorries, buses and even taxis they have spotted, via a telephone hotline or pre-paid reply cards, to the government vehicle inspection departments for possible follow-up inspections.[9]

Increasing Fuel Efficiency in Vehicles: Lean-burn Engines

The air to fuel ratio has a marked effect on the emission of pollutants. If the mixture is rich, that is too little air, combustion is incomplete, giving rise to high levels of carbon monoxide and hydrocarbons, but as combustion becomes more efficient the combustion temperature increases, so generating more nitrogen oxides. The stoichiometric ratio of 14.7:1 is the value at which conventional engines run most efficiently. However, if engines employ a higher ratio, the additional air reduces the cylinder temperature and decreases nitrogen oxide emissions. At very high ratios the benefits of lower emissions of nitrogen oxides are offset by increases in hydrocarbons because of the more difficult conditions for combustion. Lean-burn engines are designed to run at an air to fuel ratio of around 18:1 (even 20:1 in theory), a ratio which would cause conventional engines to stall. Lean-burn engines offer potential fuel savings of 5–10 per cent. Emissions from lean-burn engines are improved over a standard car, but are less effective than a car fitted with a catalytic converter, especially when operating at high speed or under strain (eg during acceleration, climbing steep hills, carrying heavy loads) when they revert to a richer mixture and then emit similarly high levels of nitrogen oxides to a standard car without a catalyst. Lean-burn engines can be fitted with an oxidation catalyst (which does not need to operate at the stoichiometric ratio), but they cannot be fitted with a three-way catalytic converter for which the air to fuel ratio of 14.7 is critical.[10]

Fuel consumption can be reduced by various improvements in engine and vehicle design. Governments can encourage such technological improvements by setting increasingly stringent average vehicle fuel consumption targets at, say, 5–10 year intervals. Penalties would then be imposed on manufacturers failing to achieve the target, whereas tax benefits could be offered to those who better the targets. Sales of less fuel-efficient vehicles could be discouraged by raising taxes on them or simply increasing fuel prices generally (which are low in the US) and undertaking a commitment to increase them each year (as has happened in the UK).

Cars sold in the US on average (sales weighted and applied to each car manufacturer) in 1993 consumed around 28 miles per gallon (mpg), nearly

9 Klausmeier and Kishan (1995) op cit

10 Mitchell, C G B and Hickman, A J (1990) 'Air pollution and noise from road vehicles', in European Conference of Ministers of Transport, *Transport Policy and the Environment*, OECD, Paris, pp 46–75

twice as efficient as cars sold in the mid-1970s, but with little improvement in recent years. President Clinton originally pledged during his campaign to increase the fuel efficiency required by law (the corporate average fuel economy or CAFE standard) from the 1990 level of 27.5 to 40 mpg by 2000 and 45 mpg by 2015. Major US car manufacturers (Chrysler, Ford, General Motors) are currently co-operating with the government on a programme using advanced technology (eg lightweight materials, improved petrol engines, fuel cell engines) aimed at achieving a fuel consumption of 80 mpg.[11]

Reducing the weight of the vehicle body (eg using aluminium, structural plastic) can save fuel by reducing the power required and making it economical to use a smaller engine. Shedding 10 per cent of a car's weight may reduce fuel consumption by about 7 per cent. Fuel efficiency can be increased by using better tyres. For example, in 1992 Michelin developed a tyre using new polymers which is claimed to reduce surface resistance by 35–50 per cent, so cutting up to 10 per cent in fuel consumption. Fuel efficiency can also be improved by better engine lubrication such as the 'zero viscosity' oils currently being developed which may increase fuel efficiency by 4-6 per cent. Finally, it should be realised that many of the technological improvements are most effective when a vehicle is new and that deterioration of the vehicle with age leads to reduced fuel efficiency. Moreover, poor maintenance, bad driving habits and congestion all also worsen fuel efficiency.[12]

Vapour Recovery: Large Canisters Versus Petrol Pump Nozzle Recovery

Evaporative emissions of VOCs can arise when tankers deliver petrol to filling stations, when cars are being filled from petrol pumps, and from vehicle fuel tanks and fuel systems when running. In addition, evaporative emissions can continue when a warmed-up engine has stopped and from the effects of high air temperatures on the fuel tank. In 1992, evaporative emissions of VOCs from the fuel tank and fuel system of vehicles accounted for about 10 per cent of total emissions of VOCs in the European Union. To control these emissions, vapour collection systems can be fitted either to petrol pumps or to the vehicles (carbon canisters).

The greatest public exposure to VOCs such as the carcinogen benzene tends to occur at petrol stations, but usually only for short periods. Attempts to reduce exposure at petrol stations include so-called stage I controls which are aimed at preventing vapour escaping during tanker deliveries to underground storage tanks. Such controls have been in force in the US since the 1970s and are currently being phased in throughout

11 'US plans 80 mpg car' and 'US car technology initiative', *The Environmental Digest*, 75, Sep 1993, p 12

12 Royal Commission on Environmental Pollution (1994) op cit, p 131; 'Michelin's green tyre to cut fuel consumption', *The Environmental Digest*, 58, Apr 1992, p 13

Europe. Austria, Sweden and parts of Germany (eg Munich and Berlin in 1987) have long required their installation and they achieve about 80 per cent recovery of toxic vapours. Installation of petrol vapour recovery devices in service stations in Los Angeles reduced emissions equivalent to 19 per cent of total hydrocarbons in California in 1980.

Stage II controls require petrol pumps to be fitted with vapour recovery equipment (vapour recovery sleeves on the nozzles of the pump hoses) as is the case in California. Currently, the European Union is debating whether to implement stage II controls or to require each new vehicle to be fitted with its own vapour recovery system, namely a large carbon canister. Petrol pumps could be fitted with recovery equipment relatively quickly, but at a cost to industry of $2 billion. In contrast, it would be less expensive to require all new vehicles to be fitted with large carbon canisters, but this would take several years before the majority of vehicles on the road have such equipment to curb VOC emissions. In 1993 Germany passed a law requiring all new petrol stations to be fitted with vapour recovery equipment. Existing stations have three to five years to comply. By 1995, Denmark, Luxembourg and Sweden had introduced similar national requirements.[13]

Carbon canisters fitted to a car allow the fuel system to breathe but absorb VOCs. A sealed cap is used on the fuel tank and a line runs from the top of the tank to a charcoal filter which absorbs and stores fuel vapour. When the engine is running, fresh air is drawn into the canister and mixed with the petrol vapours which have been absorbed onto the charcoal filter and the vapour/air mixture flows to the engine. Benzene is largely removed with a carbon canister. Small carbon canisters, standard on US cars and recently introduced in the European Union, are intended to absorb vapour from the fuel tank 'breathing', running losses when driving and from hot engines after use, whereas large carbon canisters (1–5 litres capacity) also recover vapours when refuelling.

Diesel Particulate Traps (Filters)

Particulates from diesel engines have long been of concern for their potential impact on health. Trapping exhaust particulates using a particulate trap or filter may be attempted, but if the filter cannot be regenerated (ie if the soot is not burned to form carbon dioxide) the particulates build up, causing back-pressure problems in the engine leading to possible 'blow off' of the particulates. To burn off the particulates a temperature exceeding 550°C is usually required, but the normal road temperature of diesel exhausts is only around 150°C.

Various regeneration methods have been attempted. External energy sources such as fuel or electric burners are used to burn off the particulates.

13 'Vapour recovery' *Acid News*, 2, Apr 1993, p 10; 'Stopping Petrol Fumes', *Acid News*, 4, Oct 1995, p 9

Catalytic trap oxidisers employ a catalyst to regenerate the filter by lowering the temperature required to burn off the particulates (oxidise the soot). One problem with using the catalyst is that this can lead to sulphate formation from fuel containing sulphur. This highlights the fact that plans to introduce diesel catalyst technology need to be anticipated by ensuring that low sulphur fuels are available, or that all diesel fuels have a lower content in general. Catalytic fuel additives are another approach. Tests on 110 buses in Athens claimed up to a 90 per cent reduction in particulates using a fuel additive which lowers the particle combustion threshold from around 550 to 480°C. This demonstration project proved so successful that the Greek Government has mandated the system for all buses in Athens. Generally, particulate traps can reduce particulates by more than 50 per cent, but the high temperatures used in some filter regeneration processes increase the formation of nitrogen oxides. Currently, particulate traps are relatively expensive and may cost up to 25 per cent of the vehicle engine costs (eg traps typically cost $4500 in 1992). Given this high cost there is clearly a need for governments to offer financial incentives for their installation on buses and heavy goods vehicles.[14]

Petrol-engined Versus Diesel-engined Vehicles: Which Pollutes Less?

Diesel-engined cars and vans offer better fuel economy and efficiency. In a petrol engine a mixture of air and fuel is drawn into the cylinder, compressed and ignited by a spark. In a diesel engine the fuel is injected into air which is already very hot as a result of compression and thus no spark in needed. As a diesel engine works with a surplus of air, the combustion process is more efficient. This results in a reduction in the amount of fuel consumed by at least 25 per cent by volume and 15 per cent by mass compared with a petrol engine of comparable power. Petrol engines tend to be better than diesel engines in terms of performance (eg acceleration).[15]

Assessing which type of engine is less polluting is difficult. Not only does it depend on the type of pollutant being considered, but also on whether pollution control devices (eg catalytic converters, carbon canisters) are fitted (Table 6.3). The level of engine maintenance also plays a key part. Not surprisingly, in terms of carbon monoxide, hydrocarbons, nitrogen oxides and particulates, the petrol car fitted with a three-way catalytic converter (when functioning correctly) produces lower emissions than one without a catalytic converter. Diesel emits less carbon monoxide than a car fitted with a catalytic converter, a similar amount of hydrocarbons, more nitrogen

14 Holman, C (1992) *Cleaner Buses*, Friends of the Earth, London, p 7; Quality of Urban Air Review Group (1993) *Diesel Vehicle Emissions and Urban Air Quality*, Second Report, HMSO, London; 'Cleaner diesel buses claimed', *The Environmental Digest*, 61, Jul 1992, p 14

15 Royal Commission on Environmental Pollution (1994) op cit, p 24; Quality of Urban Air Review Group (1993) op cit

Table 6.3 *Comparison of emissions from petrol and diesel cars*

Pollutant	Petrol without three-way catalyst	Petrol with three-way catalyst	Diesel without oxidation catalyst	Diesel with oxidation catalyst
Regulated pollutants				
Nitrogen oxides	****	*	**	**
Hydrocarbons	****	**	***	*
Carbon monoxide	****	***	**	*
Particulates	**	*	****	***
Unregulated pollutants				
Aldehydes	****	**	***	*
Benzene	****	***	**	*
1,3-Butadiene	****	**	***	*
Carbon dioxide	***	****	*	**
PAHs	***	*	****	**
Sulphur dioxide	*	*	****	****

Asterisks indicate which type of car typically has the highest emissions: *, lowest emissions; **/***, intermediate; and ****, highest emissions.
The table indicates only the relative importance of emissions between the types of vehicles. The difference in emissions between, say, *** and **, may be an order of magnitude, or much smaller.

Source: Quality of Urban Air Review Group (1993) *Diesel Vehicle Emissions and Urban Air Quality*, Second Report, Department of the Environment, London, p 15

oxides and considerably more particulates. If a diesel car is fitted with an oxidation catalyst, then emissions of carbon monoxide and hydrocarbons are even better. The advantages of petrol cars fitted with a three-way catalytic converter may disappear with the degrading of catalysts with age after about 60,000 km (37,500 miles). When comparing the emissions of particulates from cars using leaded petrol with diesel cars we should recognise that they are chemically different such that the health risks associated with each group of particulates may differ. Diesel particulates also have a soiling factor of around seven times that of petrol particulates. Emissions of PAHs such as the carcinogen benzo(*a*)pyrene is about 50 per cent greater from diesel than petrol cars without catalysts although this reduces when oxidation catalysts are fitted to diesel engines (eg from 1996 in the European Union).[16]

16 In the past decade, sales of diesel-engined vehicles in Europe have increased markedly and they now account for 20–25 per cent of vehicle sales. In the late 1980s and early 1990s, sales were encouraged by some car manufacturers advertising diesel-engined vehicles as 'green' or even 'pollution-free' by stressing the advantage of being more fuel-efficient and producing lower emissions of some

Fuel Improvements

Pollutant emissions can be reduced by changing the composition of the fuel. The lead, sulphur, aromatic hydrocarbons and benzene content of fuels can be reduced or eliminated. The volatility of the fuel can be lowered to reduce evaporation of VOCs. Oxygenated compounds can be added to improve combustion.

Unleaded Petrol Traditionally, lead compounds have been added to petrol to prevent knocking as this is a cheaper alternative to refining the petrol to a higher octane number. Knocking is the distinctive 'pinking' noise which occurs when there is spontaneous ignition of the petrol and air mixture in the corner of the cylinder furthest away from the spark plug. The lead allows engines to operate at higher compression ratios and under greater loads before knocking occurs. Lead also acts as an engine lubricant, reducing the wear in some parts such as valve seats. Concern over the potential health effects of airborne lead together with the recognition that catalytic converters, fitted to cars to reduce exhaust emissions of carbon monoxide, hydrocarbons and nitrogen oxides, do not function properly when lead compounds are present (the catalyst is 'poisoned' by lead) resulted in the US, Canada, Japan, then Europe and more recently many countries around the world reducing the lead content of petrol as well as making unleaded petrol available.

Health concerns focused on young children who lived near busy roads and experienced high levels of lead in their blood which may have affected their behaviour (eg attentional disorders, learning disabilities, emotional disturbances), caused dysfunction of the central nervous system (irritability, clumsiness) and affected educational characteristics (lower average IQ). Around 1970 the lead content of most European petrol was 0.84 g/l but by the late 1980s the lead content had been reduced in many countries to 0.15 g/l, the lowest level usable in petrol engines existing at the time without special adaptations. At the same time the availability of unleaded petrol increased in preparation for all new cars from 1993 which were required to be fitted with catalytic converters. These cars were designed with hardened valve seats and operated without knocking using unleaded petrol which was of a lower octane number (95) than most leaded petrol (97–98). Airborne levels of lead fell dramatically as a result of the reduced lead content of leaded petrol and with the rise in sales of unleaded petrol.

---

pollutants, especially compared with petrol vehicles not fitted with catalytic converters. However, by 1994 the concern for fine particulates (and carcinogenic compounds) as well as nitrogen oxides (linked by the public with rising asthma incidence) from diesel vehicles compared with petrol engines with catalytic converters (required on all new cars since 1993) changed the assessment.

The success of government intervention in encouraging the greater use of unleaded petrol was demonstrated in the UK. In 1986, when unleaded petrol was first introduced, public demand was small even among owners whose cars could run on unleaded petrol because it cost more than leaded petrol. It was not until the government introduced a tax differential in favour of unleaded petrol, and increased this differential each year, did sales escalate. By the start of 1993, when new cars had to be fitted with catalytic converters and therefore had to run on unleaded petrol, so ensuring sales

Table 6.4 *Unleaded petrol as a percentage of total petrol deliveries in the European Union (EU)*

Member State	1993	1994
Austria	98.1	99.8
Belgium	57.4	64.8
Denmark	75.6	98.1
Finland	87.0	99.9
France	40.8	50.0
Germany	88.7	92.3
Greece	22.9	27.6
Ireland	38.5	48.6
Italy	23.8	32.6
Luxembourg	69.0	75.6
Netherlands	75.0	80.1
Portugal	20.9	30.0
Spain	14.8	22.2
Sweden	79.5	99.4
UK	52.0	57.6
Total EU	56.1	62.4

Source: Eurostat Press Office, Luxembourg.

would continue to increase, unleaded petrol sales accounted for half of all petrol sales. By 1994, unleaded petrol deliveries reached 57.6 per cent in the UK (Table 6.4). Throughout the European Union, unleaded fuel accounted for 62.4 per cent of total petrol deliveries. Unleaded petrol accounted for more than 99 per cent in Austria, Finland and Sweden (all of whom joined the European Union in 1994 and so increased the percentage use of unleaded petrol). Motorists in the European Union's northern Member

States tend to use higher percentages of unleaded petrol than southern motorists.[17]

Oxygenated Fuels Oxygenated fuels (oxyfuels) used to lower winter carbon monoxide emissions were pioneered in the state of Colorado and led to the US Clean Air Act 1990 requiring the use of oxygenated fuels in all areas which have not attained the federal air quality standard for carbon monoxide. Oxygenated fuels with an oxygen content not less than 2.7 per cent must be used during those times of the year that are considered 'high carbon monoxide conditions'. In the US, Albuquerque, Denver, Las Vegas, Phoenix, Reno and Tucson are among those cities in which oxygenated fuels have been introduced during the winter months in an attempt to improve combustion efficiency and to reduce carbon monoxide emissions by as much as 20 per cent. In 1995 oxygenated fuels cost about 10–15 cents per gallon more than conventional fuel.

Oxygenated fuels contain small amounts of ethanol or methanol derivatives. These include ethyl-*t*-butyl ether (ETBE) derived from ether (and produced from corn) and methyl-*t*-butyl ether (MTBE) derived from methanol. The oxygen-rich additives help the fuel's hydrocarbons to burn more efficiently at low temperatures, thereby converting more of the carbon monoxide to carbon dioxide and also reducing hydrocarbon emissions. Nitrogen oxides are unaffected. The minimum 2.7 per cent oxygen by weight in US oxyfuels is achieved by adding 15 per cent by volume of MTBE or 7.7 per cent by volume of ethanol.

In those US cities where oxygenated fuels were introduced, carbon monoxide levels have fallen by 10–15 per cent (eg Denver claims a 12 per cent reduction). They benefit cars with catalytic converters (as well as older cars without) because the catalysts take several minutes to reach their operating efficiency, during which carbon monoxide and hydrocarbon emissions are uncontrolled. If the additives burn incompletely, they can form aldehydes. MTBE and methanol produce very small amounts of formaldehyde, whereas ETBE and ethanol produce acetaldehyde, both of which may cause cancer. A causal link between some people who suffer headaches, insomnia, nausea, dizziness, skin problems and coughs when driving cars using oxygenated fuels is claimed, but not yet confirmed or rejected.

In Finland, oxygenated fuels were introduced in 1991 and now account for 95 per cent of all fuel sold in the country. To achieve an oxygen content of 2 per cent, Finland uses 11 per cent of MTBE or *t*-amyl methyl ether, the latter being favoured. Finland is the only European country to manufacture oxyfuels, which are exported to Sweden for use in their cold winters. Emissions of carbon monoxide in Finland have fallen by 10–20 per cent and hydrocarbons by 5–10 per cent as a result of introducing oxygenated fuels.

---

17 Elsom, D M (1992) 'The phasing in of unleaded petrol in the United Kingdom', *Clean Air*, vol 22, pp 226–232

The European Union may consider the wider adoption of oxygenated fuels as one way to reduce the benzene content of fuel as oxyfuels, by helping hydrocarbons to burn more efficiently, offer an alternative means of maintaining a high octane content.[18]

Other Reformulated (Cleaner–burning) Fuels Reformulating the composition of petrol and diesel that can be used in all vehicles can reduce vehicle emissions and improve air quality. Lowering the volatility of fuel so it does not evaporate as readily can reduce emissions of VOCs, which react with nitrogen oxides in sunlight to produce ozone. Following the worst period of ozone pollution in the US in 1988, national regulations lowered the national average summer Reid vapour pressure of petrol, which is a measure of its volatility, by 11 per cent. A further reduction of 3 per cent took place between 1989 and 1990. A modelling analysis of New York City conditions estimated that the impact of the Reid vapour pressure reductions was a 25 per cent reduction in VOC emissions. The UK Government had intended to reduce the volatility of petrol sold during the summer months by 1993, but was delayed until 1995 due to resistance from the oil industry.[19]

However, lowering the volatility of petrol through a reduction in its butane content may give rise to other pollution problems if the octane level lost through this process is regained by increasing the aromatic content (ie giving rise to more benzene) or by the use of oxygenates (ie perhaps increasing formaldehyde depending on the additive used).[20]

The US is increasingly making the use of reformulated petrol in non-attainment air quality areas compulsory. Californian drivers began using less polluting (and slightly more expensive) phase 2 reformulated petrol all year round from March 1996 (conventional petrol no longer permitted to be sold in the area). This fuel has a minimum of 2 per cent oxygen, a maximum of 1 per cent benzene, reduced aromatic hydrocarbons (25 per cent less than before), negligible sulphur dioxide, no heavy metals and it is not allowed to result in an increase in nitrogen oxides. In addition, the emissions of ozone-forming VOCs and toxic pollutants must be reduced by 25 and 20 per cent, respectively. It is estimated that a reduction in the carcinogenic compounds will result in a fall in potential cancer cases of 35 per year from

18 Burke, M (1995) 'Are oxyfuels good for us?', *New Scientist*, 15 Jul, pp 24–27; Kiernan, V (1994) 'US says drivers must use more alcohol', *New Scientist*, 9 Jul, p 7; Miller, S S (1992) 'Carbon monoxide and oxygenated fuels in US cities', *Environmental Science and Technology*, vol 26, p 45; in 1995, 100 petrol stations in Vienna, Austria were selling petrol containing MTBE. *The Environmental Digest*, 1995/8, Aug, p 12

19 US Environmental Protection Agency (1994) *National Air Quality and Emissions Trends Report, 1993*, Report EPA 454/R-94-026, US EPA, Research Triangle Park, NC, pp 44 and 47; Her Majesty's Government (1992) *This Common Inheritance, Second Year Progress Report*, HMSO, London; 'Oil industry delays controls on petrol volatility', *ENDS Report*, 234, Jul 1994, p 33

20 House of Commons Transport Committee (1994) *Transport-related Air Pollution in London*, Sixth Report, vol 1, HMSO, London, p 26

1996 to 2010.[21] Because of its carcinogen effects, benzene has recently received much attention in Europe. Currently, the European Union has a limit of 5 per cent by volume, but there is growing pressure to lower the limit to 1 per cent. Diesel has also received attention from the European Union with the sulphur content of diesel being reduced from 0.3 per cent by weight in 1989 and 0.2 per cent in 1994 to 0.05 per cent in October 1996.[22]

Reformulated fuels can lead to small but significant improvements in air quality in an urban area. One of its attractions for air quality managers is that it can reduce emissions from all vehicles, irrespective of age. It can be used all year round, tackling summer air quality problems (eg reducing emissions of ozone-forming VOCs) and winter problems (eg reducing carbon monoxide by its increased oxygen content). There is no need to modify existing vehicles to be able to use reformulated petrol or diesel. It should not affect a vehicle's performance unless the vehicle is in a poor mechanical condition, when drivers may notice a slight increase in fuel consumption and hesitations after start-up. Unlike alternative fuels (eg methanol, electric battery), air quality improvements do not have to wait for several years until the sales of new vehicles designed specifically to use alternative fuels have begun to replace existing vehicles in significant numbers. There is no need to convert storage tanks, service station pumps or workshop equipment as when using alternative fuels. Given their higher costs of manufacturing and retail price, reformulated fuels can be used selectively if necessary – that is, in a city with poor air quality rather than throughout the country.[23]

Alternative Fuels: Biofuels

Biofuels have received increasing attention in recent years as a possible replacement for petrol or diesel or to be mixed with conventional fuels. Biofuels may be alcohols such as ethanol and methanol to replace petrol or esters such as rapeseed methyl ester to replace diesel. There are about 50–60 million cars – about 10 per cent of the global total – powered by some form of alcohol fuel such as pure ethanol or methanol or using a mixture of up to 20 per cent with petrol. As ethanol and methanol are liquids they offer a potentially convenient replacement for petrol. Alcohols emit pollutants, albeit less than petrol, and so are considered as transitional fuels in, say, California's long-term commitment to introducing cleaner vehicles.

---

21 Griffin, R D (1994) *Principles of Air Quality Management*, Lewis, Boca Raton, pp 300–301; 'California to have cleaner petrol', *Acid News*, 2, May 1992, p 6

22 Royal Commission on Environmental Pollution (1994) op cit, p 124; some fuels contain detergents to stop the build up of sooty particles in the engine.

23 Holman, C (1994) *The Effects of Petrol Quality on Emissions for Passenger Cars*, World Wide Fund for Nature, Godalming; Holman, C (1995) 'Reformulated fuels – a quick fix solution', *paper presented at the National Society for Clean Air and Environmental Protection (NSCA) Seminar on Greener Fuels for Cleaner Air?, Birmingham, Feb 1995*, NSCA, Brighton

Ethanol About 4 million cars in Brazil are powered by ethanol produced from sugar cane (hence the sickly smell of burnt sugar sometimes associated with car exhausts) using fermentation followed by distillation to recover the ethanol. Typically, as a fuel in its pure form, ethanol produces 20–30 per cent less carbon monoxide, about 15 per cent less nitrogen oxides and insignificant amounts of sulphur dioxide (petrol contains more than three times as much sulphur, although the amounts are very small anyway). Carbon dioxide release by ethanol-powered vehicles is balanced by its absorption in new sugar cane. Vehicles need alteration to run on ethanol. To prevent corrosion the inside of the fuel tank is coated with tin, the fuel lines with copper and nickel, and the carburettor with zinc. The piston needs strengthening because ethanol has a higher detonation temperature, which means the fuel–air mixture in the combustion chamber needs higher compression. The energy content is only two-thirds that of petrol so the fuel tank needs to be larger to provide the same range for a vehicle. Of significance for cold climate countries is the fact that ethanol cars are poor starters at low temperatures.

The Brazilian experiment in using ethanol (pro-alcohol) began in 1975 as a response to the high oil prices in the 1970s. Initially, ethanol was used as an additive to petrol, but all-ethanol was introduced in 1979. However, although 80–90 per cent of all new cars sold in Brazil between 1985 and 1988 were equipped to use ethanol, there has been a dramatic decline since then with only 20 per cent of all new cars being ethanol users in 1991. The reasons for this change were a combination of nationwide shortages of ethanol in 1989–1990 due to sugar cane farmers being dissatisfied with the government payments to them, and the fall in world oil prices which made ethanol too expensive without substantial government subsidies. The cost of ethanol production is up to twice that of petrol. The national trend towards using gasohol (78 per cent petrol, 22 per cent ethanol) rather than ethanol was accelerated after 1992 when the government stopped subsidising the pump price of ethanol. Brazilian car manufacturers have also put pressure on the government because they would prefer to produce only one type of car engine to run on gasohol.[24]

São Paulo illustrates some of the successes of using ethanol either in its pure form or as an additive to produce gasohol. The city has 1.1 million ethanol-powered and 1.2 million gasohol-powered vehicles. All petrol cars were phased out in the mid-1980s during a complete ban on car imports (this ended in 1990), after which high import taxes have kept imported car numbers low, although these can be converted to run on gasohol. Table 6.5 presents the air quality changes that are predicted if all the city's 2.3 million

24 Boels, L B M M (1995) *The Potential of Substitute Fuels for Reducing Emissions in the Transport Sector*, European Federation for Transport and Environment, Brussels, pp 22–23; Homewood, B (1993) 'Will Brazil's cars go on the wagon?', *New Scientist*, 9 Jan, pp 22–23; 'Brazil may abandon alcohol', *The Environmental Digest*, 70, Apr 1993, pp 14–15

Table 6.5 *Percentage air quality changes compared with the present air quality if all vehicles in São Paulo were powered by one type of fuel*

Fuel	Carbon monoxide	Hydrocarbons	Nitrogen oxides
Petrol	+120	+100	+10
Gasohol	+40	+35	No change
Ethanol	–20	–20	–10

Source: compiled from information given by Homewood (1993)[24].

vehicles were powered by petrol, gasohol or ethanol. Significant air quality improvements are predicted if all the vehicles use ethanol, whereas the replacement of the current ethanol/gasohol vehicles of São Paulo with petrol-powered vehicles would result in a major deterioration in air quality. One additional advantage of ethanol is that it does not contribute to airborne lead. Airborne lead levels in Brazilian urban areas fell from 1.6 mg/m^3 in 1978 to 0.3 mg/m^3 in 1983 following widespread ethanol adoption.

In the US, 95 per cent of ethanol is produced from corn (maize) and about 5 per cent from sugar cane or other biomass or organic matter such as wheat, potatoes and sugar beet. It is used as an additive to increase the octane rating of petrol and to reduce carbon monoxide emissions (refer to the earlier section discussing oxygenated fuels). This oxygenated fuel or gasohol, compulsory in winter months in many cities with carbon monoxide air quality problems, is subsidised by the federal government and some states exempt gasohol from their fuel taxes. In Europe, the European Union allows 5 per cent ethanol derived from cereals (wheat, maize), potatoes or sugar beet to be added to fuels (petrol and diesel). Even ethanol derived from surplus wine was permitted in 1991. Similarly, when Stockholm faced a shortage of ethanol in 1995, the city authorities were given permission by the European Commission to import 5000 tonnes of surplus red wine from Spain, from which to produce ethanol.

Methanol Methanol, also known as wood alcohol, can be produced from wood, coal or natural gas. Its high octane rating has resulted in it being used in racing cars such as the Indy 500 race cars since 1965. Unlike petrol-powered vehicles, methanol-powered vehicles emit only a few compounds, primarily unburnt methanol and formaldehyde. Unburnt methanol is much less photochemically reactive than the organic compounds emitted by petrol-engined vehicles, so ozone formation ought to be reduced when using methanol. However, the overall ozone reductions depend on how much formaldehyde is produced as this is very reactive and has a high ozone-forming potential. Formaldehyde is also a suspected carcinogen. Recognizing this concern, in 1989 California set standards of 15 mg/mile of formaldehyde as the ultimate standard needed to be achieved by vehicles using methanol. Providing formaldehyde emissions can be kept low, methanol is considered to offer useful air quality benefits compared with petrol, but only as a transitional step towards the long-term aim of the widespread use of zero-emission vehicles.

There are many practical considerations in methanol replacing petrol. Methanol produces only half the energy as the same volume of petrol, so the fuel tank would have to be twice as large to enable the same range to be driven. Methanol is highly corrosive, so petrol stations would need new storage tanks and cars would need stainless-steel fuel tanks and corrosion-resistant fuel lines and carburettors. As it is more toxic than petrol, self-service methanol pumps would pose potential problems. Pure methanol-powered cars are difficult to start in cold weather, even at 10°C. To overcome this problem M85 mixtures are used, that is 85 per cent methanol and 15 per cent petrol. Methanol's overall environmental impact would depend in part on whether it is produced from natural gas or coal. Production from natural gas would produce similar carbon dioxide emissions as petrol, but production from coal would increase emissions of this greenhouse gas by 50 per cent. The cost of production of methanol is similar to that of petrol, but the cost of converting filling stations and cars points to the need for financial support from the government if methanol is to displace petrol use significantly.[25]

Biodiesel: Rapeseed Methyl Ester The growing surplus of farmland needed to produce food crops in the European Union has increased farmers' interests in growing crops to produce fuels, using the 15 per cent of land ('set aside') required to be taken out of food production by large farms since 1992. The main focus of attention has been on producing biodiesel from oilseed rape (called canola in Canada and the US). Oil is extracted from rape simply by crushing, with 3 t of rape yielding one tonne of oil. Most diesel engines can run on unblended rape oil without modification, but they become clogged after several days. To prevent this, glycerine must be removed by separation from the oil. Each tonne of oil is mixed with 110 kg methanol in the presence of a nitrogen hydroxide catalyst and heated to 40–50°C. The glycerine settles out, leaving a clear thin liquid, rapeseed methyl ester.

Many European countries have begun building rapeseed methyl ester production plants. Austria has more than 100 petrol stations selling biodiesel. Several trials using bus fleets have been attempted. In the UK, Reading conducted trials in 1993 using buses fuelled by rapeseed methyl ester. No engine modification was necessary and emissions of sulphur dioxide, particulates, carbon monoxide, nitrogen oxides and carbon dioxide were reduced for a power loss of 2–5 per cent compared with a conventional

---

25 Boels, L B M M (1995) op cit, pp 20–22; Nadis, S and MacKenzie, J J (1993) *Car Trouble*, World Resources Institute, Beacon Press, Boston, pp 63–66

diesel engine. The trials suggested there may be problems with lubricants and the rapeseed methyl ester damages rubber pumps and hoses more than diesel. Despite the overall success of this pilot experiment, wider adoption of rapeseed methyl ester by European bus and lorry fleets is hindered by the higher cost compared with conventional but more polluting diesel fuels (eg twice as costly as diesel in the UK). This points to the need for tax concessions (eg cutting duty on biofuels to one-tenth that of diesel) and government subsidies if biodiesel is to become competitive with fossil fuels. However, producers in Austria claim that they can produce rapeseed methyl ester for the same price as diesel, so the penetration of this biofuel into the market may increase in the coming years.[26]

Compressed Natural Gas (Methane) and Liquid Petroleum Gas Gas can be used as a fuel for vehicles in the form of compressed natural gas or liquid petroleum gas. Whereas compressed natural gas is methane gas, liquid petroleum gas consists mainly of propane and butane produced as by-products from oil refineries. Liquid petroleum gas is used extensively in the Netherlands where it accounts for 15 per cent of vehicle fuels. Compressed natural gas is the cleanest fossil fuel and currently provides power for 700,000 vehicles worldwide. There are 300,000 such vehicles in Italy and 230 filling stations (the Italians have been using natural gas for 40 years), 200,000 vehicles in Russia, 100,000 in New Zealand, 100,000 in British Columbia, Canada, and 100,000 in Argentina. Currently, there are 100,000 natural gas vehicles in the US, but with the stringent emission standard targets applied in California being increasingly adopted by other states it is possible that the number of natural gas vehicles could reach 4 million by 2010. All new buses in Buenos Aires began using compressed natural gas in 1990, whereas Sydney has 250 natural gas buses operating. Budapest in Hungary intends to replace its 400 diesel buses with compressed natural gas vehicles at a cost of $6 million, but this is expected to pay for itself in four years due to the difference in petrol and compressed natural gas prices. The US Parcel Service plans to convert 2700 delivery trucks to compressed natural gas in Los Angeles and eventually all its 50,000 vehicles. Brussels introduced a fleet of 20 buses in 1994 powered by natural gas. In 1995 in the UK, there are over 300 vehicles running on natural gas and eight fast-filling stations. Mexico City has plans to convert all public transportation vehicles to run on natural gas. Almost all such vehicles have modified petrol or diesel

26 Devitt, M, Drysdale, D W, MacGillivray, I, Norris, A J, Thompson, R and Twidell, J W (1993) 'Biofuel for transport: an investigation into the viability of rape methyl ester (RME) as an alternative to diesel fuel', *International Journal of Ambient Energy*, vol 14, pp 195–218; Elvington, P (1993) 'Bio-diesel fuel: merits questioned', *Acid News*, 3, Jun, p 15; McDiarmid, N (1992) 'British buses to run on flower power', *New Scientist*, 3 Oct, p 18; Meyer, C (1993) 'Rough road ahead for biodiesel fuel', *New Scientist*, 6 Feb; Patel, T (1993) 'France placates farmers with plant fuel plan', *New Scientist*, 27 Feb

engines that run on natural gas stored in high pressure tanks located in the boot of a car or on the chassis or roof of a van, bus or lorry.[27]

The advantages of compressed natural gas are that it is often cheaper than petrol (eg half the price of petrol in the US due to no federal tax being applied) and it produces lower pollutant emissions. Carbon monoxide is reduced by 90 per cent, reactive hydrocarbons by 50 per cent and there are virtually no particulates emitted. Unlike petrol, no benzene is emitted. However, on the negative side emissions of nitrogen oxides may be higher. It emits less carbon dioxide, but methane is a greenhouse gas so this offsets this advantage with respect to the problem of global warming. It is considered a safe fuel with no fires or explosions arising from using compressed natural gas in vehicles. It is better suited to buses and trucks than cars because it offers only 25 per cent of the energy provided by a similar amount of petrol, so needs much larger storage tanks, causing the vehicles to be heavier and/or some loss of space.

Zero-emission Vehicles

Electric (Battery) Vehicles Electric vehicles using batteries have existed for many decades but they were unattractive to most potential users because the early electric motors were inefficient, the electronic devices to control the motors were unreliable and the batteries could not store enough energy to propel the vehicle very far, not helped because the batteries made the car very heavy. Today the situation has improved considerably. Current electric cars offer the greatest potential for use in urban areas where frequent stops and starts associated with commuting and deliveries (eg post and parcel deliveries) lead to a high consumption of conventional fuels.

Batteries cannot store nearly as much energy, or generate as much power, as internal combustion engines. The two key parameters which need to be considered are power density and energy density. Power density is the amount of power per kilogram of battery weight that can be extracted from a battery. Low power density translates into poorer vehicle acceleration, a reduced ability to climb hills and a slower recharge time. Energy density measures the amount of electrical energy that can be stored in each kilogram of battery. A low energy density results in a reduced range between

---

27 Compressed natural gas (85 per cent) is also mixed with hydrogen (15 per cent) to form hythane (i.e. 'Hy' from hydrogen, 'thane' from methane). It emits less hydrocarbons and nitrogen oxides compared with compressed natural gas. Biogas, like natural gas, consists of methane, but whereas natural gas is a fossil fuel, biogas comes from renewable sources. It is produced from the decomposition of organic matter, such as sewage sludge, but it can also be salvaged from waste dumps. Linkopping in Sweden, Colorado Springs in the US and Tours in France all have buses running on biogas; Elvingson, P (1994) 'Transportation fuels: exploring the alternatives', *Acid News*, 5, Dec 1994, pp 6–7

recharges. An analysis of power density and energy density reveals the advantage of internal combustion engines over batteries. Modern engines typically have a power density exceeding 400 W/kg and an energy density of more than 200 W-h/kg. In comparison, conventional lead–acid batteries offer a power density of less than 100 W/kg and an energy density less than 40 W-h/kg. The challenge is to develop a battery that approaches the qualities of the combustion engine.[28]

The conventional lead–acid battery uses alternate lead and lead oxide plates suspended in dilute sulphuric acid. Advanced lead–acid batteries (power density of 200 W/kg) are used in General Motors' successful Impact. This sporty lightweight (plastic-bodied) car offers 0 to 95 kph (60 mph) acceleration in just eight seconds – better than many sports cars – but it needs a two to eight hour recharge. In 1992, General Motors, Ford and Chrysler signed an agreement to co-operate in the development, design, testing and possible manufacture of electric vehicle components that could be used in each of the companies' electric vehicles. Other companies are testing alternative batteries. BMW uses sodium–sulphur batteries (the batteries contain liquid sodium and sulphur at a temperature of around 300°C) propelling its EI prototype introduced in 1991. It requires 12 hours for a full recharge from domestic electricity supplies and offers a range of 240 km (150 miles) and a top speed of 120 kph (75 mph). Peugeot is developing the nickel–cadmium battery and Chrysler the nickel–iron hydride battery. The nickel–cadmium battery in Nissan's Future Electric Vehicle introduced in 1991 offers a 15 minute fast recharging time, a range of 250 km (150 miles) and a top speed of 130 kph (70 mph). Zinc–air dry cells were powering 40 postal vans in Germany in 1995, using a three minute recharging time by changing electrodes for a range of 300 km; the results of this pilot study have convinced the German Post Office to use electric vehicles for 80 per cent of its fleet. Other batteries being considered by car manufacturers include zinc–bromine and lithium batteries. Generally, alternatives to the conventional lead–acid battery are more expensive, less reliable, harder to maintain and, in some cases, potentially dangerous (toxic contents).[29]

PSA (Peugeot–Citroen) and Renault are running large-scale trials in co-operation with Electricite de France which generates much of its electricity using nuclear power stations. In 22 towns, including Aignon, Bordeaux, Douai, La Rochelle and Strasbourg, battery recharging stations are being set up at the roadside and in public or private car parks. This will provide electric cars (eg models based on the Peugeot 106, Citroen AX and Renault

28 Howard, G (1992) 'Flat out for the car of the future', *New Scientist*, 7 Nov, pp 21–22; Pratt, G A (1992) 'EVs: on the road again', *Technology Review*, Aug/Sep, pp 50–59; Sperling, D (1994) *Future Drive: Electric Vehicles and Sustainable Transportation*, Island Press, Washington

29 Lossau, N (1994) 'German's post vans go electric', *New Scientist*, 22 Jan, p 20; 'BMW and Nissan launch electric cars', *The Environmental Digest*, 49/50, Jul/Aug 1991, p 17; 'Rapid recharge for batteries in Nissan's electric car', *New Scientist*, 7 Sep 1991

Clio) with convenient range-extending opportunities during the day. To maintain the momentum towards electric vehicles, the French Government announced in 1995 that it would grant a subsidy of about $1000 to anyone buying an electric car, whereas the state-owned electricity company is expected to offer a $2000 subsidy per car to manufacturers or importers of electric vehicles. These measures are aimed at securing a target of 100,000 electric cars in France by 2000.[30]

There are still many practical difficulties before electric battery vehicles gain strong favour among the wider public. The batteries have a limited lifetime and need to be replaced every two or three years. They take a long time to recharge compared with the simplicity of filling a vehicle with petrol or diesel. Typically, the rate of recharging is slow, say six to eight hours (ie overnight at home or during the day when parked at work) for a fully depleted lead–acid car battery. Energy density remains a problem, with a typical maximum range of 190 km (120 miles) before the batteries are fully depleted. The batteries, operating in series, take up significant space within a vehicle and they may represent one-third of the total weight of the vehicle and a similar proportion of its total cost. Given the need to replace batteries every few years, renting or leasing rather than buying may make more sense. Electric vehicles cost more than conventional vehicles, but this should reduce greatly as the scale of production increases. Generally, the challenge for battery manufacturers is to produce small lightweight batteries which can store large amounts of energy and can be recharged in a few minutes.

Although the benefits of electric vehicles for urban air quality are immense, it is important to recognise the huge increase in the number of batteries that would need to be manufactured for use in electric vehicles. Clearly a commitment to the recycling of these batteries, some containing toxic substances such as cadmium, needs to be adopted at the outset so that new environmental problems are not created. Electric vehicles will still cause some air pollution problems. They produce emissions of particulates from tyre wear, brake pads and clutches. A battery is not a power source: it merely stores electricity generated elsewhere. Electric vehicles do not emit pollutants directly, but the electricity to recharge the batteries does. This electricity is generated elsewhere, sometimes in power stations well outside urban areas, but pollutants are still generated and it represents a trade in emissions from one place to another, as happened with the shift from domestic coal-burning to electric and gas heating. The widespread use of electric vehicles may require increased electricity generating capacity. If these power stations are coal- or oil-fired, significant emissions of nitrogen oxides, sulphur dioxide, carbon dioxide and particulates may be produced. As a sustainable approach to tackling the air quality problem in urban areas, using electric vehicles should not be at the expense of increasing carbon dioxide emissions and so adding to global warming. In that context, an

---

30 'French boost for electric cars', *The Environmental Digest*, 1995/4, p 15; 'Electric vehicle test', *Acid News*, 3, Jun 1993, p 14

electric vehicle ought to be recharged with electricity generated by solar, water, wind or geothermal energy sources.

Hybrid vehicles are being developed as a means of reducing emissions in urban areas while offering motorists the performance advantages of existing cars. They enable less polluting electric power to be used within urban areas, but a small petrol or diesel engine offers the advantages of a conventional car for long distance travel. The Volvo ECC (environmental concept car) introduced in 1993 has a tiny gas turbine, running on diesel and driving a lightweight generator at very high speed. Even though one-fifth of the car's weight is batteries, it is not particularly heavy, has a top speed of 175 kph (108 mph) and would go 670 km (416 miles) on a tankful if you did not exceed 90 kph (56 mph). Battery power alone would take it only a fraction of that distance at a lower speed. The Canadians have developed a petrol–electric hybrid vehicle using electric motors in each wheel of the car, with the batteries being topped up by a small petrol engine which runs for a maximum of 30 minutes in every hour of driving.[31]

Hydrogen Fuel Cells Hydrogen is almost the optimum fuel in that when burned it emits only water vapour and, depending on the process, minute quantities of hydrocarbons (from the crankcase) and nitrogen oxides. Hydrogen can be used in a liquid form (requiring storage at –250°C), as a pressurised gas (but the storage tanks are heavy and bulky) or as metal hydrides. The latter consist of powdered metal mixtures including iron, manganese, nickel, titanium and vanadium. Hydrogen gas is pumped into the tank containing the metal catalysts and, cooled by water pumped in alongside the hydrogen, the metals absorb the hydrogen to form a hydride. When the hydride tanks are heated, hydrogen is released to the engine. The system is safe and cannot explode or cause explosive fires. Unfortunately, metal hydride systems are heavy, which so far limits the range of cars using this system to around 160 km (100 miles). Refuelling takes the form of feeding hydrogen gas into the storage tank through a hose. This can take 10–15 minutes, which is slow compared with filling up with petrol. A water hose is needed to remove the heat generated when hydrogen is absorbed by the powdered metals. Mercedes-Benz have 20 prototype cars and vans limited to a range of about 200 km (125 miles) between refuelling, but plan to have hydrogen-powered Mercedes buses operating in Hamburg in 1997.

Hydrogen fuel cells offer possibilities in a decade or two, especially if legislation promoting ultra-low and zero emission vehicles becomes more widely adopted in Europe, North America and Japan. A fuel cell converts chemical fuel into electricity at up to 50 per cent efficiency with no moving parts. The fuel cell was developed in 1839 by Sir William Grove in London and until the 1990s its main application for transportation has been to provide a source of electrical power and drinking water for the Apollo moon

---

31 'Canadians develop hybrid car', *The Environmental Digest*, 89/90, Nov/Dec 1994, p 15

missions in the 1960s and the Space Shuttle. The principle of the fuel cell is the reverse of the electrolysis of water in which electricity is passed through a water-based electrolyte and produces hydrogen and oxygen at the electrodes. In the fuel cell hydrogen is fed to a catalysed anode and oxygen (air) to a catalysed cathode. The electrolyte is typically a membrane capable of conducting ions. The products of this process are electricity, water and a little heat. Unlike batteries, fuel cells are not dependent on recharging, but simply use hydrogen as the fuel. Fuel cells can be powered by hydrogen which is stored or produced on-board by steam reforming from hydrocarbons or alcohol fuels (eg methanol) or ultimately directly by alcohols or hydrocarbons. The fuel cell used in a commuting vehicle could be little more than the size of two conventional batteries, but space is needed to store the fuel on-board. Prototype buses using only a solid polymer fuel cell powered by gaseous hydrogen stored on-board were introduced in the US in 1993 (eg the Los Angeles airport shuttle bus). Increasing numbers of buses and vans powered solely by fuel cells, offering double the efficiency of the internal combustion engine, are likely to be produced by the end of the century and cars next century.[32]

Solar Cars The ultimate electric-powered vehicle would use solar energy. Currently, solar panels on a roof do not provide enough power for all a vehicle's daily travel needs, although it could be used to extend an electric battery's life between, say, nightly recharging at home. In 1991, 10,000 solar panels were added to the roofs of conventional petrol-engined cars in Europe, mainly to power electronic accessories such as the ventilation of car interiors on hot days and charging batteries when sitting idle. In 1992 a demonstration project in California involved solar carports (parking spaces) which were equipped with plugs to charge electric car batteries from an array of solar cells. In 1995 the two-seater solar–electric battery hybrid car called the Hawaiian Sunray became available on the market. This comes with solar panels for use either at home or for bolting on-board. This egg-shaped mini-car is fitted with ten lead–acid batteries and has a range of up to 160 km (100 miles) between charges, achieved by either using household electricity outlets or from the solar panels. Its top speed is 110 kph (70 mph).[33]

The potential for solar-powered cars is beginning to be demonstrated. For example, the three-wheeled solar-powered car which won the annual 3000 km (1875 miles) race across Australia in 1993 managed to achieve a solar energy efficiency (the proportion of the sun's energy converted into motive power via photo-voltaic cells) of 20 per cent. This was an improvement of

32 Fisher, S (1994) 'Milestone on the road', *Financial Times*, 15 Apr, p 16; Lloyd, C (1994) 'Electric van gets clean away from batteries', *The Sunday Times*, 24 Apr, section 3, p 12

33 Essoyan, S (1995) 'Something new under the Hawaiian sun: a solar car', *Los Angeles Times*, 5 Apr

5 per cent over the winning car in 1987. Its average speed for the race was nearly 85 kph (53 mph). Unfortunately, the solar cars competing in the Darwin–Adelaide race were cramped, at times unstable and the drivers often had to suffer temperatures of 50°C.[34]

Conclusions: Promoting Cleaner Fuels and Cleaner Cars

The initial costs of developing and using reformulated and alternative fuels and cleaner vehicles can be high. This points to the need for government subsidies and tax incentives to encourage the adoption of these cleaner technologies. Governments can influence the take up of less polluting fuels by introducing fuel duties/tax according to their environmental impact. They can offer grants and subsidies to the car industry to develop and manufacture zero-emission vehicles and for the public to buy them. For example, during the mid-1980s Germany raised the annual duty for cars meeting their existing emission standards, but lowered it for cars which met the new stringent European Union standards which would come into effect in 1993 and which would require catalytic converters to be fitted. By 1988, more than 75 per cent of new cars sold in Germany already met the 1993 emission standards and by 1990 this had exceeded 90 per cent. Consequently, Germany was five years ahead of, say, the UK, and its citizens also gained five years of air quality benefits.[35]

California offers the greatest stimulus for introducing cleaner cars as it required at least 2 per cent of sales from motor manufacturers selling more than 30,000 vehicles a year to be zero-emission vehicles – assumed to be electric – in 1998 if they wished to continue selling in the state. This amounts to about 35,000 vehicles a year on Californian roads. This requirement will increase to 5 per cent by 2003 and 10 per cent of sales in 2005 (Table 6.6). This legislation is providing a model for other states to follow. California's commitment is not only for zero-emission vehicles but also for a phased strengthening of emission targets for all new vehicles. This progresses from transitional low emitting vehicle targets through low emission vehicle targets and ultra-low emission vehicle targets to zero-emission vehicles. Encouragement and requirements to introduce cleaner fuels and cleaner cars can take many forms. In 1990, Denver stipulated that fleets of 30 or more vehicles in the city must convert at least 10 per cent of their petrol-engined vehicles to alternative fuels by the end of 1992. In 1994, the UK Government made a commitment to increase road fuel duty by at least 5 per cent each year, so providing an incentive to economise on fuel and to choose more fuel-efficient vehicles. In January 1993, the European Parliament urged governments to use subsidies and tax incentives to

34 Anderson, I (1993) 'Solar dream car comes through', *New Scientist*, 20 Nov; 'Solar car race successes', *The Environmental Digest*, 77/78, Nov/Dec, p 19

35 House of Commons Transport Committee (1994) op cit, vol 2, p 55. A similar situation applied in the Netherlands where incentives were also offered.

Table 6.6 *Sales requirements for zero-emission vehicles as passenger cars and light-duty vehicles in California. Targets listed after 2010 have yet to be finalised in legislation. In 1996 the Californian Air Resources Board suggested it might relax its 1998 target but would keep rigidly to its goal of 10 per cent by 2003*

Year	Percentage of sales
1998	2
1999	2
2000	2
2001	5
2002	5
2003	10
2004	10
2005	20
2006	20
2007	35
2008	35
2009	50
2010	50

Source: South Coast Air Quality Management District (1994) *Final 1994 Air Quality Management Plan: Meeting the Clean Air Challenge*, SCAQMD, Diamond Bar, chapter 4, p 17

stimulate the sales of electric cars. In this way, it suggested electric cars could account for 7 per cent by volume of total urban vehicle traffic in the European Union by the year 2002. However, Renault consider that it will not be until 2015 that electric cars will represent 10 per cent of the total European Union market and 40 per cent of cars used in towns. Using a variety of incentives, the Japanese government aims to have 200,000 electric vehicles in operation by 2000.[36]

Traffic management in congested, polluted cities can encourage greater adoption of cleaner cars such as by banning diesel- and petrol-engined cars from city centres and requiring these to be parked at park and ride sites on the outskirts of the city. From such sites buses, trams or trains could be used to reach the city, or perhaps electric cars could be rented to travel

36 'Dutch support for electric cars' and 'Toyota and Nissan co-operate', *The Environmental Digest*, 67, Jan 1993, p 16

into the city centre.[37] Free parking and the permitted use of high-occupancy vehicle lanes even when there is only one person in the car are other incentives that can be offered to drivers of electric vehicles. The widespread use of less polluting alternative fuels and zero-emission vehicles is likely to remain a long-term objective, but reducing emissions by improved engine technologies, fitting pollution control equipment and changing fuel composition can produce a small but significant improvement in urban air quality.

Many people would like technology to solve their pollution problems and not have to change their lifestyles, habits or behaviour. They would like to continue using their car, preferably as the sole occupant, and not have any restrictions imposed on its use. Unfortunately, technology can only help the problem, not solve it. Technological solutions to air quality problems can even worsen the situation by causing other environmental pollution problems and resource depletion. Fitting cars with catalytic converters is a major step adopted by many countries, but the rising numbers of cars and the increasing distances they are forecast to be driven each year will offset some of the benefits of the expected pollution reduction. This suggests traffic-generated pollution will remain a problem despite current and planned stricter exhaust emission limits for new petrol- and diesel-engined vehicles. The limitations of technological solutions to air quality problems facing urban areas places greater responsibilities on the authorities to tackle the problem of vehicle-generated pollution in other non-technological ways. Some of these, traffic management and control policies and measures, are explored in the next chapter.

37 For motorists willing to park on the outskirts of Coventry, UK, there is a proposal to make electric hire cars available for driving into the city centre or for other uses within the city. It will use a 'dial a car' system involving mini-electric Peugeot cars.

Chapter 7

Traffic Management and Improved Public Transport

Introduction

Policies and measures which reduce the number, frequency of use and the distances travelled by vehicles and create situations where vehicle engines operate efficiently, and so emit less pollutants, all offer the potential to improve air quality in sensitive parts of an urban area, such as residential or shopping areas, or even throughout the entire urban area. To be fully effective and acceptable to the public, traffic management and restraint measures need to be combined with improving and promoting the use of public transport facilities. Indeed, given that public transport systems give rise to much lower pollutant emissions per person transported within an urban area (or have the potential to do so if given the investment in such systems), then creating a situation where public transport dominates over the car will lead to the greatest air quality improvements.

Traffic Calming

Traffic calming is an attempt to reduce vehicle speeds, particularly in residential areas, and to create an environment in which pedestrians and cyclists feel safer. Physical changes to the roads are needed in the form of road humps, extra bends, indirect routes, special paving and road surfaces, raising of side-road junctions to the level of the pavement, speed tables, road narrowings, chicanes, wider pavements, mini-roundabouts (raised structures, not simply painted circles), designated parking spaces (usually restricted to residents only) and landscaping and planting (of flower beds).[1]

1 Road humps are not, in themselves, speed reducing measures; their principle aim is to keep speeds low once this has been achieved by other physical measures such as a junction, a roundabout or a bend in excess of 70 degrees.

Maximum vehicle speed limits in areas of traffic calming are reduced from, say, 50 kph (30 mph) to 30 kph (20 mph). Traffic calming leads to a reduced severity and number of accidents as well as an improved environment. The number of vehicles using routes with traffic calming measures often decreases as such measures deter commuters from taking short cuts ('rat-runs') through residential areas and may even deter some motorists from driving into the city centre at all. Traffic calming is usually limited to residential areas rather than main routes. Improving air quality in residential areas by deterring motorists from entering these areas and diverting traffic to less sensitive areas (eg bypasses and ring roads) is to be welcomed, but not if it worsens congestion and air quality in those areas. Simply moving exhaust emissions from one location to another does not solve the overall problem of poor air quality in an urban area. Traffic calming measures have been used in countries such as Denmark, Germany and the Netherlands since the early 1970s, but towns and cities in the UK (eg Exeter, York) only began using such measures widely following the Traffic Calming Act 1992.[2]

Care must be taken to ensure that the use of road humps does not lead to bus services becoming unpopular or even being withdrawn in an area subject to traffic calming because of increased journey times, complaints of discomfort or injury from passengers and increased maintenance cost due to damage caused when travelling over the humps. This problem can be overcome by using speed cushions whose height and length are similar to road humps, but whose width is less than the axle width of a standard bus although greater than that of the average car or van.

If the traffic volume in the area is not reduced, the air quality changes resulting from traffic calming depend very much on the vehicle drivers. If traffic calming lowers a vehicle's speed, reduces the number of stops and starts along a route, and produces a smooth drive, then there should be air quality benefits. However, if it increases the aggressiveness of the driver such that he/she decelerates abruptly on approaching, say, a road hump and then rapidly accelerates away before encountering the next hump, this can lead to increased vehicle emissions. The effects of driver behaviour towards traffic calming is illustrated by a study undertaken in Buxtehude, Germany, when traffic calming measures and 30 kph (20 mph) speed limits were introduced in the 1980s (Table 7.1). The calmer drivers used third gear and travelled slightly above 30 kph, whereas the aggressive (frustrated?)

2 Centre for Research and Contract Standardisation in Civil and Traffic Engineering (1989) *Van Woonerf Tot Erf*, The Netherlands (English version); Kent County Council (1994) *Traffic Calming: a Code of Practice*, third edition, Kent County Council, Maidstone; Pharoah, T M and Russell, J R E (1989) *Traffic Calming: Policy and Evaluations in Three European Countries*, Department of Urban Development and Policy, South Bank University Occasional Paper No 2/89. The Dutch developed the woonerf concept (literally 'living area') of traffic calming in the early 1970s in residential areas. In 1988 the concept was applied to other parts of the town and the term woonerf was replaced by erf (or its plural form, erven). Denmark extended the concept by applying traffic calming on main roads through villages.

Table 7.1 *Changes in vehicle emissions from two contrasting driving styles following the introduction of traffic calming measures and 30 kph speed limits in Buxtehude, Germany. The changes are compared with the emissions produced when the speed limit was 50 kph*

Dominant gear and driver behaviour	CO (%)	NO_x (%)	HC (%)	Fuel requirements (%)
Second gear and 'aggressive'	–17	–32	–10	+7
Third gear and 'calm'	–13	–48	–22	–7

Source: Pharoah, T M and Russell, J R E (1989) *Traffic Calming: Policy and Evaluations in Three European Countries*, Department of Urban Development and Policy, South Bank University Occasional Paper No 2/89, p 48

drivers accelerated and decelerated using second gear (but at speeds less than 50 kph) and not surprisingly used more fuel in doing so. Both types of driver produced lower emissions than when the 50 kph speed limits applied in the area, but the calmer driver produced less emissions with the exception of carbon monoxide (because carbon monoxide emissions increase with decreasing speed). Generally, it seems that schemes designed to encourage steady driving speeds are more effective in reducing emissions than slow speeds per se. Thus the frequent use of shallow ramps and speed cushions seems better than schemes involving sharp changes of level or direction.

Traffic Smoothing and Lower Speed Limits

Fuel consumption and exhaust emissions are related to vehicle speed. Vehicles typically operate efficiently in the range 50–90 kph (30–55 mph). Below and above this range engines consume significantly greater amounts of fuel (Figure 7.1). Emissions of carbon monoxide, hydrocarbons and nitrogen oxides are at a maximum when vehicles travel at less than 20 kph (Figure 7.2). At high speeds both carbon monoxide and hydrocarbons decrease while nitrogen oxides increase, especially above speeds of 80 kph. This indicates that a stricter enforcement of speed limits and/or a lowering of speed limits (most countries adopt speed limits – the German autobahns are the exception) can reduce nitrogen oxides. Dutch police have the power to confiscate a vehicle found speeding at 70 kph more than the legal limit. It is suggested that if speed limits were properly enforced in the UK it would reduce nitrogen oxides emissions by 4 per cent and carbon dioxide emissions by 3 per cent.[3]

3 'Call for enforcement of speed limits', *The Environmental Digest*, 62, Aug 1992, p 12; Fergusson, M, Holman, C and Barrett, M (1989) *Atmospheric Emissions from the Use of Transport in the UK*, vol 1, *The Estimation of Current and Future Emissions*, World Wide Fund for Nature, Godalming

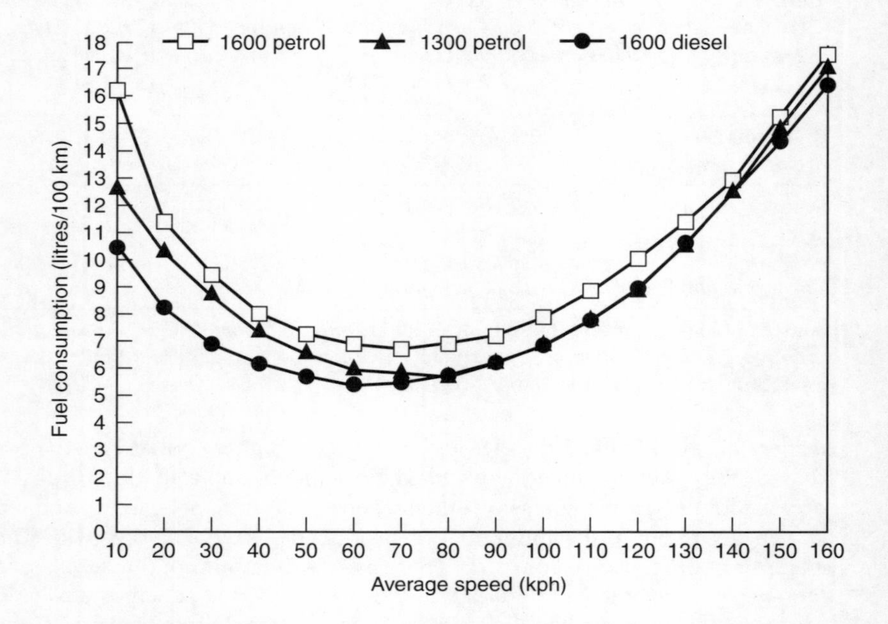

Figure 7.1 *Variation of fuel economy with speed of car*

Source: Fergusson, M, Holman, C and Barrett, M (1989) *Atmospheric Emissions from the Use of Transport in the United Kingdom*, vol 1, *The Estimation of Current and Future Emissions*, World Wide Fund for Nature – UK, Godalming

Creating a freer flow of traffic and reducing traffic jams during rush hours results in vehicles operating more efficiently which, in turn, lowers exhaust emissions. This can be achieved in a variety of ways. Stringent parking restrictions along major routes, called priority red routes, have been shown to reduce congestion and improve air quality in London and Paris, providing the traffic volume does not increase. A pilot scheme in London reduced emissions of nitrogen oxides up to 2 per cent and hydrocarbons and carbon monoxide by about 10 per cent.[4]

Traffic signal co-ordination throughout an urban area, termed urban traffic control, can increase the proportion of vehicles travelling in the fuel-efficient range and reduce the proportions in ranges below and above these speeds, which can result in a reduction in exhaust emissions by 3–6 per cent or even more. In congested parts of urban areas, careful scheduling of traffic light signals can ensure that fewer traffic queues occur alongside crowded shopping areas compared with less sensitive areas. Phasing a sequence of traffic lights to create 'green waves' helps to promote a smoother traffic

4 References to priority red routes are listed in Note 20, Chapter 9

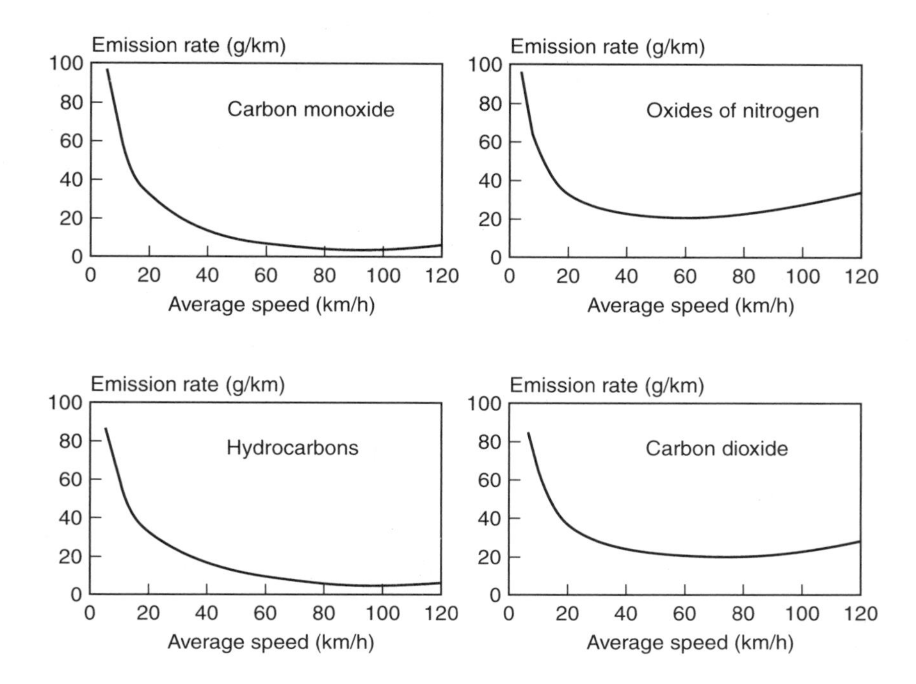

Figure 7.2 *Speed-related emission factors for petrol-engined cars without catalytic converters*

Source: Department of Transport (1994) *Design Manual for Roads and Bridges*, vol 11, *Environmental Assessment, Section 3*, HMSO, London

flow, although this can hinder buses which have to stop between lights and so get caught by a red light. Adjusting freeway entry meters can help smooth the traffic flow at busy times.[5]

Congestion can be reduced through rapid dissemination of advice to drivers about accidents and traffic jams ahead using roadside electronic signs or computer links inside the car, so enabling drivers to take alternative routes. Computer links to vehicles can be used to inform drivers of the least congested route to follow to reach a given destination. Berlin is testing such a system called LISB (Leit-und-Information-System) which provides drivers of 700 vehicles with an on-board computer which informs the driver verbally of the best route to take to reach their desired destination. Volkswagen are developing a system which displays information in the driver's field of view

5 Butterwick, L, Harrison, R and Merritt, Q (1991) *Handbook for Urban Air Improvement*, Commission of the European Communities, Brussels, p 169; House of Commons Transport Committee (1994) *Transport-related Air Pollution in London*, Sixth Report, vol 1, pp 19, 20 and 23, and vol 2, p 96

(on the windscreen) linked to sensors which can give route instructions, warn of pedestrian crossings and alert the driver if they are driving too close to the vehicle in front. It could be extended to notify the driver of the availability of parking places to reduce the time wasted and the fuel consumed when searching for a parking space.

Research is being undertaken into the use of a collision control radar system in vehicles which senses a vehicle ahead and automatically adjusts the speed of the car and brakes the car if necessary. Providing motorists were confident in such a system this could reduce the distance between cars and could lead to a doubling or even tripling of road capacity. The long-term aim of such a system would be to make major routes such as motorways and ring roads automated such that as soon as a driver entered such roads the vehicle would be under computer control.[6] Whether such a system improves air quality is debatable, especially as it is a measure directed towards enabling the number of private cars to increase rather than a measure to discourage this trend. The safety and stress reduction aspects of the system are to be welcomed, but it encourages the view that roads can cope with an unlimited expansion in the numbers and use of cars (frequently occupied by only one person). This message does not help campaigns concerned with improving air quality.

Traffic Bans

Traffic bans can be used to reduce the total volume of traffic or specific types of vehicles along specific streets or in a designated area. Reducing traffic volumes is intended to reduce exhaust emissions in targeted areas and, if supported by improvements in public transport, can also improve air quality throughout the urban area. Traffic bans can be applied according to a type of vehicle (eg heavy goods vehicles, vehicles not equipped with catalytic converters, vehicles with odd or even licence plates on alternate days), time of day (eg at times of potential congestion) and type of movement (eg through journeys or access).

Bans can encourage a more rapid phasing-in of cleaner vehicles by banning all but 'clean technology' vehicles such that there is greater incentive for people to purchase such vehicles. Prague, Czech Republic intended to ban all non-catalyst vehicles from its historic centre from October 1992, but later had to revoke the regulation when it was realised that there was too little time for vehicles to be updated. In March 1993 Hungary introduced a ban on heavy trucks at weekends and holidays. In the capital, Budapest, the authorities decided to ban all two-stroke engined vehicles such as Trabants and Wartburgs from the city centre unless they were fitted with a catalytic converter. The authorities offered to pay half the cost of fitting the catalytic converter. Following the IRA terrorist bombing of an office block in London in 1993, the UK Government decided the police

6 Mullins, J (1994) 'Cars that drive themselves', *New Scientist*, 15 Oct, pp 37–40

should block off roads into the City centre with checkpoints. This measure reduced the traffic volume and reduced traffic emissions by 15–16 per cent in the cordoned-off area, although there was a slight increase immediately outside the cordon. Aachen, Germany reported that a ban in traffic in the city centre has reduced carbon monoxide levels by 40 per cent, nitrogen oxides by 50 per cent and benzene by more than 50 per cent. The plan was initially opposed by local shopkeepers worried about loss of trade, but this fear proved unfounded.[7]

Many cities such as Athens, Bologna, Lagos, Mexico City, Milan and Santiago have introduced short-term bans on traffic using odd and even last digit numbers on licence plates during smogs but some have extended this to entire smog seasons by banning cars for one day a week depending on the last digit of the car's licence plate.[8] This strategy can fail if better-off commuters simply buy a second car – often an older more polluting vehicle – which allows them to alternate their cars according to the number plate. Employers may even offer company cars for this purpose. The development of a market in fake licence plates is another problem. The air quality effectiveness of any ban on private cars can be diminished if commuters switch to alternative types of transport such as taxis and motorcycles which, in some cases, can be equally polluting (eg Athens).

Traffic Routing, Bypasses and Traffic Cells

Without necessarily having to impose a traffic ban, through traffic can be encouraged to avoid a congested city centre by building a bypass or a ring road. Such roads usually provide a higher quality, simpler and quicker route past a city than using city centre streets, especially for heavy goods vehicles. Once a bypass or ring road exists many city authorities then impose city centre restrictions on heavy goods vehicles. Many cities have expanded since their bypasses or ring roads were built such that these major roads now often lie adjacent to suburban residential areas and can pose a serious risk to local air quality because of the high traffic volumes using them. Local traffic adds to the traffic volume on ring roads, originally built to cope with through traffic, as local drivers often find it quicker to reach another part of the city via the ring road than by wending their way through congested city centre streets.

---

7 'Hungary's traffic pollution', *The Environmental Digest*, 67, Jan 1993, p 15; 'Car free cities club formed', *The Environmental Digest*, 81, Mar 1994, p 14. References for the London traffic management cordon are given in Note 22, chapter 9

8 Bonnel, P (1994) 'Urban car policy in Europe', in *Proceedings of Car Free Cities Conference, Amsterdam, March 1994*, pp 131–137; French, H F (1990) 'Clearing the air', in Brown, L R et al (eds) *State of the World 1990*, W W Norton, New York, pp 98–118; São Paulo introduced a voluntary scheme for drivers not to use their cars on one day a week depending on the last digit of the car's licence plate in 1995, and may make this compulsory in 1996. *The Environmental Digest* 1995/8, Aug, p 15

Encouraging local traffic to use ring roads when travelling from one suburb to another within an urban area has been a strategy adopted in several cities. The authorities divide the city into a small number, say, five, traffic cells. Only public transport, taxis and emergency vehicles are allowed to cross a cell boundary. Other traffic has to go via the ring road. Air quality benefits have occurred because traffic volumes throughout the city have generally decreased. This is in part due to many city residents recognising the time advantage that public transport, walking and cycling have in being able to cross cell borders. However, some deterioration of air quality may have been experienced locally due to increased traffic emissions at the access junctions to and from the ring road and because some vehicles consume more fuel travelling from cell to cell. Selective access using traffic cells has been applied in Bologna in Italy, Bremen in Germany, Copenhagen in Denmark, Groningen in the Netherlands, and Vienna in Austria.[9]

Many countries attempt to solve traffic congestion problems in cities by building more roads to cope with the traffic. This policy can be self-defeating, however. New roads, including bypasses, encourage more cars to use them. New roads continue the cycle of continual traffic growth whose drivers demand new roads. A bypass built to reduce traffic congestion in a city centre may within a few years become congested itself, while traffic in the city centre simply returns to its original pre-bypass and congested levels. Part of the reason for this is that traffic congestion deters some drivers from using their cars. If travel times are cut by building a new road it seems that the roads act as a magnet to increase traffic levels. This recognises Anthony Downs' so-called 'fundamental law of traffic congestion', which is that it is impossible to reduce city centre traffic jams and other vehicle externalities by investing solely in road and transit infrastructure.[10]

Road (Congestion) Pricing

Increasing attention is being directed towards making drivers pay for the environmental costs of using their vehicles in relation to how much use is made of the vehicle. This could be achieved by transferring taxation from vehicle ownership to vehicle use according to the distance travelled each year (perhaps even related to measured end of year exhaust emissions), the type of vehicle (eg higher taxes for less fuel-efficient cars, lower taxes for cars fitted with pollution control devices) and where it is driven (eg city centres, motorways/freeways, over bridges, through tunnels). In congested urban areas this can take the form of setting higher parking charges and even fuel taxes.

One environmental pricing approach which is more frequently discussed than it is implemented is road (congestion) pricing. This scheme charges

9 Butterwick, L *et al* (1991) op cit, pp 193-196

10 Downs, A (1992) *Stuck in Traffic: Coping with Peak Hour Traffic Congestion*, Brookings Institution, Washington DC; Hamer, N (1995) 'Report slams official traffic forecasts', *New Scientist*, 7 Jan

drivers for entering the city centre or even charges for the amount of time spent driving within the city centre. In its simplest form motorists wanting to use the 'cordoned' city centre would have to display permits on windscreens like tax discs. Those not displaying a current permit would have their licence plate noted by traffic wardens or police and would subsequently be fined. The cost of the permits would need to be high enough to deter significant numbers of motorists from entering the city. Instead of using permits, or in addition to using permits, charges could be made at toll stations either manually (for the convenience of visitors and tourists) or electronically. The latter method requires vehicles to be fitted with some form of charge card (smartcard), like a telephone card, which can be scanned and the appropriate charges deducted. Ideally, this would take place without vehicles having to stop or slow down at toll collection points. This provides a challenge for technology given that 10,000–15,000 vehicles per hour may use some urban motorways such the London Orbital Motorway (M25). Nevertheless, Austria experimented using the smartcard system on an autobahn near Salzburg in 1994 and plans to extend it subsequently to many routes. Both manual and electronic collection methods are able to vary the charge according to the time of day (eg morning and afternoon rush hours) or day of the week (eg lower charges at weekends, no charge on a Sunday or public holidays).[11]

Singapore introduced road pricing in 1975 in the form of an area licensing scheme for cars. This required drivers to display daily or monthly permits during morning traffic peaks. It quickly produced a reduction in cars during the morning peak of 76 per cent, although this subsequently fell to 44 per cent. Traffic reduction also produced an increase in vehicle speeds of 22 per cent – that is, less congestion. In 1989 the scheme was extended to include all private vehicles including also charging for afternoon traffic peaks. In the early scheme cars carrying four or more people were exempt, which produced a new trade in youngsters offering themselves for hire as passengers and, in a small part, this contributed to half the cars entering the restricted area being exempted from the charges. Singapore plans to replace its system of displaying permits with electronic road-pricing using smartcards by late 1997.[12]

Hong Kong's experimental scheme in 1983–1985 began using electronic licence plates which were recorded by an inductive loop installed in the road at the toll collection points. A central computer registered each time the vehicle passed and a bill was sent to the vehicle owner each month. Vehicles without special licence plates were photographed and enforcement measures taken against them. The scheme was discontinued in the face of

11 Butterwick, L *et al* (1991) op cit, pp 180–192; Department of Transport (1993) *A Review of Technology for Road Pricing in London*, Report prepared by University of Newcastle-upon-Tyne, HMSO, London; 'Austria swipes lead on electronic tolls', *New Scientist*, 11 Dec

12 'Singapore launches electronic road-pricing', *The Environmental Digest*, 83/84, May/Jun 1994, p 19

strong concerns over civil liberties when the public realised that the system gave police and other government agencies information on their movements. The scheme produced a 20–24 per cent reduction in cars at peak times (commercial vehicles were exempt) but as use of public transport increased by only 3 per cent, the benefits of the scheme were offset by increased car use at off-peak times. However, carbon monoxide emissions were reduced by 14–17 per cent, hydrocarbons by 3 per cent and nitrogen oxides by 6 per cent. The concern over civil liberties is not a problem using modern systems because they use pre-paid smartcards from which charges can be deducted electronically without the need to identify the vehicle or its owner providing a valid card is carried in the vehicle.[13]

Milan, Italy introduced a peak entry licence for the city centre which produced a 50 per cent reduction in traffic. Of those drivers who changed their behaviour, 16 per cent delayed their journey, 36 per cent parked outside the control area and 41 per cent switched to public transport. Bergen, Trondheim and Oslo in Norway have introduced a 'toll ring' during weekday morning periods aimed at raising revenue for road building (70–80 per cent of the tolls go towards road investment). The road pricing scheme introduced in Oslo in 1990 involves a combination of 19 toll booths and electronic tags fitted to windscreens, which allows automatic billing of vehicles as they enter the city. Stockholm has outlined plans to introduce a fully electronic road pricing system aimed at reducing traffic emissions of nitrogen oxides. It is estimated that if the road pricing scheme is combined with a public transport fare reduction of 50 per cent, it could achieve the goal of a 30 per cent reduction in nitrogen oxides five years earlier than using the road pricing scheme alone.[14]

Charging for access to downtown city areas in the US may receive greater attention in the future. In 1988, Mayor Edward Koch of New York City welcomed the suggestion of charging a $10 fee for all vehicles entering the southern part of Manhattan. In the UK, road pricing as a means of reducing traffic congestion and improving air quality in city centres is being explored by Bristol, Cambridge, Edinburgh, London and Sheffield. In September 1993, Cambridge demonstrated its approach to road pricing whereby vehicles are fitted with on-board equipment carrying an electronic smartcard which is scanned automatically using microwaves from roadside beacons. Unlike most road pricing schemes which impose fixed city centre entrance charges, the Cambridge system proposes to charge vehicles only when the road is congested – that is, when the vehicle speed falls below a predetermined speed averaged over, say, 0.5 km. Cambridge's scheme forms part of the EC ADEPT – Automatic Debiting and Electronic Payment for Transport – project which involves experiments in Greece and Portugal and is also concerned with providing traffic information to an on-board computer, so enabling

13 Hurdle, D (1990) *Road Pricing for London*, London Boroughs Association
14 Organisation for Economic Cooperation and Development (OECD) (1990) *Environmental Policies for Cities in the 1990s*, OECD, Paris, pp 74–76

drivers to avoid traffic jams and accidents as well as receiving parking information.[15]

Electronic road pricing schemes may be costly to implement but the costs can be quickly recouped. Road pricing is intended to give motorists a free choice of either paying to drive into the city centre, or parking their cars outside the city centre and then transferring to public transport, or sharing cars to share the costs, or simply using public transport in the first place. However, there are many key questions which need addressing before road pricing is introduced. For example, how effective will a scheme be in reducing traffic emissions and improving air quality? Will it simply displace the pollution as drivers attempt to get as close to the restricted area as possible before parking? Will people living in city centres be exempt as well as those living near the cordon who may need to criss-cross the toll point frequently? How would city centre businesses be affected? Will investors choose to locate in areas not affected by road pricing? With regard to these questions about business it is hoped that by reducing traffic congestion the city centre becomes a far more attractive environment for shoppers and tourists such that trade and investment improves.

One critical question concerns the fairness of road pricing: does the measure simply create less congested roads for better-off motorists? With regard to this question, it is vital that the tolls collected are directed towards improving and subsidising public transport facilities in the area rather than being used for road investment or simply added to government revenue. Road pricing should benefit all urban residents and should not penalise those of lower incomes who cannot afford to pay the tolls, own a car or live in a part of the city which is less polluted by vehicles. Before traffic tolls for access into many major city centres become commonplace, it will be necessary to persuade the public that road charging is indeed a better approach to improving air quality than the many other measures available.

Controls for Engine-idling Stationary Vehicles

A stationary vehicle left with its engine idling produces high levels of carbon monoxide and hydrocarbons emissions as the engine is not working efficiently. Engine-idling stationary vehicles are found in traffic jams and queues at traffic lights. Buses waiting at bus stops, coaches and taxis waiting at collection points and commercial vehicles loading and unloading add to the numbers of such vehicles. In many cases education of drivers is all that is needed to get drivers to switch off their engines if they are likely to be stationary for longer than a few minutes.

In Switzerland drivers are required to switch off their engines if more than fifth in line at traffic lights. Failure to do so may result in fines. Blue 'eco

---

15 Cambridgeshire County Council (1993) *Demand Management: the Cambridge Approach*, Transportation Studies, Cambridgeshire County Council; 'Road pricing experiment launched in Cambridge', *The Environmental Digest*, 75, Sep 1993, p 13

lights' have been tried which are placed next to the traffic signal to inform drivers when to switch off and switch on their engines. The blue light flashes as long as the red phase has enough time left to make it worthwhile switching off the engine. Other versions of these lights tell drivers exactly how many seconds remain before the light changes to green. Where traffic queues are likely to be lengthy or where road bends obscure the traffic lights, advance signalling may be needed to ensure drivers receive information about the need to switch off engines. This measure reduces fuel consumption and vehicle emissions considerably in the vicinity of traffic lights. In a very small number of cases poorly maintained vehicles may fail to restart and congestion can be worsened. One problem which offsets the air quality benefits resulting from this measure is that restarting the engine consumes large amounts of fuel and this may produce high levels of hydrocarbons when restarting an engine. In other words, the air quality improvements, proportional to the length of time the engine is switched off, must be balanced against the increase in emissions occurring when switching on, especially in the case of badly maintained or older vehicle engines. On average, tests suggest that vehicles save fuel when a car engine is switched off for more than 15 seconds. Similarly, emissions were less when the engine was switched off for more than 20–30 seconds.[16] A recent advance for diesel cars (which could be adapted to petrol engines) is idling control which switches off the engine when the vehicle is stationary or coasting and restarts it at a touch on the accelerator.[17]

Diesel emissions from buses are often a cause of concern in city centres. Buses waiting at bus stops can be a particular problem when they are left with their engines running (though in cold weather the engine is needed to provide heat for passengers). To tackle this problem, Denver requires that vehicles stationary for ten minutes must switch off their engines.[18] Increased recognition of urban air pollution problems has resulted in some bus companies in the UK now instructing bus drivers to switch off engines when standing for more than five minutes. It would help improve air quality if drivers of all commercial vehicles agreed a code of conduct to switch off engines when stationary for more than a few minutes. However, making this compulsory with the threat of fines would probably be more effective and it would not be difficult for traffic wardens to implement if they were given the powers to do so.

---

16 Butterwick, L *et al* (1991) op cit, pp 197–198; Brilon, W and Wiebusch-Wothge, R (1989) *Effects of Environmental Traffic Lights on Fuel Consumption of Vehicles, Energy Efficiency in Land Transport*, Proceedings of a Seminar, May 1988, Report Cd-Na-12284-EN-C, Commission of the European Communities, Luxembourg

17 Freeman, V (1993) 'VW decides to turn green', *The Times*, 8 Oct; Royal Commission on Environmental Pollution (1994) *Eighteenth Report: Transport and the Environment*, HMSO, London, p 132

18 Local Government Task Force (1991) *Local Government Air Quality Programs in the Denver Metropolitan Area*, Regional Air Quality Council, Denver, p 6

Parking Controls

In many cities, demand for city centre parking will outstrip supply over the next decade, if it has not already done so. Car parking charges (eg higher for all day parking), controlling access to parking by time of day (eg only open after 9.30 am to give preference to shoppers rather than commuters), controlling the number of private workplace parking spaces, redistributing parking spaces from town centres to peripheral park and ride sites, and stricter enforcement of illegal parking (eg more traffic wardens, higher fines, use of wheel clamping) can reduce traffic volumes and focus the attention of commuters on public transport options. City authorities may need extended powers to tackle some problems. For example, Cambridge in the UK copes with 90,000 vehicles entering the small city each day, but with 40,000 privately owned workplace parking places available there is little to discourage many people driving into the city centre.[19] In the US, 80 per cent of all employees receive free parking and it is estimated that a parking charge of $30–35 per 20 day working month would more than double the cost of the drive-alone journey and lead to a reduction in such commuting by 10–30 per cent. Since 1993 in California, in order to discourage car use, employers with more than 100 employees are required by law to offer cash to their employees in lieu of subsidising their public parking charges. Thus employees have an incentive not to drive to work. It is claimed this 'cash out' scheme could reduce commuting trips by 50 per cent.[20]

Following the Swiss Federal Court's ruling in 1993 that the management and reduction of parking spaces can be used as a legally enforceable means of air pollution abatement, Fribourg, which experiences 23,000 vehicles per day causing nitrogen dioxide levels to be above the national standard, plans to adopt this approach. The current parking needs of employers were determined in three city zones, defined according to the quality of public transport available. Parking spaces for employers in each zone were then reduced, with the city centre zone reduction being about 30 per cent. It was estimated that the parking policy would decrease current traffic volumes by 28 per cent and projected traffic volumes by 46 per cent in the city centre, which would decrease nitrogen dioxide levels significantly. The success of the strategy depends on expanding and promoting public transport facilities.[21]

---

19 Elsom, D M and Crabbe, H (1995) 'Practical issues involved in developing effective local air quality management in the United Kingdom', in Power, H *et al* (eds) *Air Pollution*, Vol 2, Computational Mechanics, Southampton, pp 483–492

20 Royal Commission on Environmental Pollution (1994) op cit, p 192; 'Paid for not parking', *Acid News*, 4, Oct 1994, p 20

21 Gygax, H (1995) 'Parking strategy in the pollution control program of an urban area', *Proceedings of the 10th World Clean Air Congress, Espoo, Finland*, Finnish Air Pollution Prevention Society, Helsinki, paper 547

Improving and Favouring Public Transport

Public transport systems emit far less pollution per person transported than private cars. Helping buses move more freely by the use of bus-only streets and bus priority lanes (bus lanes) improves public transport efficiency. To counteract persistent abuse of bus lanes by other drivers special concrete kerbs may be installed along some or all of the bus lanes. These kerbs not only prevent motorists from entering the bus lanes but can act as a guide rail for buses. A small guide wheel attached to the wheels of the bus and in contact with the kerbs provides a safety guidance system. Successful schemes operate in Essen, Germany and Adelaide, Australia with Leeds, UK planning to implement a similar scheme.

Giving buses priority at traffic lights can be achieved by fitting buses with electronic devices (transponders) which delay a red light until the bus has passed through or brings the green light forward. Once the bus has passed through the intersection, the timings are adjusted back to the original cycle. Studies suggest when road junctions are operating at around 80–90 per cent of capacity this measure can reduce bus delays by about 10 per cent without increasing delays to other vehicles significantly. However, when roads are at full capacity prioritising may cause much greater delays to other traffic and so no priority to buses may be given in such situations. Bus lanes and priority at traffic lights as well as introducing computerised displays at bus stops (as used frequently for metros) telling waiting passengers how long before the next bus will arrive all help to improve the efficiency and acceptability of public transport.[22]

Light rail systems or metros have the advantage over buses in operating on protected routes which are subject to fewer delays and so offer a faster and more reliable service. Metro systems, involving the construction of underground lines, require a huge investment even if the network of routes is phased in over a number of years. Beijing, Cairo, Mexico City, Shanghai and Singapore have built metros in recent years but because of the high construction and operating costs involved many cities have opted for light rail systems instead. One-quarter of all cities with over 200,000 inhabitants and half with a population of over 600,000 in Austria, Belgium, France, Germany, Italy, the Netherlands, Sweden and Switzerland have a light rail or tram system. Many other countries have recognised the potential advantages of such systems and are now developing or planning to introduce them. In the UK, Manchester opened the $190 million Metro Link in 1992 which uses existing rail track for part of its journey, switching to tramlines on city centre streets. Sheffield's Supertram opened in 1994. Blackpool, Glasgow, Tyne and Wear, and London (Docklands) also operate light rail systems, whereas over 40 other UK towns, cities and conurbations have undertaken feasibility studies or are awaiting government finance for

22 Hamer, M (1994) 'Buses to get green light through city traffic', *New Scientist*, 7 May, pp 20–21

the go ahead (eg the West Midlands Metro scheduled to begin in 1997). It should be remembered that electric-powered transport systems do use electricity generated by coal- or oil-fired power stations so they do create pollution, albeit not in the city centre. However, their overall role in improving air quality is that they give rise to considerably less pollutant emissions per person transported than cars.[23]

Implementation of traffic management measures which discourage the use of private vehicles must be linked with measures to make public transport cheap (eg subsidised fares), convenient, comfortable, safe (eg for women at night) and efficient (eg minimal waiting time, reliable, dense network of routes). Efficiency can be achieved with commitment and investment. For example, Besancon in France (population 120,000) claims a 95 per cent coverage of urban population by public transport within a radius of 300 m from a boarding place. Convenience extends to enabling travellers to switch readily from one mode of transport to another (including park and ride schemes offering free car parks at the city outskirts and frequent buses with cheap fares into the city). Pre-paid integrated fares ('travel cards') which are interchangeable when transferring between buses, metros and light rail systems make public transport convenient. Currently too many commuters in cities throughout the world rely on cars rather than public transport and the situation has become accentuated in recent years. For example, in the UK in 1991, 67 per cent of men and 52 per cent of women travelled to work by car or van compared with 59 per cent and 37 per cent in 1981 (and the proportion of households with two or more cars rose from 26 per cent to 42 per cent). In contrast, the use of buses fell from 11 to only 6 per cent for men and from 24 to 15 per cent for women. Vehicle emissions are the major reason why so many cities now experience poor, and perhaps worsening, urban air quality. For the sake of achieving and sustaining healthy urban air quality, city authorities need to encourage, persuade and push commuters to use public transport instead. If that policy is to succeed it will need massive investment in public transport systems after so many years of underfunding.[24]

Ride Sharing, Changing Public Attitudes and Lifestyles

Too many vehicles in urban areas have only one occupant. If people could be persuaded to share cars, especially when commuting to and from their place of work, traffic volumes and associated exhaust emissions could be reduced substantially. For example, in Birmingham, UK, if car sharing could be promoted so that average occupancy increased from say, 125 to 150

23 Holman, C (1991) *Transport and Climate Change: Cutting Carbon Dioxide Emissions from Cars*, Friends of the Earth, London, p 56; Whitelegg, J (1992) *Traffic Congestion: Is There a Way Out?* Leading Edge, Hawes, p 116

24 Nijkamp, P and Perrels, A (1994) *Sustainable Cities in Europe*, Earthscan, London, pp 120–121; 'Strong growth in car use', *The Environmental Digest*, 87, Sep 1994, p 14

people per 100 cars (ie vehicle occupancy of 1.25 to 1.50), more than 8000 cars (17 per cent of the total) would be taken off the region's roads each day, saving energy, reducing vehicle emissions and improving traffic speeds. Even increasing the average vehicle occupancy from say, 1.4 to 1.5 may reduce vehicle emissions by 5 per cent. However, many people are reluctant to share and suffer the condition known as NIMF (not in my frontseat). Motorists like the freedom offered by travelling alone: one person's hours of work may be irregular or not coincide with another person's hours because of overtime, and a driver may have to make other journeys on the way to or from work (eg shopping, collecting children).

Journey-matching services are sometimes offered by authorities, agencies or employers to bring together prospective car sharers. Commuter Computer in Los Angeles was set up in 1974 and has worked with 1800 companies and has assisted about 45,000 people to share rides. In Los Angeles in 1990 about 83 per cent of all journeys to work were by lone drivers but the long-term aim is to reduce that to 20 per cent. Edinburgh, UK launched a journey-matching scheme in 1992 following a survey which showed that 80 per cent of cars entering the city carried only one occupant and identified 20,000 people who could be pooling their cars, so saving money, lessening congestion and reducing vehicle emissions. However, with no incentives offered very few people were attracted to the scheme (only 100 people were registered on the scheme in 1993). In 1993, in the Netherlands, around half a million people are ride sharing. It began with companies offering the use of minibuses that could be shared by several employees travelling from the same suburban commuter area. The government then set aside 275 roadside car pool locations where drivers leave their cars, call a central number and pick up a lift. On any working day, 60 per cent of the 7000 places at the car pools are taken up by commuters.[25]

A wide range of incentives can be used to persuade people to share cars. Los Angeles introduced a special freeway lane as well as car parks reserved exclusively for ride sharers (vehicles carrying two or more people). However, it is not always easy to build additional high vehicle occupancy lanes in congested cities, especially in Europe, and only Amsterdam has attempted this, without success. In August 1994 the Dutch Transport Ministry was forced by court order to close the experimental car pool lane opened in October 1993 on the A1 road into Amsterdam as it was declared to be illegal to discriminate against lone drivers. Sydney, Australia, has operated high vehicle occupancy lanes since 1974. It is important to ensure that reserving a lane for high occupancy vehicles does not result in greater congestion in the remaining lanes, otherwise emissions from the slower stop and go traffic in those lanes could offset the gains from ride sharing. Inducements for ride sharers include offering cheap, well-situated car parks for exclusive use by ride sharers, even allowing high occupancy vehicles

25 Eason, K (1993) 'Car-sharing Dutch show the way to ease clogged roads', *The Times*, 27 Oct, p 7

to use certain bus priority routes, and for employers to offer higher distance allowances for ride sharers. The latter can come about by the authorities offering employers tax benefits. Single-occupant cars can be discouraged and ride sharing encouraged by increasing the charges for parking and reducing the number of car parking spaces.[26]

Ride sharing is most successful when it is a legal requirement. In the US this measure is directed at large employers. Denver introduced a trip reduction ordinance which requires large businesses to reach a 35 per cent ride share goal within five years. In this case, ride share refers to any method of commuting other than single-occupant vehicles (eg employers can provide mass transit pass subsidies). A similar requirement could be applied to schools to develop plans to reduce the number of single children, usually 11 years or under, who are brought to and from school by car even over relatively short distances (mostly because of safety concerns about the dangers of traffic or for fear of molestation). Schools and education authorities could be made responsible for organising safe alternatives such as ride shares, school buses, escorted cycling and guided walking.

Widespread education is needed to help commuters realise that their cars are the major cause of the poor urban air quality they and their families experience and that by using their cars less they will begin to remedy the problem. Many cities have used campaigns in an attempt to increase public awareness of the damage to the environment by vehicle exhausts and road congestion. In Albuquerque, New Mexico, problems of carbon monoxide pollution in winter prompted a campaign 'Don't drive one in five' to encourage motorists to refrain from driving their cars one day a week and to use alternate modes of transport. In the Netherlands in 1991, the government launched a campaign based on the advertising campaign slogan 'Your car can survive a day without you: can you survive without your car?' The West Midlands in the UK campaigned 'Don't choke the city' in 1992 and it urged people to leave their car at home at least once a week and switch to public transport, share lifts, walk or cycle to work. Also in the UK, West Yorkshire buses carry the message 'Cars are bad news for the environment; you're looking at an alternative', whereas Southampton campaigns for 'People first, cars second'. Nottingham is exploring ways of offering incentives to its council employees in an attempt to persuade them to use public transport, car shares, car pools or to cycle to work. Denver city employees are encouraged to live close to their place of work by being paid a starting salary which reflects how far their residence is from their work. Percentage increases or reductions are applied ranging from +7.5 per cent if less than a mile, +5 per cent at 1–2 miles, par for 2–5 miles, –2.5 per cent for 5–10 miles, –5 per cent for 10–20 miles and –7.5 per cent if more than 20

26 Albersheim, S R (1982) 'An assessment of transportation control measures for improving air quality', *Transportation Quarterly*, vol 36, pp 451–468; 'Europe's first car-pool lane closes', *The Environmental Digest*, 86, Aug 1994, p 15

miles. A housing allowance is also provided as houses close to the city centre are more expensive.[27]

Traffic congestion increases pollution emissions so the introduction of 'flexitime' and staggered working hours can reduce traffic volumes during peak commuting times. In the UK, Hertforshire's 'travelwise' campaign is aimed at encouraging motorists to 'avoid the rush hour and think what you're missing'. However, work rescheduling in very congested cities can simply extend the period of congestion and it does not address the key issue of too many cars being used overall. Authorities in Bangkok, Thailand, are not only staggering the office hours of civil servants but are introducing a four-day week for these employees. It is estimated that the number of cars on the streets could be reduced by 20 to 30 per cent if civil servants worked four 10-hour days rather than five 8-hour days. Improved communication systems now offer more opportunities for people to work at home using computer links to offices. In a US survey in 1992 it was found that 7 per cent of the working population was telecommuting for all or part of the working week. In the UK in 1995 there were estimated to be more than 2 million (and by the year 2000 there will be around 5 million) 'teleworkers' enjoying a more productive and less stressful lifestyle while not adding to the vehicle-generated pollution problems of urban areas. In the Los Angeles basin, policies promoting telecommuting aim to reduce work trips by almost 30 per cent by 2010. The main obstacles to a rapid expansion of telecommuting are more social than technical, as workers are reluctant to give up socialising in the workplace.[28]

Setting Traffic Reduction Targets

National governments, and city authorities if they have the powers to do so, should set targets for reducing the commuting use of private cars and increasing the use of public transport or alternatives such as cycling. The existence of appropriate targets would highlight to everyone that there is a clear commitment to tackling the problem of vehicle pollutants within a set timetable. Targets provide a basis for assessing the likely effectiveness of proposed transport planning measures to achieve those targets. Intermediate targets help to monitor progress towards the final goal. In the Netherlands the government has set a target to restrict traffic growth to 35 per cent between 1986 and 2010 compared with a forecast of 70 per cent. In the UK, the Royal Commission on Environmental Pollution has urged the government to set targets. The Commission recommends reducing the proportion of urban journeys undertaken by car from the current 50 per cent in the London area to 45 per cent by 2000 and 35 per cent by 2020;

27 Foute, S and Andrew, S (1991) 'Denver, Colorado's carbon dioxide transportation strategies', *Proceedings of the Conference on Cities and Climate Change, Toronto, Canada, June 1991*, Climate Institute, Washington DC, pp 169–173

28 Wickham, T (1994) 'Teleworking: a remote chance of success', *The Sunday Times*, 4 Dec, p 14

and from 65 per cent in other urban areas to 60 per cent by 2000 and 50 per cent by 2020. The Commission suggests setting a target for increasing the proportion of passenger-kilometres carried by public transport from 12 per cent in 1993 to 20 per cent by 2005 and 30 per cent by 2020. In addition, cycle use ought to rise to 10 per cent of all urban journeys by 2005, compared with 2.5 per cent now. Such targets are the means of achieving and sustaining an overall air quality target for the UK which, states the Commission, should be to achieve full compliance with WHO health-based air quality guidelines by 2005.[29]

Promoting Cycling

In 1993, worldwide production of bicycles (cycles) reached 108 million, exceeding motor vehicle production by nearly three to one. Currently, there are around 800 million cycles in the world. In China there are around 70 cycles for every motor vehicle and cycling is the principal means of travel. Many people in Africa, Asia and Latin America depend heavily on cycles and load-carrying three-wheelers to commute to work and for transporting produce to market. In many cities in Asia, cycling accounts for 20–60 per cent of people's trips. The situation in Europe, Australasia and North America is very different. The increased use of cars in urban areas during the past 50 years has been partly at the expense of cycling. Relatively few people cycle to work now. This is a situation that is likely to occur in cities in Africa, Asia and Latin America as the number of motor vehicles increases rapidly. If vehicle emissions in cities in both the North and South are to be reduced, then more commuters have to be encouraged to use less polluting forms of transport: cycling offers that alternative for some people. Where cycles are already used widely, as in many Asian cities, it is important that their contribution to commuting is sustained.[30]

Cycling can offer advantages over cars for some people, especially those who commute short distances. In European and American cities those people who do cycle to and from work give reasons for doing so such as it is cheap, healthy, quick, more convenient than using a car for parking, and even it is enjoyable. Given these perceived advantages of cycling, more effort should be made by the authorities to enhance the positive qualities of cycling to encourage a significant shift towards cycling. Inducements for people to cycle rather than use the car include improved facilities such as more dedicated cycle lanes, traffic-free cycle routes, covered and burglar-proof cycle parks (even including cycle lockers equipped with a secure compartment in which to store shopping), changing facilities and showers at their place of work, advanced stop lines at traffic lights, priority to turn

29 Royal Commission on Environmental Pollution (1994) op cit

30 Brown, L R, Kane, H and Roodman, D M (1994) *Vital Signs: the Trends that are Shaping Our Future 1994–95*, Earthscan, London, pp 18, 88–89; Replogle, M (1992) *Non-motorised Vehicles in Asian Cities*, World Bank Technical Paper No 162, Washington DC

right against a red light at junctions, exemption along one-way streets, better facilities for taking cycles on public transport (at no cost) and traffic management schemes which give priority to cyclists. Cycling needs to be considered in all new developments and road schemes. Employers should be encouraged, even required, to give travel allowances ('cash outs') for those who cycle to work in lieu of the free car parking that many employees enjoy.

Extensive cycle hire facilities at rail and bus stations can encourage the integration of cycling with public transport. Copenhagen, Denmark, makes available 5000 cycles on loan, in the same manner as luggage trolleys at railway stations or supermarket trolleys, with a coin needed to detach a cycle from a rack which can be reclaimed when the cycle is returned. A special design and built-in radio transmitter are intended to discourage theft. In the UK, Bristol encouraged people to use cycles more often by offering the free use of cycles through its Green Bike Scheme launched in 1991 to promote its network of cycle routes. In the UK some cities operate successful cycling policies. For example, in the historical city of York 20 per cent of journeys to work were by bicycle in 1991, whereas in Oxford and Cambridge, both with high numbers of students, the figures were 19 and 27 per cent, respectively. However, such figures are low compared with what can be achieved. In Munster, Germany, 43 per cent of journeys to work are undertaken by cycles, whereas in Delft and Groningen in the Netherlands the figures are 43 and 50 per cent, respectively. Even larger numbers use cycles as the means to reach bus and railway stations and the promotion of such a 'bike and ride' policy offers great potential to reduce the use of commuter cars.[31]

Land Use Policies: Minimising the Need to Travel

Planners have a key part to play in promoting and adopting policies that reduce vehicle emissions. Too many cities have been designed to encourage the use of the car rather than to use buses, cycles or even to walk: it is estimated that two-thirds of all urban space in Los Angeles serves the need of cars. The traditional policy of separating home from work – reflecting that many workplaces were once major sources of pollution so segregation reduced pollution exposure – has increased the distances that employees now have to commute, which gives rise to increased fuel consumption, traffic congestion and poor air quality. Today in many cities, workplaces are no longer polluting or visually intrusive and a policy of separating home from work is no longer needed on this basis. Other policies that have

---

31 Harrison, J, Smorenburg, K, and McClintock, H (1993) 'Success stories in cycle planning', *Town and Country Planning*, vol 62, 328–335; Lowe, M D (1990) 'Cycling into the future', in Brown, L R *et al* (eds) *State of the World 1990*, W W Norton, New York, pp 119–134; Snelson, A, Lawson, S D and Morris, B (1993) 'Cycling motorists – how to encourage them', *Traffic Engineering and Control*, vol 34, 555–559

encouraged a dependency on cars are the siting of large leisure and shopping centres at the edge of or even outside a town. A reversal of this policy such that these facilities are located in existing city or suburban centres which are highly accessible by means other than the car will lead to reduced vehicle emissions. According to the UK Government, planning policies which reduced the need for people to travel could cut air pollution and fuel consumption by up to 15 per cent over the next 20 years. [32]

Although air pollution problems may become more severe as a city's physical size increases, there is no clear evidence that physical expansion alone leads to a worsening of air quality. Rather it is the nature of the transport systems, land use patterns, and spatial layout of a city that are more crucial. The 'compact city' is only one model for planners to consider. What is important is that planners adopt land use policies that result in homes, shops, leisure facilities, schools and workplaces being planned and sited in ways that encourage people to reach them by public transport, cycle or on foot.

Conclusions: Reducing Dependence on Private Vehicles

The principal cause of poor air quality in many towns and cities around the world is motor vehicle emissions. Traffic management policies and measures such as traffic calming, traffic smoothing, road pricing and parking controls can create situations in which emissions from existing traffic are kept as low as possible, they can divert traffic to less sensitive parts of the city, and they can reduce the number of cars in congested city centres. However, the number and use of cars are increasing at such a rapid rate that many of the air quality gains from these policies and measures will be offset in the future. What are needed are policies and measures which reduce the dependence on private vehicles and enable alternative means of mobility within urban areas to dominate, namely the use of buses, metro, light rail and cycles as well as walking.

---

32 Ecotec (1993) *Reducing Transport Emissions Through Planning*, Report to the Department of the Environment, HMSO, London; Department of the Environment (1994) *Planning Policy Guidance: Transport*, PPG13, HMSO, London; Department of the Environment (1994) *Planning Policy Guidance: Planning and Pollution Control*, PPG23, HMSO, London; Wood, C M (1990) 'Air pollution control by land use planning techniques: a British–American Review', *International Journal of Environmental Studies*, vol 35, pp 233–243; 'Planning policies to shun the car', *The Environmental Digest*, 70, Apr 1993, p 15. UK legislation now allows local authorities to resist the development of out of town shopping centres which reinforce the dependence on the car.

Chapter 8

Controlling Industrial and Residential Emissions

Introduction

Emissions from industrial plants, power stations, businesses and households can make significant contributions to urban air pollution problems. Electricity generating stations are major sources of pollutant emissions in both developed and developing countries as more than half the world's consumption of coal and one-third of fossil fuel consumption go to generate electricity. In the 1980s, electric power generation rose by 60 per cent in The North and by more than 110 per cent in The South. Without altered policies, pollution from the fossil fuel generation of electrical power will rise ten-fold in the next 40 years. A wide range of industrial plants can give rise to high concentrations of pollution in their vicinity. The current intensification of industrial activities in Southern countries is exposing more and more people to harmful emissions. Moreover, as these countries develop their industry often shifts from manufacturing textiles and wood products and food processing, towards far more polluting industries such as processing and manufacturing chemicals, petroleum, metal and paper. Industrial emissions and wastes are expected to increase more than five-fold in the next 40 years as demand for industrial goods escalates.[1]

Household emissions expose large numbers of people, especially women and children, to poor indoor air quality as well as adding pollutants to the ambient urban atmosphere. About half the world's people cook all or some of their meals using biomass fuels (wood, agricultural and forestry residues, and dung). Biomass fuels used in cooking, heating and small-scale industries account for about 14 per cent of the world's energy demands. In Southern

1 World Bank (1992) *World Development Report 1992: Development and the Environment*, Oxford University Press, New York

countries biomass supplies 35 per cent of energy needs and contributes significantly to the high levels of suspended particulates experienced in their cities. The transition from biomass fuels to commercial fuels such as kerosene, low-grade coals and lignite (often in the form of briquettes) can result in a worsening of particulate and sulphur dioxide pollution problems. As shown by the experience of many cities in the western world, air quality improvements can be achieved by increasing the efficiency of cooking stoves and heating systems and shifting to fuels such as anthracite, oil, electricity and natural gas. Increased attention has been given to district heating systems in recent years. They use the waste heat from power stations by tapping the steam when it leaves the steam turbine, leading the steam through a heat exchanger, and enabling heat to be provided to households, schools, businesses and hospitals via a network of pipes forming a district heating system. Currently in Europe only 6 per cent of the power plants recover their surplus heat to supply heating systems. If all suitable cities in the EU were to have district heating systems using heat from cogeneration it would save 15 per cent of energy use and reduce pollutant emissions significantly. Governments can encourage cleaner household heating systems by offering grants for converting heating systems to burn cleaner fuels and through legislation (eg designating areas in which only smokeless fuels may be burned). Ultimately, improved building insulation, energy conservation measures and more energy efficient household appliances can reduce energy consumption.[2]

Industrial plants and electricity generating stations can cause serious air pollution problems locally (as well as contributing to acid deposition in remote areas), but there are many ways of reducing emissions from these sources such as by using less polluting fuels, increased efficiency in the production and consumption of energy, and more widespread installation of effective pollution control equipment (Table 8.1). Land use planning policies can help minimise the exposure of urban residents to industrial emissions. Legislation can require strict emission standards and minimum technological standards to be met. The authorities can encourage the adoption of good practices through economic instruments. Managers of

---

2 Minimum energy efficiency standards need to be set for domestic appliances (refrigerators, dishwashers, washing machines and driers) and fittings (eg light bulbs). Such products should be required to display their energy efficiency (ecolabelling) for the benefit of consumers. To reduce emissions of volatile organic compounds which give rise to photochemical pollution, regulations need to be introduced requiring paints, glues and varnishes to be water-based or low in solvents. Bans on some activities undertaken in residential areas are appropriate in some cases such as restricting when garden bonfires may be lit or garden incinerators used. Even a complete ban on the use of petrol-powered lawn mowers and solid-fuel barbecues was introduced in Los Angeles. For progress on district heating installations in Europe, refer to Nijkamp, P and Perrels, P (1994) *Sustainable Cities in Europe*, Earthscan, London and 'Cogeneration to reduce energy consumption', *Acid News*, 2 Apr 1995, p 5. Half of all households in Denmark are connected to district heating systems.

Table 8.1 *Measures to reduce emissions from industrial sources*

Cleaner fuels		Technological Advances		Legislation and Planning Controls	Economic Instruments
Use less polluting fossil fuels	Use alternative and renewable energy sources	Post-combustion removal	Improved combustion and fuel efficiency		
Low-sulphur coal and oil	Hydro	Electrostatic precipitators	Low nitrogen oxides burners	Licensing	Emission charges
	Solar			Emission standards	Taxes on energy use
Natural gas	Wind	Flue gas desulphurisation	Fluidised bed combustion	Buffer zones	Grants
Coal cleaning (physical and chemical)	Biomass	Flue gas denitrification	Combined cycle gas plants	Minimum stack heights	Fines
	Fuel cells				Emissions trading
		Selective catalytic reduction	Integrated gasification – combined cycle plants	Land use planning and relocation	
		Selective non-catalytic reduction		Prescription of technology and practices	
				Spraying of coal stock piles	

industrial plants can be given some flexibility in their choice of meeting legislative requirements by allowing emissions trading to take place.

Cleaner Fuels

The sulphur content of coal varies from below 0.5 per cent to over 10 per cent by weight, the majority of coals currently in use being within the range 1–3 per cent. The sulphur dioxide released when the coal is burned is proportional to the sulphur content of the coal, although about 10 per cent is retained in the ash. Pyritic sulphur can be removed by relatively inexpensive physical cleaning, whereas organic sulphur, chemically bound in coal mineral matter, can be removed by chemical or biological processes, although the technologies are not yet well developed commercially. Physical coal cleaning can reduce sulphur dioxide emissions by up to 40 per cent and it can also reduce the amount of particulates (ash) produced.[3] Greater reductions in sulphur dioxide emissions can be achieved by switching from high-sulphur coal to less polluting fuels such as low-sulphur coals (less than 1 per cent), oil and natural gas (which contains no sulphur). The ultimate aim of a policy advocating cleaner fuels would be to use alternative energy sources such as geothermal, hydro, solar and wind energy and fuel cells.

Flue-gas Scrubbers

Particulate emissions from coal- and lignite-fired power stations can be removed from emissions using mechanical collectors and electrostatic precipitators, whereas flue gas desulphurisation and flue gas denitrification scrubbers (FGD) can remove a high percentage of sulphur dioxide and nitrogen oxides from stack emissions.[4]

Flue gas desulphurisation scrubbers can remove up to 95 per cent of the sulphur depending on the technique employed. Various methods and sorbents are available to capture the sulphur dioxide, with the most appropriate methods being those that produce marketable end products

---

3 Physical coal cleaning can be achieved by grinding the coal and washing it with water to remove the coal particles (which tend to float) from the rock and soil fractions (which fall to the bottom of the water). Pyritic sulphur has a specific gravity of about 5.0, whereas coal has a maximum specific gravity of around 1.8.

4 Flue gas desulphurisation was first installed at Battersea power station in London in the 1930s, but later removed. Only in the 1970s in Japan and the US did FGD systems begin to be used more widely. Not until the mid-1990s, under pressure from the European Union, did the UK begin installing FGD systems at the 4000 MW Drax coal-fired power station, the largest in Europe. Elsom, D M (1992) *Atmospheric Pollution*, second edition, Blackwell, Oxford, pp 313–316 and 327–330; Cochran, J R and Ferguson, A W (1993) 'Selective catalytic reduction for NO_x emission control', in Zanetti, P, Brebbia, C A, Garcia Gardea, J E and Ayala Milian, G (eds) *Air Pollution*, Computational Mechanics, Southampton, pp 703–718; Griffin, R D (1994) *Principles of Air Quality Management*, Lewis, Boca Raton, pp 159–206; Tavoulareas, E S and Charpentier, J-P (1994) *Clean Coal Technologies for Developing Countries*, World Bank, Washington DC

rather than sludge requiring disposal that simply results in an air pollution problem becoming a land or water pollution problem. Flue gas desulphurisation systems using wet scrubbing with limestone produces gypsum (calcium sulphate) used in making plaster, plasterboard, cement and concrete. After wet scrubbing the flue gases are reheated to improve their thermal buoyancy before being emitted to the air. Other methods produce sulphuric acid, elementary sulphur or ammonium sulphate, which are of commercial value.

Selective catalytic reduction (SCR) was pioneered by Japan in the 1970s, but is now being taken up more widely. It is a post-combustion process that reduces nitrogen oxides to form nitrogen and water by chemically reducing the nitrogen oxides with vaporized ammonia in the presence of a catalyst to nitrogen gas and water. Selective catalytic reduction is the most effective post-combustion nitrogen oxides control technology available and is capable of achieving reductions in nitrogen oxides of 80 to 90 per cent. There are also less expensive selective non-catalytic reduction systems available in which the reaction between nitrogen oxides and vaporized ammonia or urea (which decomposes at high temperature to ammonia, water and carbon dioxide) is achieved, not using a catalyst, but by thermal conditions. It is less effective than SCR, reducing emissions by 30–75 per cent.[5]

The capital cost of installing flue gas scrubbers is high, more so if retrofitting rather than if incorporating them into a new plant at the outset. Typically the cost of an FGD system may represent 15–20 per cent of the total capital costs for a new power station and it can add 5–10 per cent to the costs of electricity generation. Not surprisingly, given the cost and level of technology, most of the world's industrial and power station plants fitted with flue gas scrubbers are found in Japan, Europe and North America.[6]

Improved Combustion Processes

Improved efficiencies in combustion processes through the modification of existing plants or new technologies for new plants can offer significant reductions in the emissions of sulphur dioxide and nitrogen oxides from fossil-fuelled power stations. The most highly developed technologies are low nitrogen oxides burners, fluidised bed combustion (FBC) and integrated coal gasification/combined cycle systems.

Low nitrogen oxides burners separate combustion in the furnace into two stages. During the first stage, the conversion of fuel-bound nitrogen to nitrogen oxides is controlled by forcing the fuel nitrogen compounds into the gas phase using a fuel-rich condition. Under this condition, there is a

5 In Germany by 1992 there were 200 FGD systems, 140 SCR systems and 10 selective non-catalytic reduction systems fitted to power stations. Agren, C (1992) 'Flue-gas cleaning: big German gains', *Acid News*, 5, Dec, pp 15–16

6 In 1988, the percentage of national coal-fired generating capacity fitted with FGD systems varied from 20 per cent in the US, 40 per cent in (West) Germany, 50 per cent in Sweden, 60 per cent in Austria and 85 per cent in Japan.

deficiency of oxygen and the intermediate nitrogen compounds decay at a maximum rate into molecular nitrogen. The remaining combustion air is admitted in the second stage. This slow burning rate reduces the flame temperature, thereby limiting the amount of thermal nitrogen oxides formed during the latter stages of combustion. There are various designs of such burners but they all share the requirements for a much tighter control of the combustion process than was typically achieved with the previous generation of burner and combustion air system designs.

Fluidised bed combustion, developed since the 1960s, uses crushed coal fluidised with sand, its own ash or limestone in which the particles are supported by a strong rising current of air. Sulphur is removed through reactions with the limestone such that it can then be taken directly from the furnace as a solid residue which needs disposal. Better control of the furnace temperature means that emissions of nitrogen oxides are also reduced significantly (and FGD is not needed). Fluidised bed combustion enables a wide range of fuels to be burned, including those with a high ash and moisture content. Pressurised FBC is a further development in which the unit is enclosed in a pressure vessel enabling greater energy efficiency to be achieved.

Combined cycle gas (CCG) plants produce electricity by burning natural gas to drive a turbine while using the waste heat, which is usually discarded in single gas turbine plants, to produce steam to power a second turbine. Integrated gasification combined cycle (IGCC) plants generate electricity by transforming coal into a gas which then operates in a similar way to CCG plants. Although 10 per cent of the coal's potential energy is lost in this conversion, it is a much less polluting method of generating electricity from coal. The IGCC units have a high thermal efficiency (the proportion of energy converted into electricity from the fuel), achieving 45–50 per cent compared with 33–37 per cent in most conventional coal-fired plants or 40 per cent in new plants. Disregard for the efficient use of energy in central and eastern Europe and in Southern countries, together with weak enforcement of construction and operating standards, has meant that some coal-fired power stations achieve as little as 20 per cent efficiency, giving rise to excessive pollutant emissions. The best available commercial technology for natural gas currently is a CCG plant with a gas to electricity efficiency of 58 per cent. It represents a spinoff from aircraft engine technology and promises 60 per cent efficiency in the future.[7]

Planning Control

Land use planning can be used to separate major industrial sources from residential areas to reduce the impact of the high pollution levels often found

7 Geake, E (1992) 'Clean burn brightens coal's image', *New Scientist*, 7 Nov; 'Natural gas: a better option', *Acid News*, 4, Oct 1993, pp 9–11; 'Attempt to make coal a more acceptable fuel', *Acid News*, 1 Feb 1994, p 10. The world's largest IGCC in 1994 is located at Buggenum in the Netherlands with a capacity of 250 MW.

in the immediate vicinity of an industrial plant. Housing would not be allowed in the area around such a plant, being termed the buffer (or sanitary clearance) zone. Planting trees in the buffer zone not only screens the industrial plant, but the leaves of the trees provide increased surface areas on which particulate and gaseous pollutants can adhere or be absorbed, thus limiting the local spread of pollution directly. The width of buffer zones varies from a few hundred metres to 2 km. Unfortunately, in many cities in Southern countries the planning authorities experience difficulty in implementing this control measure as squatter settlements develop in the buffer zone.

During the past century the trend in Northern countries has been for industry to move out of the inner city where it developed originally and to be located in urban–peripheral industrial parks. Planning controls have encouraged this by advocating the deliberate separation of industrial areas from residential areas. This applies particularly with respect to residential areas of middle- and high-income dwellings rather than low-income dwellings, some of which form squatter settlements in the less attractive land close to industrial areas. Urban planning policies have long advocated the zoning of land in terms of industrial parks being located away and often downwind from suburban residential areas.[8] This separation has been maintained even though many commuters cannot use the urban core-oriented public transport network to get to work, even if they wanted to. Home and place of work are often long distances apart. However, as countries have developed, heavy industry has declined such that industrial or business parks often contain many businesses which create little pollution other than that connected with employees travelling to work. In other words, the original reasons for separation (eg toxic emissions, noise, visual intrusion) are no longer valid. What is now needed is a change of policy that will lead to a reduction in the energy consumed by employees travelling to and from work. There may remain a case for isolating potentially hazardous industrial plants, but industrial plants and businesses emitting little or no pollution directly should be relocated into areas well served by public transport and closer to where people live. Such a policy will

8 Land use zoning policies often locate industrial sources on the leeward side of an urban area, that is downwind in relation to the prevailing winds. The aim is to ensure that the pollutants are carried away from the city. However, wind direction is less critical than wind speed. The poorest dispersal of pollution occurs with light winds and these usually blow from non-prevailing wind directions. Locating industry on the windward side of an urban area in relation to the prevailing winds may be more effective providing these winds are strong and can encourage dispersal of the pollutants. Siting of industry in relation to topography can help minimise pollution impacts by choosing exposed, windy sites in preference to valleys and basins where pollution is liable to be trapped by temperature inversions. Wood, C M (1990) 'Air pollution control by land use planning techniques: a British–American Review', *International Journal of Environmental Studies*, vol 35, pp 233–243

encourage the use of public transport systems which are far more energy efficient and less polluting per passenger kilometre than cars. It will also encourage more people to cycle and walk to work.[9]

Licensing of Industry

One of the most important actions that countries, or city authorities if they have the powers, need to take concerning industrial plants, power stations and businesses is to set stringent emission standards, specifying the maximum amount or rate of pollution allowed to be released from each source type. This can then be followed up by requiring that each emission source obtains a licence both for its construction and operation (renewed annually), confirming that it has adopted the best available technology and practices for minimising emissions and meeting emissions standards. The strictness with which emission standards are set and licences granted varies greatly from country to country at present. Some countries such as the US have set stringent technology forcing standards giving companies a set time, usually several years, to meet an emission standard which can be met only by technological innovation. It is good practice to ensure that construction and operating licences, specifying the type of technology needed to be installed to achieve emission standards, are revised periodically as new technology becomes available. Less strict emission standards and technology requirements are usually applied to existing industrial plants as it is more expensive to retrofit control technology than new plant. Terms used to indicate what emission standards, level of technology and type of pollution control equipment are to be used by industry include the traditional UK best practicable means (BPM) and its replacement, the European Union's best available technology/techniques not entailing excessive cost (BATNEEC). Some of the US requirements include maximum achievable control technology (MACT), the best available control technology (BACT), the generally available control technology (GACT) and the reasonably available control technology (RACT). Such phrases indicate that careful consideration is given to the cost of the technology and the state of technology available.

Some countries set minimum heights for industrial stacks (chimneys) on the assumption that the taller the stack the greater the dispersion of pollutants away from the point of origin. Wind speeds normally increase with height, so tall stacks emit pollutants into stronger winds, which encourage dispersion and dilution. Tall stacks are needed for industrial plants located in valleys and basins because these locations are prone to low-level temperature inversions. The tall stacks enable emitted plumes to penetrate an inversion. Unfortunately, the wider dispersion achieved by tall

9 White, R R (1992) 'The international transfer of urban technology: does the North have anything to offer for the global environmental crisis?', *Environment and Urbanization*, vol 4 (2), pp 109–120

stacks has contributed to the widespread and worsening problem of acid deposition (by sulphates and nitrates), which has had serious adverse effects on many ecosystems even in remote areas. Concern for this problem has resulted in a discouragement of the (very) tall stack policy in recent years on the basis that emissions should be reduced at source rather than be simply spread further afield.

Stringent planning controls need to be applied to potentially hazardous industrial plants. The operators of such plants should be required to draw up on-site and off-site emergency plans to deal with an accidental release of toxic emissions as well as to adopt strict day to day safety practices and procedures. The devastating consequences of inadequate safety and lack of emergency plans were clearly demonstrated by the chemical accidents at Seveso, Italy in 1976 and at Bhopal, India in 1984, as well as by the nuclear reactor accident at Chernobyl in the former Soviet Union in 1986, which resulted in the world's most serious release of radiation. Although countries such as the US and European Union Member States have introduced legislation concerning hazardous industrial plants (eg the European Union's Seveso Directive), most countries in The South have yet to implement the necessary legislation.

Emissions Trading: Selling Pollution Permits

The US Clean Air Act 1990 encouraged the establishment of trading markets for sulphur dioxide emissions following its requirement that the total annual emissions of sulphur dioxide from power stations and industrial plants exceeding 25 MW capacity had to be cut by 10 Mt by the year 2000. The most polluting 110 plants had to attain the reductions by 1995 and the rest by 2000. In 1993 an emissions trading market was initiated in which companies were given permits equivalent to about half of their average emissions in the 1980s. If companies wanted to continue emitting pollutants at existing levels beyond the deadline of 1995 or 2000, they would need to buy emission credits. Alternatively, they would have to halve their emissions. In 1993 the government auctioned off 275,000 t of permissible pollutants to begin the trading. Those companies deciding to delay fitting of flue gas scrubbers or changing to cleaner fuels bought some emission credits at $122–450 per tonne – significantly less than most estimates of fitting scrubbers. Companies exceeding their emission limit are liable for fines of $2000 per excessive tonne. Companies fitting scrubbers or switching to low-sulphur fuel and so reducing their sulphur dioxide emissions can trade these 'permits to pollute' on the market. A new industrial plant must purchase credits that will permit its sulphur dioxide emissions. When a plant closes, its stock of credits becomes non-transferable and is effectively retired. Where a company replaces an older plant by a newer one, the company receives one credit for every two credits held by the old plant. To stimulate the trading (although it is allowing an increase in pollution), Congress set aside 300,000 sulphur dioxide credits in 1995 to reward energy-efficient utilities who could then bank, sell or use the credits as appropriate.

Emissions trading is a market-based approach to air quality management which sets out to meet the dual goals of environmental protection and economic growth. It is estimated to save industry $2 billion per year in implementation costs over traditional command and control measures. It is a relatively easy system to implement, although it requires careful monitoring of emissions to ensure companies comply with their allowances, and it offers the regulator the option of withdrawing or devaluing the permits to reduce national emissions of a pollutant. The scheme operates nationally rather than within a city. There is concern that trading might lead to air quality in one area worsening or that this scheme fails to recognise that one area may be more vulnerable to pollution emissions than another. The concern to date has mainly centred around acid deposition effects on ecosystems, but could equally apply to the numbers of people at risk in different parts of an urban area from, say, acid aerosols. Legislation does exist which requires that new sources do not led to significant deterioration of air quality, even if air pollution standards are not violated (ie non-attainment area), but this does mean that air quality is allowed to worsen slightly.[10]

In 1994 emissions trading in the US extended to trading between different pollutants, with an Arizona company exchanging 25,000 t of sulphur dioxide credits for 1.75 Mt of carbon dioxide credits from a New York State company. Emissions trading between countries may take place in the future under a scheme called Joint Implementation, whereby nations trade carbon dioxide quotas as part of the UNEP Climate Change Convention. Although this scheme concerns carbon dioxide emissions it may have implications for other pollutants. For example, three American electricity companies have agreed to help fund the conversion of a power station at Decin, Czech Republic, from lignite to natural gas as well as to improve its energy efficiency in exchange for 40 per cent of the carbon dioxide emission–reduction credits. In other words, residents of the city of Decin will benefit from the virtual elimination of sulphur dioxide and particulate emissions from their power station and the US companies hope they can offset these (less costly) greenhouse gas reductions against any they have to make at their own plants.[11]

---

10 Combs, R and Selwyn, J (1993) 'Emission permits', *Acid News*, 5, Dec, pp 11–13; Goldburg, C B and Lave, L B (1992) 'Progress on market incentives for abating pollution: trading sulphur dioxide allowances', *Environmental Science and Technology*, vol 26, pp 2076–2078; Kiernan, V (1993) 'What am I bid for two tonnes of sulphur dioxide?', *New Scientist*, 10 Apr, p 10; 'US pollution futures market', *The Environmental Digest*, 69, March 1993, p 14; 'Pollution trading starts in US', *The Environment Digest*, 59/60, May/Jun 1992, p 12; Tiger, A (1995) 'Emissions trading: slow in getting going', *Acid News*, 3, Jun 1995, p 6. Canada, concerned about emissions from US industrial plants near its border, may be able to buy up permits of these plants and then retire them.

11 Kiernan, V (1994) 'Market forces clean up in the US', *New Scientist*, 26 Nov, p 11; Kiernan, V (1994) 'US trades green points in Bohemia', *New Scientist*, 7 May, p 5

The South Coast Air Quality Management District launched the Regional Air Incentive Market in 1994. Emission limits were set for sulphur dioxide and nitrogen oxides (and later for VOCs) and the 1000 participating companies received baseline emission credits. They could then choose to reduce their emissions below their allocated limit and sell the excess credits at twice yearly auctions to companies who prefer to pay for the right to emit more. Air quality improvements are achieved by an annual reduction in emission limits of between 5 and 8 per cent. If the California scheme proves successful then it may gain wider adoption in Canada, Mexico and the European Union.[12]

Conclusions: the Government's Role

Governments have a key part to play in requiring and encouraging industry, businesses and householders to become less polluting by improving energy efficiencies, adopting cleaner technologies, using cleaner fuels and minimising energy consumption in general. Given the high costs involved in cleaning up industry alone, it may be appropriate for Southern nations to initially target the worst polluters.[13]

12 'California markets air pollution', *The Environmental Digest*, 77/78, Nov/Dec 1993, p 16; South Coast Air Quality Management District (1995) *Annual Report 1994: Clean Air is Everybody's Business*, SCAQMD, Diamond Bar, 16 pp

13 Weak enforcement of emission standards in China in the past, in part due to the government's encouragement of industrial production at the expense of environmental quality, has resulted in large numbers of industrial plants exceeding emission standards. In a bid to tackle this situation not only are fines being used to try to clean up industry, but in 1993 the government took the unusual step of trying to shame the gross polluters by publicly naming 3000 polluting businesses. These businesses represented only 4 per cent of all polluters but were responsible for over 60 per cent of the country's total industrial pollution. 'China lists polluters', *The Environmental Digest*, 71, May 1993, p 12

Chapter 9

Smog City Case Studies

Illustrating the Seriousness of the Urban Air Pollution Problem

Most of the world's cities are suffering some serious air pollution problems which are being tackled with varying degrees of success. Four case studies are examined here: Los Angeles, London, Mexico City and Athens. Los Angeles was chosen because it is the city which first experienced serious photochemical smogs and where the authorities have applied some of the most radical and stringent pollution control policies in the world in an attempt to rid the city of air pollutants. London is where the term smog was first coined, being used to describe the polluted smoky fogs it had been experiencing for centuries. London highlights the fact that the successful elimination of one major air pollution problem does not necessarily mean that others will not emerge requiring even more stringent pollution control policies and measures. Unlike the other case studies, Athens is not a megacity (commonly defined as urban agglomerations with a population exceeding 10 million), but it highlights how even a medium-sized city generating sizeable pollutant emissions in an unfavourable topographical setting and climate can suffer pollution problems as severe as any megacity. Mexico City is the final case study explored. It offers a dire warning of the unhealthy air quality that many other cities in rapidly developing countries may have to cope with in the near future – if they are not already having to do so – unless economic, social and planning policies can be followed which check the phenomenal surge in pollutant emissions that has characterised most urban development in the world until now.

Los Angeles: Car City, Smog City

Los Angeles – car city, smog city. To many people, linking these two descriptions of Los Angeles explains why the region experiences such poor air quality. Indeed, emissions from 9 million motor vehicles in the Los

Angeles basin are responsible for many of its air pollution problems but industry, businesses, urban planners and the climate have all also played a part in creating the serious air quality problem facing Los Angeles today.

Los Angeles first experienced the yellow pall of photochemical smogs in the 1940s. Ever since, these smogs have been stinging eyes, burning throats and lungs, and causing tightness in the chests of residents and visitors to the city. Moreover, the effects can be long term as children growing up in the city have been shown to have suffered a 10–15 per cent reduction in lung function. Autopsies of more than 100 Los Angeles County teenagers and young men who died suddenly between 1987 and 1989 showed that three out of four had some lung damage. The autopsies did not identify causes, but air pollution was believed to a factor. The human health costs of the basin's air pollution have been estimated at around $10 billion. Even if concentrations of only one pollutant, PM_{10}, could be reduced to meet federal standards, this would prevent 1600 premature deaths annually among those who suffer from chronic respiratory disease.[1]

The Los Angeles basin or South Coast Air Basin (comprising four counties) contains nearly 14 million people, 9 million vehicles and 40,000 industrial sources of pollution. Road transport accounts for 44 per cent of reactive organic gas emissions (VOCs), 55 per cent of nitrogen oxides and 87 per cent of carbon monoxide emissions. Around 70 per cent of the surface of Los Angeles is devoted to the car in the form of roads, driveways, parking and petrol stations. This includes the Santa Monica Freeway (I-10) from Los Angeles to Culver City which is the busiest highway in the US with 288,000 vehicles a day. Pollution emissions become trapped within the basin, which is bounded by mountain ranges on three sides and with the Pacific Ocean forming the fourth side. Air pollution problems are made worse in the basin by the presence of frequent temperature inversions, whereby cool air from the Pacific Ocean underlies warm air aloft. This inversion layer traps pollutants and limits the amount of clean air into which pollutants can dilute while, at the same time, the mountains prevent the pollutants from escaping the basin. Long periods of intense sunshine and high temperatures favour photochemical reactions which produce ozone. Land and sea breezes cause the pollutants trapped in the basin to be recirculated around the basin. The effect of the sea breeze circulation is evident in the spatial distribution of the number of days when ozone exceeds federal standards in that the highest exceedances occur well inland away from downtown Los Angeles, which is the major source of the precursor emissions (Figure 9.1). A similar

1 Hall, J V, Winer, A M, Kleinman, M T, Lurman, F W, Brajer, V M and Colome, S D (1992) 'Valuing the health benefits of clean air', *Science*, vol 2655, pp 812–816; Krupnick, A J and Portney P R (1991) 'Controlling urban air pollution: a benefit-cost assessment', *Science*, vol 252, pp 522–528; Lents, J M and Kelly, W J (1993) 'Clearing the air in Los Angeles', *Scientific American*, vol 269 (4), pp 18–25

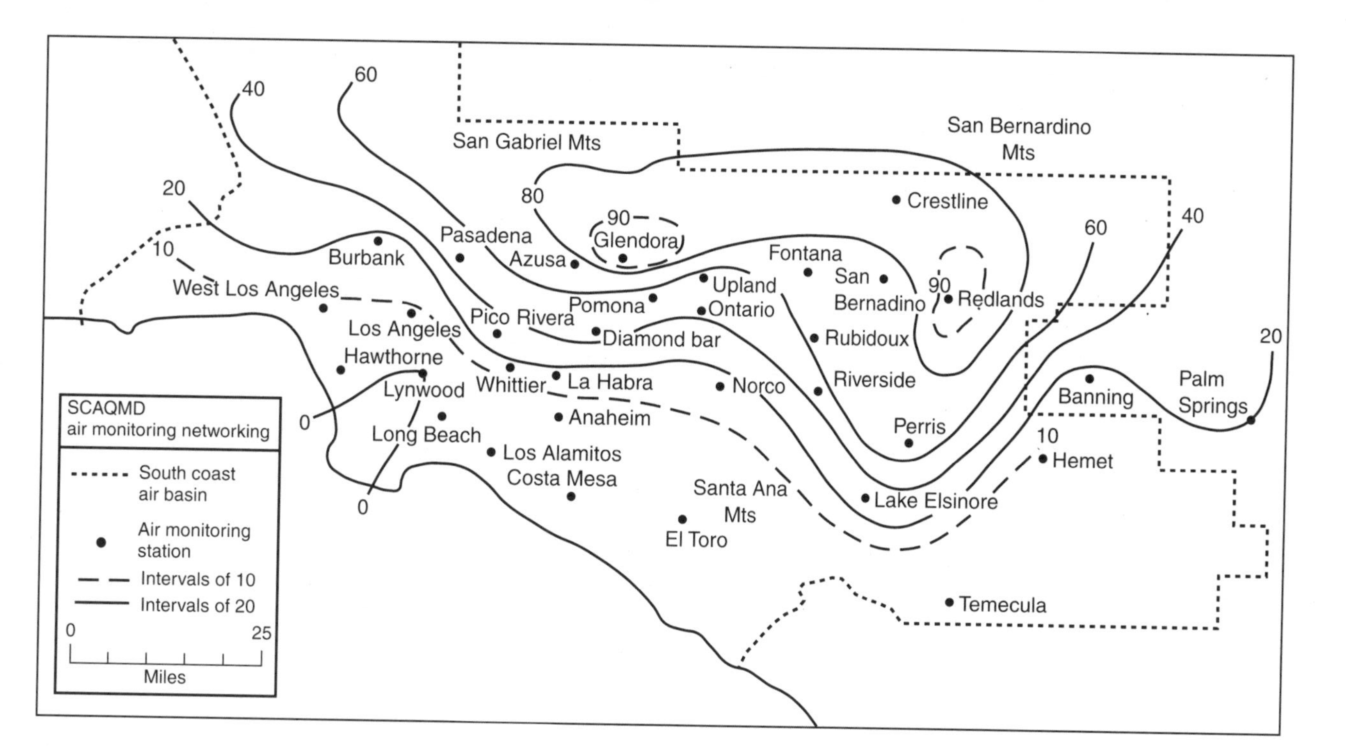

Figure 9.1 *Number of days on which the federal one-hour ozone standard of 120 ppb (240 μg/m³) was exceeded in the South Coast Air Basin in 1993*

Source: South Coast Air Quality Management District (1994) *Final 1994 Air Quality Management Plan: Meeting the Clean Air Challenge*, SCAQMD, Diamond Bar, ch 2, p 10

spatial pattern occurs for peak hourly ozone concentrations.[2] Some pollution does escape from the basin. For example, of the 90 days in San Diego in 1993 when state standards were exceeded, 51 days (57 per cent) were caused by the transport of pollution from Los Angeles, about 190 km (120 miles) to the north.

The seriousness of California's air quality problem, not just Los Angeles but Sacramento, San Diego and San Francisco, has long allowed it to adopt stricter standards and control policies than those applied nationwide. California claims to have the strictest air quality standards and control programme in the world. A range of standards and alert levels has beeen adopted for health protection purposes. The state standard for average hourly ozone concentrations is 90 ppb (75 on the Pollutant Standards Index; PSI) whereas the federal standard is 120 ppb (100 PSI). California established a health advisory reporting level of 150 ppb (138 PSI) in September 1991 after medical research showed that ozone posed a health threat at this lower concentration (Figure 9.2). Sensitive individuals are advised to avoid all outdoor activity and athletes are advised to avoid strenuous outdoor activities at this level. A stage 1 episode (commonly called a smog alert) is issued at 200 ppb (200 PSI) and sensitive people are advised to go indoors, and the general public are told to avoid vigorous outdoor activities. A stage 2 episode, when all physical activity should stop, is issued at 350 ppb (275 PSI). Once stage 2 alerts were commonplace (eg 15 in 1980), but none has occurred since 1988. A stage 3 episode, last called in 1974, when everyone should stay indoors, is set at 500 ppb (400 PSI).

Despite several decades of pioneering and increasingly stringent control legislation, Los Angeles experienced the worst air quality in the US in 1993 with respect to carbon monoxide, nitrogen dioxide and ozone, together with very high levels of fine particulates. Table 9.1 highlights that Los Angeles–Long Beach and Riverside–San Bernardino are very much worse than other cities in the US with regard to the number of days when ozone exceeded the federal standard from 1984–1993. Interpreting long-term trends from this table is difficult due to the confounding factors of meteorology and emission changes. For example, just as the worsening in 1988 can be attributed in part to meteorological conditions being more conducive to ozone formation than previous years, the 1992 decrease was due, in part, to meteorological conditions being less favourable for ozone formation than in other recent years. Also, since the worst year of 1988, the volatility of petrol has been lowered by federal and state regulations, so leading to a reduction in emissions of ozone precursors. Trends which attempt to adjust for meteorology do show a downward trend during the past decade. For

2 Blumenthal, D L, White W H and Smith, T B (1978) 'Anatomy of a Los Angeles smog episode: pollutant transport in the daytime sea breeze regime', *Atmospheric Environment*, vol 12, pp 893–907; Elsom D M (1992) *Atmospheric Pollution: a Global Problem*, second edition, Blackwell, Oxford, pp 41–42 and 226–231; GEMS (1992) *Urban Air Pollution in Megacities of the World*, Blackwell for WHO/UNEP, New York, pp 25, 135–146

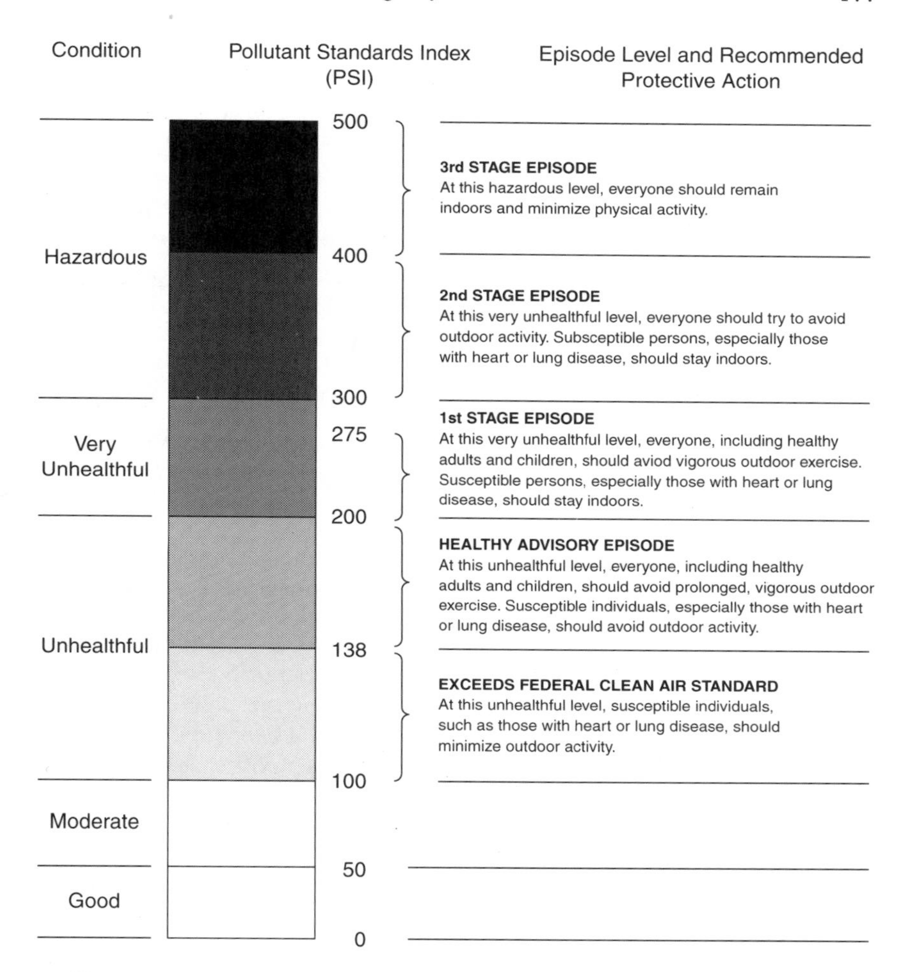

Figure 9.2 *Health advice associated with various Pollutants Standards Index numbers used in the South Coast Air Basin*

example, the number of days in the Los Angeles basin exceeding the federal standard showed an overall decrease of 22 per cent over the period 1976 to 1991 (from 155 to 121 days). Similarly, the number of basin days with stage 1 episodes showed a 64 per cent decrease over the same period (from 111 to 40 days).[3]

3 Davidson, A (1993) 'Update on ozone trends in California's South Coast Air Basin', *Air and Waste*, vol 43, pp 226–227; California Air Resources Board (1992) *Ozone Air Quality Trends in California 1981–1990*, California Air Resources Board, Sacramento; South Coast Air Quality Management District (1994) *Air Quality Trends, 1976–1993*, South Coast Air Quality Management District, Diamond Bar

Table 9.1 *Number of days when hourly ozone levels exceeded the federal standard of 120 ppb (240 µg/m³) for the period 1984–93 for selected locations in the US*

Area	1984	1985	1986	1987	1988	1989	1990	1991	1992	1993
Houston	49	48	43	52	48	34	48	40	30	26
Los Angeles	152	154	159	145	165	138	118	111	130	102
New York	17	19	7	15	32	10	13	19	3	6
Philadelphia	22	25	19	32	34	17	11	24	3	20
Riverside	164	142	151	149	163	146	121	119	126	112
San Diego	51	50	42	40	45	54	39	25	19	14
Washington	12	12	10	20	35	4	5	16	2	12

Source: Extracted from US Environmental Protection Agency (1994) *National Air Quality and Emissions Trends Report, 1993*, US EPA Report 454/R-94-026, Research Triangle Park, NC, pp. 124–125

Almost like a boxer throwing one last heavy punch aimed at dealing with its pollution problems once and for all, the South Coast Air Basin adopted the radical Air Quality Management Plan initially in 1989, with the final version being approved in 1994. This remarkable plan has three tiers or stages based on the anticipated availability of levels of technology. The first tier relies on existing technology, the second on breakthrough technologies and the third tier relies on technology that has not yet been fully developed, but is considered attainable. Through this plan the South Coast Air Basin is intended to attain federal standards for nitrogen dioxide by the end of 31 December 1995, carbon monoxide by 31 December 2000, fine particulates (PM_{10}) by 31 December 2001 with provisions for a five year extension (ie a target of 2006 being most likely) and ozone by 15 November 2010. The target date for achieving state standards for nitrogen dioxide is the end of 1997, carbon monoxide the end of 2000, PM_{10} post-2010 and ozone post-2010.[4]

One of the key measures in the plan is to require that 40 per cent of cars, 70 per cent of freight vehicles and all diesel buses convert to cleaner fuels such as methanol by 1998. However, the most radical requirement is that 2 per cent of cars sold in the state in 1998 and 10 per cent by 2003 must be zero emission vehicles (ZEVs). With subsequent re-examination this requirement may be extended to 20 per cent by 2005, 35 per cent by 2007 and 50 per cent by 2009 (see Table 6.6). By 2003, not only will 10 per cent

4 Lloyd, A C, Lents, J M, Green C and Nemeth, P (1989) 'Air quality management in Los Angeles: perspectives on past and future emission control strategies', *Journal of Air and Waste Management Association*, vol 39, pp 696–703; South Coast Air Quality Management District (1989) *Air Quality Management Plan*, South Coast Air Quality Management District, El Monte; South Coast Air Quality Management District (1994) *Final Report Air Quality Management Plan: Meeting the Clean Air Challenge*, South Coast Air Quality Management District, Diamond Bar

Table 9.2 *Californian emission standards for motor vehicles (g/mile, US test cycle)*

Type of vehicle	Carbon monoxide	Nitrogen oxides	Reactive Organic gases*
Conventional	3.4	0.4	0.250
Transitional low emission	3.4	0.4	0.125
Low emission	3.4	0.2	0.075
Ultra-low emission	1.7	0.2	0.040
Zero emission	0	0	0

* Non-methane hydrocarbons (VOCs).

of all new vehicle sales have to be ZEVs, but 15 per cent will have to be ultra-low emission vehicles and 75 per cent low-emission vehicles. Emission limits are given in Table 9.2. By 2007 all new cars must use clean-burning fuels such as methanol or electric power. Major motor and oil manufacturers have expressed doubts that technology can meet these demands, but after several years of trying to get the pollution control agencies to weaken and delay their proposals they appear to have accepted the need to try to meet the stringent fuel and vehicle requirements. It may have helped some manufacturers to have accepted the decision, albeit reluctantly, because California is the largest car market in the world and failure to comply would mean large fines or being barred from selling in California. Chrysler has opted for advanced lead–acid batteries for its ZEVs, although it considers that nickel–metal hydride batteries have shown much promise when production costs can be reduced. Using 27 connected batteries, Chrysler's minivan can travel 96–112 km (60–70 miles) before recharging is needed (eight hours for full recharge using conventional household current). Each battery pack will cost between $4500 and $6000 and last about three years. Chrysler must produce about 1500 electric vehicles in California in 1998, rising to 7500 by 2003.[5] General Motors launched its $35,000 two-seater EV-1 in 1996. It uses lead-acid batteries (nearly 40 per cent of the car's weight) and has to be recharged every 140 km (88 miles). California's decision to insist on sales of a small but growing number of ZEVs has boosted interest and investment in developing electric cars, not only in other US states such as New York and Massachusetts, but throughout the world. Many other cities in the US and elsewhere in the world may follow the technology forcing policy example set by California. There were 12,600 clean-fuelled vehicles in California in 1994. The LA Metropolitan Transit Authority operates 330 methanol-powered buses and has ordered 196 compressed natural gas buses. The Orange County Transit Authority plans to purchase 70 propane buses. Smaller electric shuttle buses are growing in numbers throughout the state.

5 Nauss, D W (1995) 'Chrysler to sell electric van battery choice', *Los Angeles Times*, 6 April; Reeves, P (1994) 'LA recharges its batteries', *The Independent*, 17 May

Tighter federal and state emission standards for vehicles are only fully effective in tackling pollution problems if vehicle owners ensure that their vehicles meet these standards. In 1984, vehicle inspection tests were introduced to ensure they did. These smog checks are required for motor vehicles once every two years or after a change of ownership. However, an undercover investigation found that only one in four of all vehicles was receiving a reasonably thorough inspection. This has prompted California to introduce centralised inspection stations (test only) as well as the current decentralised system of garages (test and repair) licensed to undertake smog checks. Older vehicles or vehicle makes with a higher than average frequency of smog check failures may be assigned to centralised stations to ensure the highest standard of test is applied. As found in many other cities around the world, it is the 10 per cent high-emitting vehicles that contribute more than half the total vehicle emissions. To help identify gross polluters there is the 1-800-CUT-SMOG line to report polluting vehicles so as to encourage these vehicle owners to clean them up. Vehicle scrapping programmes have been explored as a means of dealing with some of the older vehicles which have high emissions. Payments are made to scrap these cars or loans are offered for replacement (5000 were scrapped in 1993 and 1994).

The pollution potential of petrol has been examined critically in recent years and reformulated petrol has been introduced. Reformulated petrol is petrol whose composition has been changed to reduce emissions of VOCs and benzene and it contains an oxygenate such as ethanol or MTBE. Whereas oxygenated fuels are intended to reduce carbon monoxide levels (and to a lesser extent hydrocarbons) during cold days, reformulated fuels are aimed at reducing smog-forming emissions in warm weather. Phase 1 reformulated petrol became available in 1992 and is intended to reduce reactive organic gases by 7 per cent. Further reductions are expected with the improved phase 2 reformulated petrol from 1996. Reformulated petrol is compatible with modern car engines and fuel systems, although in poorly maintained cars it may lead to a slight reduction in distance travelled and increased hesitations after start-up. The federal Clean Air Act 1990 mandated the use of reformulated petrol in all areas that failed to meet air quality standards for ozone. Conventional petrol may not be sold in those areas. The federal Environmental Protection Agency classified non-attainment areas for ozone into five classes according to the extent of their problem. These five classes ranged from marginal (relatively easy to clean up) to extreme (which will take a lot of work and a long time to clean up). Los Angeles is the only area to be classified as extreme. The 1990 act uses this new classification to tailor clean-up requirements to the severity of the pollution and set deadlines for reaching clean-up goals.[6] California adopted

6 Griffin, R D (1994) *Principles of Air Quality Management*, CRC Press, Boca Raton, pp 283–297; Klausmeier, R and Kishan, S (1995) 'World-wide developments in motor vehicle inspection/maintenance (I/M) programs', *Proceedings of the 10th*

its own Clean Air Act two years earlier (in 1988). It has often been the case that federal pollution control legislation follows California's lead. This Act sets guidelines for the strategies and specific measures to tackle its extreme air pollution problems and aims to reduce emissions of carbon monoxide, nitrogen oxides and reactive organic gases (VOCs) by 5 per cent every year.

Control of emissions from industry and businesses is through the use of operating permits. To provide some flexibility and market incentives an emissions trading scheme was set up in the Los Angeles area in 1994 for 1000 of the biggest polluters. It is called RECLAIM (Regional Clean Air Incentives Market). Permits are issued for a specified value in emissions of hydrocarbons and nitrogen oxides and, more recently, for VOCs. Companies that reduce emissions below the permitted level can sell the credits so gained to others for whom similar action would be uneconomic. Each year the emission value of the permit for each company is reduced by 5–8 per cent, forcing companies to reduce their emissions and so leading to a steady improvement in air quality from year to year. By 1997, if the scheme continues to expand, it may have saved companies about $670 million.[7]

Vehicle emissions are being cut down by reducing the number of solo commuters and increasing the number of workers who take transit, car pool, van pool, walk, cycle or telecommute (eliminating 3 million worktrips by 2010 is the telecommuting target). Employers with 100 or more employees at a work site are required to take part in the trip reduction programme. An average vehicle ridership (AVR) is calculated by dividing the number of employees reporting for work in working hours by the number of vehicles driven by the employees over the working week. If there are 300 employees reporting for work each day making 1327 journeys by vehicle during the week, the AVR is 1500 divided by 1327, which equals 1.13. In 1988, the regional AVR was about 1.15. AVR targets are set which are 1.75 in the downtown area, 1.5 in intermediate areas and 1.3 in outer areas. It is likely that these targets will be raised in the coming years. Employers are required to have a plan approved which outlines how the AVR target will be achieved and maintained. Trip reduction plans are expected to include a list of incentives such as preferential parking for ride sharers, subsidies for car pools or use of public transport and facilities to encourage the use of bicycles. Adoption of non-standard work schedules (eg 40 hours over four days or 80 hours over nine days) may also help reduce the number of trips. Employers failing to submit plans have been fined such that total fines amounted to $2 million in 1992. By 1994, around 6000 companies employing

---

World Clean Air Congress, Espoo, Finland, vol 3, Finnish Air Pollution Protection Society, Helsinki, paper 546

7 South Coast Air Quality Management District (1995) *Annual Report 1994: Clean Air is Everybody's Business*, South Coast Air Quality Management District, Diamond Bar, 16 pp; 'Smog exchanges', *Acid News*, No 2, May 1992, p 14; 'South Coast Air Quality Management District', *Journal of Air and Waste Management Association*, vol 42, 1992, pp 704–705; 'Smog trading gets green light', *Journal of Air and Waste Management Association*, vol 42, 1992, p 402

nearly 2 million commuters had set trip reduction plans. Although this tackles commuters employed by large companies, it does not tackle other work-related journeys, shoppers and many other journeys.[8]

Four out of five employees throughout the US enjoy free parking either through parking spaces made available to them or through public parking costs being paid by employers. Los Angeles intends to limit free parking and require employers to offer employees cash equivalent to the value of their parking perks so that more employees may choose to share transport, walk or cycle, or use public transport. Los Angeles once had an extensive tram system (using the Red-cars), but the motor manufacturers bought it and closed it down. In 1990 a new light railway network began with the Blue line running between downtown Los Angeles and Long Beach for 32 km (20 miles) and in 1993 the 27 km (17 miles) Red Line was added, running north from downtown to Hollywood. Expansion of the network will add the Busway and the Green Line such that in 30 years time there may be 590 km (370 miles) of light rail network. The 150-mile metro network being developed at a cost of $5 billion may encounter problems in persuading some people to travel underground in an earthquake-prone area. Nevertheless, public transport is at last receiving the attention it has needed for several decades. Plans for a fully integrated public transport system for southern California are estimated to cost up to $100 billion. Some of the potential benefits of a public transport system will not be realised because the Los Angeles Basin is so vast, about 95 km (60 miles) wide. This means that mass transit systems can serve only a limited number of commuters, especially given that many commuting journeys in the basin are not to or from downtown Los Angeles.

Los Angeles is attempting to improve air quality using a wide range of measures. Although technofixes involving the introduction of less polluting fuels and vehicles are an essential part of the long-term air quality control strategy for the basin, increasing attention is being given to try to modify the lifestyle of residents, such as through ride sharing and telecommuting programmes, staggering working hours, encouraging greater participation in park and ride commuting, and even moving businesses closer to residential areas. Air quality is better than it was in the 1950s and 1960s, but it is still poor even after implementing the most stringent air quality standards and pollution control policies in the US. Rapid population growth, the expanding size of the urban area and the distance travelled by vehicles continue to partially offset progress towards clean air. Consequently, doubt remains as to whether the Los Angeles basin will attain federal and state air quality standards within the next 10 years as the Air Quality Management Plan intends. The decades that have passed during which Los Angeles residents have had to suffer poor air quality with only limited improvements

8 Bae, C-H C (1993) 'Air quality and travel behaviour; untying the knot', *Journal of American Planning Association*, vol 59, p 65-74; Grant, W (1994) 'Transport and air pollution in California', *Environmental Health and Management*, vol 5, pp 31–34

having been achieved during that time offer a warning, or perhaps a lesson, to other megacities both in the Northern and the Southern world.

Smogs Return to London

In the late 1980s, residents of London realised they had been mistaken to believe that smogs were part of their history and would not return. The smogs returned, though not in the same form. London was once infamous for its thick, yellow–green polluted fogs (sometimes called 'pea soupers'). These enveloped London each autumn and winter when a high-pressure system (anticyclone) brought low-level temperature inversions, very light winds and subfreezing temperatures lasting several days. Vast amounts of suspended particulates and sulphur dioxide from millions of domestic chimneys serving inefficient coal-burning household fires together with emissions from thousands of wasteful industrial plants spewed into the foggy and stagnant atmosphere of the River Thames basin (Figure 9.3). The result was inevitable: dense, health-threatening smog. One of the worst London smogs occurred from 4 to 10 December 1952, being the culmination of a long sequence of such smogs that had been experienced for more than a century. Sooty smoke from coal burning produced peak daily concentrations of black smoke exceeding 5000 μg/m^3 and average daily

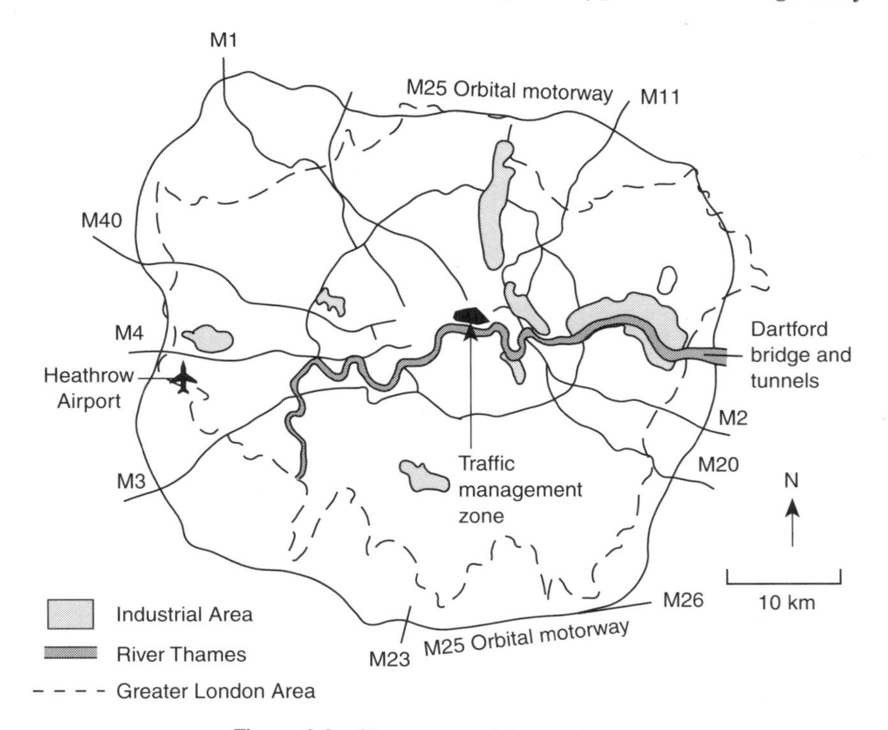

Figure 9.3 *Sketch map of Greater London*

sulphur dioxide concentrations of between 1000 and 1400 ppb (3000–4000 μg/m^3), leading to a highly acidic fog (with a pH of perhaps 1.6, as acid as the electrolyte in a car battery) and with visibility reduced to 5 m at times. This air pollution episode resulted tragically in nearly 4000 premature deaths among the elderly and those with heart and respiratory diseases.[9]

The 1952 smog prompted the government to introduce the Clean Air Act of 1956 (with an update in 1968). It permitted local authorities in London and other urban areas to designate smoke control areas within which only smokeless fuels were allowed to be burned. Financial assistance was given to householders to convert their domestic heating appliances to use smokeless fuels. The Act also strengthened industrial emissions standards and set minimum stack heights so that industrial emissions would be dispersed away from the local vicinity more effectively. Other London smogs followed the disastrous 1952 smog, but they never caused so many deaths again.[10] Since the late 1950s, smoke and sulphur dioxide concentrations have fallen dramatically as Londoners converted heating appliances to burn smokeless fuels initially and then, in later years, installed more convenient gas, electricity and oil central heating systems. Industrial emissions fell as electricity generation became consolidated into large 2000 MW power stations which were located away from the city. The extensive industry around the docks to the east of the city also declined or relocated further eastwards along the Thames estuary as London's role as a port declined. In the 1970s the fall in domestic and industrial emissions of sulphur dioxide levels was being offset by emissions from new development office block developments heated by fuel oil with a high sulphur content (3.5 per cent). Consequently, the City of London introduced legislation limiting the sulphur content of fuel oil to 1 per cent within its administrative area, the central business district of London. This policy initiative was subsequently taken up nationally with powers to restrict the sulphur content in fuel oil to 1 per cent being offered to other local authorities in the UK Control of Pollution Act 1974.[11]

9 Brimblecombe, P (1987) London air pollution, 1500–1900, *Atmospheric Environment*, vol 11, 1157–1162; Brimblecombe, P (1987) *The Big Smoke*, Methuen, London; Elsom D M (1992) op cit; Elsom, D M (1995) 'Atmospheric pollution trends in the United Kingdom', in Simon, J (ed) *The State of Humanity*, Blackwell, Oxford, pp 476–490; Pearce, F (1992) 'Back to the days of deadly smogs', *New Scientist*, 5 December, pp 24–28

10 On the tenth anniversary of the 1952 smog, in December 1962, daily average sulphur dioxide concentrations again exceeded 1400 ppb (4000 μg/m^3). This smog was held responsible for several hundred deaths. However, it marked the last of London's 'pea soupers' such that with similar meteorological conditions in December 1975 the smog produced peak daily smoke and sulphur dioxide concentrations of 800 μg/m^3 and 450 ppb (1200 μg/m^3), respectively: Greater London Council (1983) *Thirty Years On: a Review of Air Pollution in London*, GLC, London

11 Laxen D P H and Thompson M A (1987) 'Sulphur dioxide in Greater London, 1931–1985', *Environmental Pollution*, vol 43, pp 103–114. Although industrial sources of pollution play a small part in London's air quality problems now, there are

Through the 1980s and 1990s pollutant emissions from domestic, industrial and commercial sources declined while vehicle emissions increased rapidly. By 1988, London had about 2.7 million motor vehicles serving its population of nearly 7 million in Greater London (or over 10 million if the urban agglomeration is used to designate its area). Motor vehicles became the most important single source of fine particulates (black smoke), carbon monoxide, nitrogen oxides and VOCs (including benzene) in London (Table 9.3).[12] It was only a matter of time before the occurrence of unfavourable meteorological conditions made Londoners realise that smogs had returned.[13] Not surprisingly, surveys of public opinion on environmental issues showed that the percentage of respondents who were 'very worried' about traffic exhaust fumes and urban smog rose from 23 per cent in 1986, through 33 per cent in 1989 to 40 per cent in 1993, whereas there was a slight fall in concern for issues such as acid rain, ozone layer depletion and global warming between the last two survey years.[14]

Table 9.3 *Road transport contributions to total emissions in the UK and in London in 1990*

Pollutant	Percentage of UK emissions	Percentage of London emissions
Black smoke	46	96
Carbon monoxide	90	99
Nitrogen oxides	51	76
Sulphur dioxide	2	22
VOCs (hydrocarbons)	41	97

occasions when sulphur dioxide plumes from coal-fired power stations located to the east, in the Thames estuary, become grounded in the London area, causing a sudden rise in sulphur dioxide concentrations for brief periods (exceeding WHO ten-minute and one-hour guidelines).

12 House of Commons Transport Committee (1994) *Transport-related Atmospheric Pollution in London*, sixth report, vols 1 and 2, HMSO, London; London Research Centre (1993) *London Energy Study*, London Research Centre

13 'Smogs Return to London' was the message broadcast by the news media in November 1988 and November 1989. On 15–16 November 1988, carbon monoxide eight-hour concentrations reached 17 ppm (19.8 mg/m^3) and one-hour nitrogen dioxide levels 345 ppb (660 µg/m^3). Elsom, D M (1992) op cit, pp 250–251; Laxen, D (1989) 'Winter smogs return to London?', *London Environmental Bulletin*, autumn, pp 6–7; London Scientific Services (1990) *London Air Pollution Monitoring Network Fourth Report – 1989*, LSS, London, 12 pp

14 One of the successes in reducing pollution in London, and in the rest of the UK, during the 1980s concerns airborne lead. The national reduction in lead content in petrol from 0.40 to 0.15 g/l which took place at the end of 1985, together with the increased use of unleaded petrol, resulted in lead levels falling by over 80 per cent in London between 1980 and 1989. Elsom, D M (1992) op cit,

The worst winter smog of recent years took place between 12 and 15 December 1991. Nitrogen dioxide one-hour concentrations reached 423 ppb (809 μg/m³). The smog may have been responsible for 160 excess deaths. However, there was no breach of the European Union Directive on nitrogen dioxide because, although hourly means exceeding 105 ppb (200 μg/m³) were recorded at the urban background sites at which compliance is measured, the requirement in the Directive is for 98 per cent compliance over a year. Concentrations of benzene increased to six to seven times its usual level during the episode.[15]

Even before the winter smogs returned in the late 1980s, London began experiencing photochemical smogs. These became noticeable initially during the exceptionally hot summers of 1975 and 1976, but from the late 1980s onwards high concentrations of ozone occurred during any warm sunny anticyclonic spell. Typical peak hourly values during the worst ozone episodes each year in central London since the mid-1970s lie in the range 100–150 ppb (200–300 μg/m³), with occasional exceptional values around 200 ppb (400 μg/m³). Nitrogen dioxide levels are also high during these episodes. Generally, nitrogen dioxide concentrations over London are higher than other cities in the UK. As may be expected, nitrogen dioxide levels are highest in central London, whereas ozone concentrations tend to be lower in this area and higher in the suburbs. This pattern is due to ozone being used up in the central area of London in converting fresh nitric oxide emitted from vehicles into nitrogen dioxide. Higher ozone concentrations occur not only in the outer suburbs, but in surrounding rural areas and in that sense London (as well as continental Europe) exports its pollution to the rest of the country. Even so, ozone may still reach relatively high and health-threatening levels throughout the London area. Ozone levels may worsen in central London in the coming years as the proportion of cars fitted with catalytic converters rises because these reduce nitrogen oxide emissions which currently lead to the removal of some ozone from the urban atmosphere. Only about 22 per cent of cars had catalysts by mid-1995 and

---

pp 263–268; Annual average lead concentrations in central London fell from 480 ng/m³ in 1985 to 270 ng/m³ in 1986 according to the Department of the Environment (1995) *Digest of Environmental Protection and Water Statistics*, No 16, HMSO, London (table 2.16); increased concern for vehicle emissions is in part related to the public's concern for the rise in asthma rates. It is likely that the total number of Londoners in vulnerable groups at risk from air pollution exceeds one million. The number of hospital consultants, hospital admissions and prescriptions for asthma-related drugs has doubled in the past 15 years in London, with the bulk of the increase being among children under five years. House of Commons Transport Committee (1994) op cit

15 Bower, J (1992) *Initial Analysis of Nitrogen Dioxide Pollution Episode, December 1991*, Warren Spring Laboratory, Stevenage; Brown, W (1994) 'Deaths linked to London smog' *New Scientist*, 25 Jun, p 4; Connor, S (1994) 'Health advisers meet in secret over deadly smog of 1991', *Independent on Sunday*, 26 June, p 4; Royal Commission on Environmental Pollution (1994) *Eighteenth Report: Transport and Environment*, HMSO, London, p 28

it is likely to be 2015 until the annual turnover of cars will mean that all cars are fitted with this pollution control equipment. One other consideration with regard to ozone episodes is that significant amounts of precursor emissions are imported from continental Europe such that solutions to this pollution problem will have to involve an international approach, not be simply limited to London or the UK.[16]

In the past, London commuters relied heavily on its radial rail and Underground (metro) systems for commuting, but changes in the nature and location of employment have meant that rail and metro networks no longer fully reflect public needs and this has encouraged the growth in reliance on cars.[17] As the road network has grown it has produced additional pressures to rely on cars, as shopping centres, hospitals and sports facilities have been located further away from residential areas and suburban centres. The government at last recognised this problem in 1994 and urged local authorities to redress the balance by locating workplaces, schools and shopping complexes closer to residential areas and areas served well by public transport to reduce the need to travel by car.[18] Nevertheless, 70,000 cars per hour (with four out of five carrying only one occupant) crawled into central London each weekday morning at an average speed of 13 kph (8 mph) in 1993 (it was 21 kph or 13 mph in 1972), which is half the speed of commuters in cities such as Birmingham, Bristol, Leeds and Manchester, with the prospect of gridlock never far away. Most drivers are commuting with some sort of employer assistance (eg company car, free parking space at work or subsidised off-site parking at a private car park). Car journeys in London have risen by 20 per cent since 1981 and now account for 43 per cent of all journeys to work, while cycling has decreased by 30 per cent since 1981. The government forecast an increase in road traffic of 83–142 per cent by 2025 compared with 1988. Two-thirds of car journeys in London are under

---

16 Ball D J (1987) 'A history of secondary pollutant measurements in the London region 1971–1986' *The Science of the Total Environment*, vol 59, 181–206; UK Photochemical Oxidants Review Group (1990) *Oxides of Nitrogen in the United Kingdom*, Second PORG Report, Department of the Environment, London; UK Photochemical Oxidants Review Group (1993) *Ozone in the United Kingdom 1993*, Third PORG Report, Department of the Environment, London. Examples of peak hourly ozone values for central London include 150 ppb (26 June 1975), 212 ppb (27 June 1976), 153 ppb (27 July 1979), 124 ppb (14 June 1989) and 112 ppb (22 July 1989).

17 Few new rail or Underground lines have been built in recent years except for the Docklands light rail system and the link to Heathrow Airport. There is an urgent need for a rail link between the east and west parts of central London, the so-called Cross Rail Link between Paddington and Liverpool Street stations. The Underground, with 400 km (250 miles) of track serving 270 stations, is in need of expansion and modernisation. It is so congested that at peak times at some stations passengers are regulated in their access to the platform for safety reasons.

18 Department of the Environment (1994) *Planning Policy Guidance: Transport*, PPG13, HMSO, London; Department of the Environment (1994) *Planning Policy Guidance: Planning and Pollution Control*, PPG23, HMSO, London

8 km (5 miles), which means that engines and catalysts operate inefficiently for much of those journeys (the cold start penalty) emitting large amounts of pollutants. Many of these short journeys could be undertaken readily by walking, cycling or public transport instead.[19]

Only in last few years has the UK Government begun to recognise that its transport policy of building new roads may not be the solution to growing congestion problems and that new roads simply generate more traffic. However, the UK Government's long-standing commitment to road building was highlighted in its proposal in 1993 that the M25, London's 190 km (119 mile) orbital motorway completed in 1986, was to be widened to 14 lanes along its busiest sections. This would form an eight-lane motorway with two three-lane link roads either side for local traffic undertaking short journeys. The original rationale for this motorway was to serve long distance traffic, but it has become part of the daily commuting network, with motorists using it for short distances. In August 1995 variable speed limits, when the current 100 kph (70 mph) limit is cut to 95 kph (60 mph) or 80 kph (50 mph), were introduced at times of congestion on the M25 near Heathrow airport. This 16 km (10-mile) segment is the busiest road stretch in the UK, carrying up to 200,000 vehicles per day even though it was designed to take only 88,000 vehicles. This Controlled Motorway Initiative involving variable speed limits is similar to that which operates near Frankfurt, Germany and Amsterdam, the Netherlands. It is intended to smooth traffic flows, reduce congestion and so decrease the number of stop–start occasions when vehicles are slow moving or stationary with engines idling and emitting higher emissions. However, it can only be considered a short-term measure as projected annual increases in traffic volume will soon lead to congestion returning.

Around 500 km (315 miles) of Priority Red Routes, urban clearways along which stopping is banned during working hours, are to be implemented along existing London roads by 1997. This initiative follows a pilot scheme implemented in north London in January 1991. During the first few months of the pilot scheme, some peak car journey times were shortened by 25 per cent, but this soon fell to around 10 per cent as the faster journey times encouraged new traffic to use the route. Vehicle emission reductions of 1–2 per cent of nitrogen oxides and 10 per cent hydrocarbons and carbon monoxide were achieved. Bus journey times were quicker along the pilot

19 Department of Transport (1989) *National Road Traffic Forecasts (Great Britain)*, HMSO, London; Department of Transport and London Research Centre (1992) *Travel in London: the London Areas Transport Survey 1991*, Department of Transport, London (61 per cent of Greater London households have access to at least one car); Eason, K (1994) 'Why Londoners are slower than others', *The Times*, 8 September; 'London car journeys rise', *The Environmental Digest*, 81, Mar 1994, p 14. To encourage cycling as a viable alternative to driving for short journeys, there are plans for a 1600 km (1000 mile) cycle network throughout London.

route, but the proposed Red Routes Network has been criticised for not incorporating many more bus lanes.[20]

Policies to limit all-day parking to encourage commuters to use public transport are not as effective as desired in London because private off-street parking used by commuters accounts for 60 per cent of all spaces in the centre. Stricter control of the maximum number of parking spaces incorporated into new developments is needed and the density of such developments needs to be more closely related to the public transport accessibility in that area – that is, the poorer the public transport development, the lower the development density permitted. Policies which guide new commercial and industrial development to locations already well served by public transport can minimise any increase in the number of people who commute by car. Restricting and taxing the parking spaces of existing companies would encourage a shift from commuting by cars to public transport.[21]

Following a terrorist bombing of Bishopsgate in the financial heart of London, a cordon was established in July 1993 to control the entry and exit of vehicles in the City of London. The effect of this 1.6 by 1.4 km cordon was to reduce traffic flows by diverting it onto other surrounding routes. This led to a reduction of vehicle emissions (carbon monoxide, hydrocarbons, nitrogen oxides, particulates and carbon dioxide) of around 15–16 per cent inside the cordon, but an increase immediately outside the cordon of 2 per cent. When the security reasons for the 'Ring of Steel' no longer applied (due to the IRA ceasefire in August 1994), the pollution and other environmental benefits that this scheme had produced resulted in the City of London making the cordon permanent, with the possibility of later doubling its area by extending it westwards.[22]

Congestion charging (road pricing) has been considered for London but not yet implemented. A 1989 study suggested that charging a fixed fee for entry into central London at peak times would reduce traffic terminating

---

20 Red Routes (Axes Rouges) were implemented in Paris in 1990; Traffic Director for London (1993) *The Network Plan: Executive Summary*, Traffic Director for London. Vehicle flows have increased along the Haringey–Islington–Tower Hamlets pilot Red Route by 8–11 per cent since the scheme was implemented; House of Commons Transport Committee (1994) op cit, p 55, para 4.9

21 Only following the Road Traffic Act 1991 did London's local authorities gain powers of enforcing on-street parking with the transfer of traffic wardens from the police to local councils in 1993–1994. One borough, Westminster, in 1995 offered free parking at any of its 10,000 kerbside spaces to drivers of electric vehicles.

22 Corporation of London (1993) *The Way Ahead: Traffic and the Environment*, Draft Consultation Paper, Corporation of London, 5 pp; Corporation of London (1994) *Vehicle Emissions in the City of London: Effects of London's Traffic Management Scheme*, Executive Summary, Corporation of London; Wood, K and Smith, R (1993) *Assessment of the Pilot (Red) Route in London*, TRL Report PR31, Transport Research Laboratory, Crowthorne; 'Traffic pollution decreased by London cordon', *The Environmental Digest*, 79, Jan, 1994, p 14

there by 30 per cent and reduce through traffic by 75 per cent. This would ease congestion, create smoother traffic flows and increase demand for buses by around 15 per cent and trains/Underground by 7 per cent. Congestion charging is favoured by central government because it can be introduced relatively quickly and can be self-financing compared with the time and cost of building more infrastructure such as new Underground or even light rail lines. Nevertheless, if congestion charging is to be introduced it needs to be linked with major improvements in the reliability, convenience, safety and comfort of public transport, together with cheaper fares which integrate all forms of public transport systems.[23]

Many London buses are operating beyond their design life. For example, 490 Routemaster buses in London Transport's 5000 bus fleet were designed to last up to 17 years yet their average age is now around 30 years. Although these vehicles receive newer engines to eke out their life, many now operate with engines over ten years old. This highlights that setting increasingly stringent emission standards for new buses has little effect on existing bus emissions. Even though one full bus can take up to, say, 50 cars off the streets, the difference in emissions from 50 new cars and one old bus has narrowed over the years. Stringent emission standards for existing buses are needed, together with government incentives to encourage bus and haulage companies to replace old, polluting vehicles with new, cleaner ones as well as to use alternative fuels. However, the proposed deregulation of London's buses, a policy applied to other parts of the UK in 1986, discourages companies from investing substantially in new vehicles. Retrofitting London's buses with diesel particulate traps, following trials in some London buses, was considered but rejected because of the huge cost involved ($37 million or £25 million) without government financial assistance. Policies which give buses priority over other traffic are being pursued. Experiments were undertaken in 1994 giving buses priority at traffic lights by fitting buses with transponders which can extend the green light long enough for the bus to get through or advance the green light so the bus is delayed as little as possible. Even so, many more bus lanes are needed with stricter enforcement to prevent cars using them or parking on them. Currently there are 90 km (56 miles) of bus lanes, which represents only 3 per cent of the total bus route length compared with 300 km (188 miles) in Paris (12 per cent of route length) and 234 km (146 miles) in Tokyo (23 per cent of route length). Electronic information boards at bus stops

---

23 Hewitt, P (1989) *A Cleaner, Faster London: Road Pricing Transport Policy and the Environment*, Institute for Public Policy Research, Green Paper No 1; Hurdle, D (1990) *Road Pricing for London*, London Boroughs Association; Parliamentary Office of Science and Technology (1993) *Road Pricing*, Briefing Note 43, London; Moore, T (1994) 'Drivers may be charged to enter cities', *Daily Telegraph*, 22 Aug, p 1. Some road pricing does exist in the form of tolls charged for using the Dartford tunnels and bridge crossing the River Thames on the M25 at the eastern edge of Greater London (with 20 per cent of weekday traffic now making payment using smart cards).

giving the time to wait until the next bus (linked to sensors on the buses) were piloted in 1994 with a view to improving the quality of the service. However, with 600 bus routes and 17,000 bus stops in London, the financial outlay for full implementation would be enormous.[24]

UK Government spending on public transport has been far less forthcoming than spending on roads. Sixty years ago London had 2600 trams, but scrapped them because they were too old, slow and inflexible compared with buses (the last tram ran 1952). Some limited progress in reintroducing light rail systems is being made with a 27 km (17 mile) network of light rail, called Tramlink, being built to serve the suburban area of Croydon by 1998. This follows successful light rail systems introduced in Manchester and Sheffield. London needs massive investment by the government in public transport systems linked to clear transport policies. The London Planning Advisory Committee has put forward a strategy to make public transport a realistic alternative to the use of cars by urging a commitment to ensure that nobody lives more than 0.8 km (0.5 miles) from two Underground/rail stations or four bus routes.[25] The Royal Commission on Environmental Pollution has suggested that the government adopts targets to reduce the proportion of urban journeys undertaken by car from 50 per cent in the London area to 45 per cent by 2000 and 35 per cent by 2020. A more demanding target for reducing commuter car traffic by 3 per cent per year and total vehicle emissions by 5 per cent per year has been suggested by the London Boroughs Association.[26]

The application of national or European Union pollution control legislation and economic instruments cannot solve the air quality problems of London on their own. For example, although total vehicle emissions are expected to decline as the proportion of cars with catalytic converters rises, increased numbers and use of road vehicles will eventually offset the benefits of

24 Holman, C (1992) *Cleaner Buses*, Friends of the Earth, London; Hamer, M (1994) 'Buses to get green light through city traffic', *New Scientist*, 7 May, pp 20–21; London Boroughs Association (1990) *The Scope for Bus Priorities in London*, London Boroughs Association (and 1991 update supplement); Hurdle, D and Bell, S (1993) *All Aboard! Attractive Public Transport for London*, London Boroughs Association; London's buses are estimated to produce 2500 t of particulates, 2600 t of carbon monoxide and 6900 t of nitrogen oxides annually according to the London Energy Study (1993) ibid

25 Hamer, M (1995) 'A growing desire for streetcars', *New Scientist*, 28 Jan, pp 14–15; London Planning Advisory Committee (1995) *State of the Environment Report for London*, London Planning Advisory Committee

26 Similar national targets were set by the Commission for increasing the proportion of passenger-kilometres carried by public transport from 12 per cent in 1993 to 20 per cent by 2005 and 30 per cent by 2020 as well as to increase cycle use by 10 per cent of all urban journeys by 2005, compared with 2–5 per cent now. Targets for the reduction in the number of short journeys made by car (eg local shopping, transporting children to and from school) are similarly suggested. Royal Commission on Environmental Pollution (1994) op cit; London Boroughs Association (1993) *Capital Killer II: Still Fuming over London's Traffic Pollution*, London Boroughs Association, p 35

catalysts. Modelling the effects of current vehicle emission control measures suggests that nitrogen dioxide levels in central London will decline by only 5 per cent by the year 2000 from levels in the 1980s. In other words, air quality problems will continue unless other actions are taken. Indeed, emissions of nitrogen oxides in London need to be cut by half to ensure that one-hour nitrogen dioxide concentrations never exceed 100 ppb (190 $\mu g/m^3$), which is the government's public information threshold for 'poor' air quality (there were 40 hours of such poor air quality in Westminster during 1994).[27] One of the limitations London faces in trying to deal with its air quality problems has been the limited powers the 33 London authorities, which form the Association of London Government, have compared with central government. Local authorities have a better understanding of the problems the city faces as well as a clearer grasp of the solutions to deal with those problems than central government, yet they lack the legislative powers and resources to be able to take effective action. Subsidiarity (the transfer of responsibility for action from central to local government) is needed with regard to tackling air quality problems, especially with regard to transport policy.[28]

In 1995 the UK Government at last recognised the need to give local authorities a greater role in managing local air quality by passing the Environment Act 1995 (which, in some ways, anticipated the European Union Framework Directive on Ambient Air Quality Assessment and Management). This introduced the National Air Quality Strategy, which not only requires local authorities to assess air quality within their area, but it offers a range of powers to tackle air quality problems to ensure that all urban areas in the UK will meet new national and European Union air quality standards by 2005. Banning traffic temporarily along certain routes during poor air quality is one new power, although the consequences of doing so will need careful examination so that the ban does not divert the vehicles, simply displacing

27 Munday P K, Timmis, R J, and Walker C A (1989) *A Dispersion Modelling Study of Present Air Quality and Future Oxides of Nitrogen Concentrations in Greater London*, Report LR 731, Warren Spring Laboratory, Stevenage; Quality of Urban Air Review Group (1993) *Urban Air Quality in the United Kingdom*, First Report, Department of the Environment, London, pp 53 and 56; Quality of Urban Air Review Group (1994) *Urban Air Quality in the United Kingdom*, Second Report, Department of the Environment, London, pp 13, 62–63

28 Whitelegg, J (1993) *Transport for a Sustainable Future*, Belhaven, London, pp 158–160. Public campaigns and voluntary schemes to reduce the use of cars and increase the use of public transport are insufficient on their own to tackle poor air quality. For example, a voluntary scheme whereby motorists with odd and even licence plates would be asked to leave their cars at home on alternate days has been proposed but it is unlikely to be adopted sufficiently to make a significant difference. Ghazi, P (1994) 'City car ration plan', *The Observer*, 28 Aug, p 1. Until the introduction of the Environment Act 1995, there was an attempt by London local authorities to obtain new powers to carry out daily roadside emissions testing of vehicles and issue penalties to make enforcement self-financing for infringements through the London Local Authorities Bill (No 6) submitted to Parliament.

the area suffering poor air quality. Previously, temporary traffic bans may have been possible under the Road Traffic Regulations Act 1984 when 'there is a likelihood of danger to the public' but no local authority in the UK had attempted this when air quality was poor because of legal uncertainties (although parents of children with asthma launched a legal case in May 1995 to force Greenwich council to close or severely curtail traffic along a congested road where they live). A wide range of other powers may be made available by the new Act in areas with air quality problems (Air Quality Management Areas). Local authorities have long urged central government to allow them to undertake random roadside testing of vehicle exhausts to identify the gross polluters (the worst 10 per cent of vehicles being responsible for 57 per cent of total vehicle carbon monoxide emissions and 66 per cent of total vehicle hydrocarbon emissions in London). They have asked for powers to require such motorists to rectify badly tuned or poorly maintained engines or face a fine. Other powers that London authorities could employ include requiring the compulsory retrofitting of particulate traps to the older buses, the fitting of vapour recovery equipment to petrol station pump delivery nozzles, the use of reformulated or alternative fuels (especially in public service diesel vehicles) and setting large employers ride sharing targets which reduce the number of single-occupant car commuter trips.[29]

Unlike many other major cities in the world, London has had to rely for too long on national (and European Union) pollution control powers and measures to tackle its air quality problems rather than have its own powers to deal with them. Yet it is the 33 local authorities which form the Association of London Government who are better placed than the national government to recognise and respond to the pollution problems faced by Londoners. The Environment Act 1995 marked a turning point, with London authorities beginning to gain some of the powers they need to tackle London's episodic and long-term air quality problems more effectively than at present. Whether these powers, and the resources needed to apply them,

---

29 Association of London Government/South East Institute of Public Health (1995) *Air Quality in London 1994*, Second Report of the London Air Quality Network, South East Institute of Public Health, Tunbridge Wells; Cawley, C (1994) 'Exhaust watch – the Westminster initiative way', *Clean Air*, vol 24, pp 13–19 (some of London's 19,000 taxis and 5000 buses are included in the gross emitter category which is of concern in semi-pedestrian areas, such as Oxford Street, which is closed to all traffic but buses and taxis); Department of the Environment (1994) *Improving Air Quality: Discussion Paper on Air Quality Standards and Management*, DoE, London; Department of the Environment (1995) *Air Quality: Meeting the Challenge*, DoE, London; Elsom, D M and Crabbe, H (1995) 'Practical issues involved in developing effective local air quality management in the United Kingdom' in Power, H *et al* (eds) *Air Pollution*, vol 2, Computational Mechanics, Southampton, pp 483–492; Muncaster, G (1994) 'Experience with remote sensing', *paper presented at the National Society for Clean Air and Environmental Protection Seminar on Targeting Traffic Pollution – Options for Local Air Quality Management, 8 December 1994*, NSCA, Brighton

are sufficient to produce acceptable air quality by say, 2005 remains to be seen. Measures to reduce the use of cars, especially single-occupant cars, will not work without central government investing substantially in expanding and modernising public transport systems in London.

Athens and the Nephos

Athens is blighted by the nephos. Athens, a city of more than 4 million people, traps pollutants within its basin, which is surrounded by the Saronic Gulf (Mediterranean Sea) on one side and mountain ranges on the other

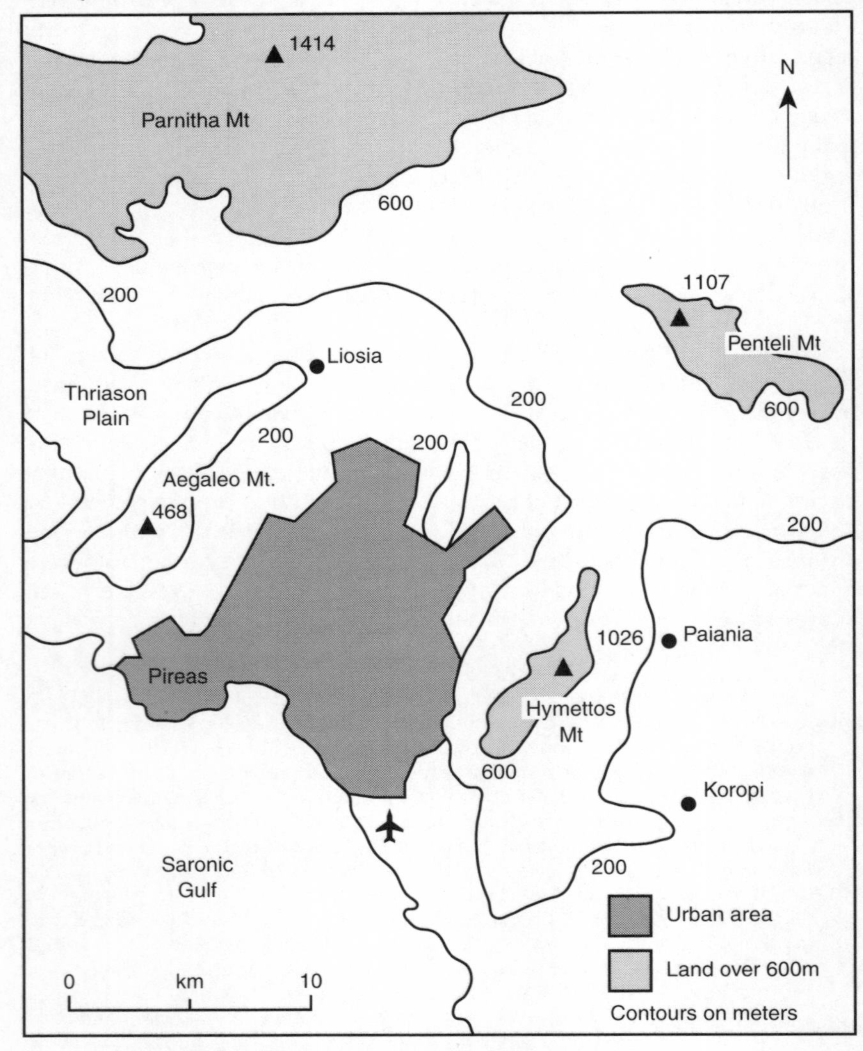

Figure 9.4 *Map of Greater Athens*

three sides (Figure 9.4). Since the late 1970s, traffic emissions have escalated greatly, giving rise to frequent photochemical smogs, known locally as the nephos (from the Greek word meaning cloud). Emissions come from 800,000 cars and trucks – many a decade old – as well as 17,000 antiquated diesel-powered taxis, 5000 poorly maintained buses and 230,000 motor cycles. Its Mediterranean climate of frequent temperature inversions, intense sunshine and high temperatures together with light winds combine to produce high concentrations of pollutants, especially the photochemical pollutants of ozone and nitrogen dioxide. Like Los Angeles, the sea breeze circulation exerts a significant influence on ozone formation in the Athens basin. Ozone formed over the city one day can be transported out to sea by the night-time land breeze and kept aloft, preventing it from being depleted. It is then brought back over the city by the sea breeze early the next day and then atmospheric mixing causes surface ozone levels to rise rapidly.[30]

In 1991, there were 180 days when air quality exceeded health-based standards and posed a threat to health. Fine particulates, carbon monoxide, nitrogen dioxide and ozone can reach very high levels, triggering smog alerts (Table 9.4). Photochemical pollution problems got steadily worse during the

Table 9.4 *Smog alert levels in Athens. Values are ppb(μg/m³) except for CO [ppm(mg/m³)]*

	NO_2 (one-hour)	CO (eight hours)	SO_2 (24 hours)	Black smoke (24 hours)	O_3 (one-hour)
Safety alert	105 (200)	13 (15)	75 (200)	250	100 (200)
Stage 1 restriction	262 (500)	21 (25)	150 (400)	400	150 (300)
Stage 2 restriction	366 (700)	30 (35)	188 (500)	600	250 (500)

1980s as nitrogen dioxide and ozone levels increased by 35 per cent and 20 per cent annually, respectively. Stage 1 alerts were called 18 times during the 1980s and the situation has worsened through the 1990s. In June and October 1991 hourly nitrogen dioxide levels reached 357 ppb (683 μg/m³) and 364 ppb (696 μg/m³), respectively. Ozone levels have frequently exceeded the European Union health protection alert level of 90 ppb (180

30 Gusten, H, Heinrich, G, Cvitas, T, Klasinc, L, Ruscic, B, Lalas, D P and Petrakis, M (1988) 'Photochemical formation and transport of ozone in Athens, Greece', *Atmospheric Environment*, vol 22, pp 1855–1861; Katsoulis, B D (1988) 'Some meteorological aspects of air pollution in Athens, Greece', *Meteorology and Atmospheric Physics*, vol 39, pp 203–212; WHO Regional Office for Europe (1991) *Impact on Human Health of Air Pollution in Europe*, WHO Regional Office for Europe, Copenhagen, 18 pp (figure 2 presents the spatial distribution of the maximum one-hour ozone concentrations for 36 stations in Europe during the 1980–1989 period highlighting that Athens experienced the highest value).

μg/m³) as well as on several occasions exceeding the alarm level of 180 ppb (360 μg/m³). Ozone concentrations in the Athens basin are among the highest values reported throughout Europe. The influence of the sea breeze as well as scavenging of ozone by vehicle emissions of nitric oxide often leads to ozone levels being higher in the northern suburbs than in the city centre or southern parts of the city. In contrast, nitrogen dioxide levels are highest in central Athens. Although sulphur dioxide from diesel-powered vehicles and industry is not a serious threat to health in Athens, it is causing irreparable damage to historical monuments such as the temple of the Parthenon on the Acropolis, which rises above the dirty brown pall shrouding the city below. The sulphur dioxide converts the marble into gypsum which cracks and flakes off. Corrosion of the marble by nitrogen oxides is also of growing concern and may have reached the same order of magnitude as sulphur dioxide. Traffic emissions account for virtually all of the carbon monoxide, 75 per cent of nitrogen oxides, 68 per cent of VOCs, 8 per cent of sulphur dioxide and 1 per cent of suspended particulates (but 64 per cent of black smoke).[31]

When high levels of nitrogen dioxide, ozone or fine particulates coincide with exceptional summer air temperatures, the result is that hundreds of people may be admitted to hospital. More than 100 premature deaths each year are attributed to poor air quality. During the summer of 1987, when high pollution concentrations coincided with air temperature exceeding 40°C (104°F) on seven days in a 10-day spell, more than 2000 excess deaths occurred, with possibly up to half of those deaths being attributed to air pollution. However, separating out the effects of heat and pollution, particularly on elderly people with heart and lung diseases, is difficult, so the deaths triggered by pollution may be much less than sometimes claimed by the news media. Nevertheless, smogs do cause ill health, with coughs,

31 Boucher, K (1990/91) 'The monitoring of air pollutants in Athens with particular reference to nitrogen dioxide', *Energy and Buildings*, vol 15/16, pp 637–645; Eliou, C (1991) 'Choking Greeks look to the gods for help', *The Times*, 2 Oct, pp 1 and 17; Kirby, H (1992) 'Dying for a breath of fresh air', *The Times*, 29 May, p 5; McCormick, J (1989) *Acid Earth*, second edition, Earthscan, London, pp 124–125; Moussiopoulos, N (1993) 'Photochemical air pollution in Athens', in Zanetti, P, Brebbia, C A, Garcia Gardea, J E and Ayala Milian, G (eds) *Air Pollution*, Computational Mechanics, Southampton, pp 255–280; Moussiopoulos, N, Gusten, H, Asimakopoulos, D N and Cvitas, T (1993) 'The Thessaloniki 1991 photochemical pollution measurement campaign' *EUROTRAC Newsletter*, no 11, pp 20–24; Sabatakakis, M (1990) 'Air quality monitoring in Greece', *World Health Organisation Newsletter*, no 7, Dec, pp 2–4; Sikiotis, D and Delopoulou, P (1992) 'The corrosion of Pentelic marble by the dry deposition of nitrates and sulphates', *The Science of the Total Environment*, vol 120, pp 213–224; UNEP/WHO (1993) *City Air Quality Trends (GEMS/AIR Data)*, vol 2, UNEP, Nairobi, pp 9–12; Ziomas, I C, Zerefos, C S, Bais, A F, Proyou, A G, Amanatidis, G T and Kelessis, A G (1989) 'Significant increasing trends in surface ozone in Greece', *Environmental Technology Letters*, vol 10, pp 1071–1082; 'Rome and Athens suffer pollution crises', *The Environmental Digest*, 72/73, Jun/Jul 1993, p 16

watery eyes, dizziness and pounding hearts being common symptoms experienced by residents and tourists during the smogs.

Between 1982 and 1995 a scheme was operated to try to halve the number of vehicles entering the central area (inner ring road) of Athens. At the beginning of the scheme cars with licence plates ending in an odd or an even number were allowed access on alternate days: vehicles with odd-numbered digits gained access on odd-numbered dates. This prompted many Athenians, those who could afford it, to purchase a second car with a licence plate that allowed them access on the days when their other car was banned. The response from the authorities in 1983 was to change the regulations. Access on one day was given to vehicles where the last digit on the licence plate was zero to four, and on the next day to vehicles with digits from five to nine. To discourage further purchases of old cars by people trying to overcome the restrictions, the authorities warned that they might change the regulations again. They did. In 1988, they reintroduced the odd and even regulation for alternate day access. Restrictions did not apply at weekends and on major holidays. Taxis were exempt, although an attempt to include taxis in the ban in 1988 (when it was shown that taxis were responsible for 30 per cent of exhaust emissions) resulted in strikes, boycotts and deliberate staging of traffic jams until the taxi drivers' exemption was restored in 1989. Different times during the day when the restrictions applied have been tried, with the aim being to halve the use of cars in the central area. The authorities eventually settled on 6.00 am to 8.00 pm. Enforcement of the restrictions was the responsibility of 50 police positioned at major roads on the inner ring road boundary, but evasion levels were high.

The government assessed the effects of the scheme in 1985. It was found that the number of private cars was reduced by 22 per cent compared with the situation before the restrictions were imposed, but the number of taxis increased by 26 per cent in the inner ring. Increased emissions from the diesel taxis caused monitored levels of black smoke to increase. Nitrogen dioxide concentrations fell by 38 per cent and sulphur dioxide by 16 per cent, while carbon monoxide levels remained unchanged. The traffic flow and air quality benefits of this scheme were not as great as expected for several reasons. Firstly, car ownership rose rapidly during the 1980s. Economic growth, combined with the ban, has encouraged families to own two cars which they can use on alternate days. Often the second car is older and more polluting than the first. Secondly, public transport services are so limited that many commuters have taken to using taxis and motorcycles, with both types of vehicles being as polluting, if not more polluting, than private cars.[32]

---

32 Butterwick, L, Harrison, R and Merritt, Q (1991) *Handbook for Urban Air Improvement*, Commission of the European Communities, Brussels, pp 173–174, 330–331; Giaoutzi, M and Damianidias, L (1990) 'Greece', in Barde, J-P and Button, K (eds) *Transport Policy and the Environment*, Earthscan, London, pp 157–176

During stage 1 smog alerts the odd/even restriction on cars is extended to the outer ring road. During stage 2 alerts a total ban is applied to all private vehicles within the inner ring road and the odd/even restriction applied to taxis within the inner ring road. During smog alerts, cars carrying less than three people are banned from the inner traffic ring. After more than a decade of temporary or partial traffic bans in Athens, a ban on cars, motor cycles and taxis was made permanent in April 1995 in the 2.5 km^2 of the city centre within the inner ring road. Streets have been made into pedestrian areas, traffic redirected and free bus services offered. The ban, initially for a three month experiment, applies from 8.00 am to 8.00 pm, but delivery vans and residents' cars are exempted.[33]

Traffic emissions are excessive because of the high average age of cars in the city (averaging about 11 years due to high taxation suppressing sales of new cars during the late 1980s), their poor maintenance and their use of low-grade fuels. Policies being adopted to improve the situation involve the introduction of less polluting fuels (eg reduction of sulphur in diesel and lead in petrol), offering incentives to use cleaner fuels (eg to taxi drivers opting to use unleaded petrol or liquid propane gas), and inspecting exhaust emissions from vehicles regularly. Vehicle inspection programmes produced limited success in the 1980s because of corruption or a lack of enforcement of standards (eg a motorist whose car failed at one testing station found it easy for it to pass at another) and too few testing stations, which created a massive backlog of cars awaiting testing. However, in 1995 annual emission tests were introduced and drivers now have to carry a valid certificate of approval otherwise they are fined.[34] The European Union Directive requiring all new vehicles since 1993 to be fitted with catalytic converters will help to reduce emissions in the long term, but the air quality effectiveness of this measure depends on a high turnover of vehicles. Because of high import duties on cars and a lack of a major car manufacturing industry, the rate of purchase of imported new cars was very low throughout the 1980s. Cars cost two or three times more than in other European countries and so cars were scrapped at an annual rate of only 0.5 per cent compared with 5 per cent in many other European Union Member States. The government belatedly recognised this problem and the cost of vehicles is coming into line with other European Union Member States. Incentives are being offered to scrap old cars by offering reduced car and road taxes for new vehicles.[35]

Lifestyle changes are being attempted. Staggering working hours is hoped to reduce traffic flows at peak times. For example, since 1995 some civil

33 'Car(e)free Athens', *Acid News*, no 3, Jun 1995, p 4; 'Athens bans vehicles in city centre test', *Los Angeles Times*, 11 Apr 1995

34 'Early to work to cut traffic fumes', *Clean Air*, vol 24 (2), summer, p 95; Economopoulos, A P (1987) 'Development of the five-year air pollution abatement plan for the Greater Athens area', *JAPCA – Journal of Air & Waste Management*, vol 37, pp 889–897

35 Pelekasi, K and Skourtos, M S (1991) 'Air pollution in Greece: an overview', *Ekistics*, vol 348/349, pp 135–155

servants are required to start work early, at 7.00 am or 7.30 am during the summer, while shop workers begin at 9.30 am. Since the 1980s the authorities have encouraged the city to adopt the same business hours as the rest of Europe. This means operating continuous shopping hours rather than the traditional times of 9.00 am to 2.00 pm and 5.00 pm to 8.00 pm, with a three hour lunchtime siesta. Removing the three-hour break in the day reduces traffic flows by replacing four rush hours a day with only two.

Urban planning has not helped the pollution problem in Athens. It is a high-density city with only 4 per cent consisting of parks and green spaces (about eight times less than Paris or London) which offer little non-polluted air to dilute transport emissions in the city's street canyons. Congestion occurs due to an inadequate road network which feeds traffic into the vicinity of two main squares. Modernising the traffic light system and reorganising traffic routes has been an important consideration in attempting to lessen congestion and so reduce excessive emissions from lengthy queues of engine-idling vehicles.

Improvements to the small capacity public transport system is a long-term priority. Plans include building two new metro lines (90 km or 56 miles of track opening in 1997 to carry 450,000 passengers daily), increasing the existing carrying capacity of the metro by 20 per cent and the trolley bus network by 30 per cent, introducing park and ride schemes along the inner and outer routes, renewing the bus fleet (600 new buses to replace the old and heavily polluting Hungarian-made buses), fitting particulate traps to all buses, and giving street priority to buses (eg bus lanes, bus ways). Dedicated bus lanes have produced average bus speeds of 20 kph (13 mph) compared with only 9 kph (6 mph) along congested streets where bus lanes are not available.[36]

Although transport emissions are mainly responsible for the nephos, industry and central heating units also contribute significant emissions. Many of the 3500 industrial plants are located near the harbour of Piraeus in the southwestern part of Athens. The long-term plans to improve air quality include relocating more industry, ministries and public corporations away from the city centre using tax incentives where appropriate. The airport may be moved from Hellenikon in the Athens Basin to Sparta in the Messogia Plain. The sulphur content in fuels is to be reduced as required by a European Union Directive. During smogs, industries are required to reduce emissions by 30 per cent during a stage 1 alert and to stop production completely during a stage 2 alert. Similarly central heating units have to be reduced during a stage 1 alert and are prohibited during a stage 2 alert.

The nephos began obscuring the clear azure summer skies of Athens in the 1970s. During the early 1980s, when the city was gaining the reputation as the most polluted city in western Europe, politicians promised that

36 Organisation for Economic Co-operation and Development (OECD) (1991) *Environmental Policies for Cities in the 1990s*, OECD, Paris, p 78

solutions could be found within a few months. Traffic restrictions were introduced in the central area and plans were made to use cleaner fuels throughout the basin and for major improvements in public transport. Unfortunately, the weakening of stringent pollution control proposals and delays in implementing plans due to economic and political circumstances, together with the rapid rise in the number of vehicles, mean that poor air quality problems will continue in Athens for some time. Model predictions for ozone levels suggest that unless radical measures are introduced to reduce vehicle emissions in this medium-sized city, then no significant improvement is likely until 2020.[37]

Mexico City: Megacity, Megapollution

Many claim that Mexico City is the most polluted city on this planet. Its residents suffer very poor air quality due to a combination of considerable emissions (generated by 20 million people, 35,000 industries and nearly 3 million vehicles), its topographical location and subtropical climate. The city's high altitude (2250 m, 7400 ft), where oxygen is one-quarter that of sea level, means that combustion is much less efficient. Even new vehicles can produce unacceptable levels of pollutants. The city is enclosed by mountains and volcanic peaks with air entering or leaving the high-altitude basin only in the southeast of the city (Figure 9.5). It experiences frequent temperature inversions during its winter dry season between November and April or May. Cool air drains down the mountain sides into the city basin and becomes capped by the warm air generated by the urban heat island, so strengthening the inversions. Daily temperature inversions last regularly until mid-morning. The city experiences plentiful winter sunshine because of its elevation and latitude (19°N), which leads to strong photochemical activity. With frequent occurrences of calm or very light wind conditions it is not surprising that any pollutants generated in the city stagnate and build up to very high levels.

Mexico City experiences exceptional ozone levels, especially in the southwest residential parts of the city. Air movements during the day cause precursor emissions from the city centre to drift towards the southwest, by which time photochemical reactions have had the opportunity to produce high concentrations of ozone and other photochemical oxidants. With no exit from the basin in this direction the polluted air becomes trapped up against the mountains and it lingers in this area. The city also suffers from very high concentrations of carbon monoxide, lead, particulate matter and sulphur dioxide. Air quality deteriorated rapidly in the late 1980s. In 1992, unacceptable levels were registered for ozone, particulates and carbon monoxide on an astonishing 358 days (354 days in 1991). Breathing

37 Moussiopoulos, N (1989) 'Three-dimensional simulation of the photochemical air pollution in Athens, Greece', in Brasser, L J and Mulder, W C (eds) *Man and his Ecosystems. Proceedings of the 8th World Clean Air Congress, The Hague, The Netherlands, September 1989*, vol 3, Elsevier Science, Amsterdam, pp 419–425

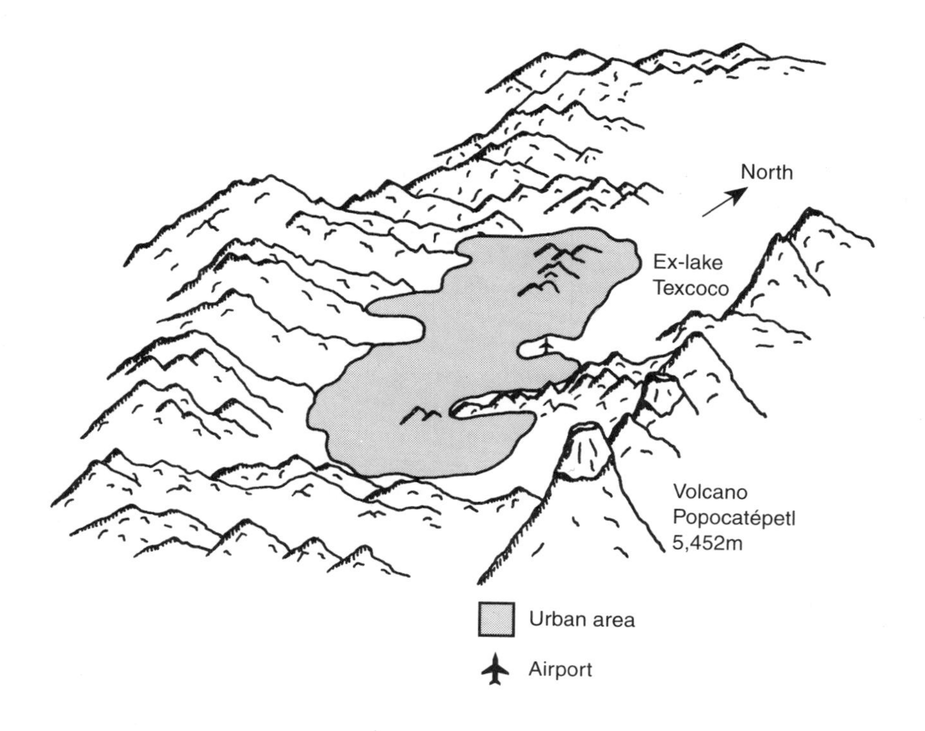

Figure 9.5 *Sketch showing Mexico City located in a high-altitude basin (approximately 2250 m) and surrounded by mountains and volcanic peaks, some reaching over 5000 m*

the air is said to be the equivalent of inhaling pollutants from 40 cigarettes a day. Visitors complain of burning eyes, sore throats, heart palpitations and respiratory problems. It is not surprising therefore that oxygen booths, supplying oxygen at a cost of $2 per minute, are planned to be installed around the city centre for use by people with breathing difficulties. Foreign visitors recognise the health threats posed by living in the city, with some foreign diplomats even having their tour of duty shortened from three to two years and told to take their children out of the city. It is claimed that two million people are suffering from diseases caused or aggravated by air pollution.[38]

38 Cody, E (1992) 'Choking city gasps even more', *International Herald Tribune*, 27 Mar; *The Economist*, 18 Feb 1989, p 69; 'World's first pay-as-you-breathe kiosks installed in Mexico', *The Environmental Digest*, 44, Feb 1991, p 13; Gilbert, A (1994) 'Viva the city', *Geographical*, vol 56, Jun, pp 17–20; Thomson, I (1990) 'Mexico City', *Sunday Times Magazine*, 9 Dec, pp 29–35

Ozone levels reached a staggering 600 ppb (1200 μg/m^3) in November 1992 in southwest Mexico City. Some months see ozone levels exceeding WHO guidelines nearly every day, with more than half the days reaching twice the WHO guideline. In 1991, there were 192 days when ozone levels reached twice the WHO guidelines.[39] Although ozone has long been regarded as the most serious air pollution threat to human health in Mexico City a recent study suggests that health costs associated with suspended particulates are potentially as much as $800 million a year – more than eight times greater than those attributed to ozone.[40] Part of the particulate loading of Mexico City comes from the tolvaneras (dust storms) which blow dust particles from the dried bed of Texcoco Lake to the northeast of the city as well as from extensive landfill (domestic rubbish), construction and dried sewage disposal sites. Extensive planting of trees is being undertaken to try to reduce wind-blown dust and to add to the oxygen levels of the city.[41]

Transport is a major source of air pollution in Mexico City, contributing 97 per cent of carbon monoxide, 66 per cent of nitrogen oxides, 54 per cent of VOCs and 48 per cent of total emissions on a toxicity weighted basis. Cars and taxis dominate motor vehicle emissions, being more polluting than buses and minibuses.[42] The average age of cars is 10 years and 60–90 per cent are in poor repair or badly maintained. Vehicles traditionally run on a very rich air–fuel mixture (8:1) which would not allow three-way catalytic converters to function (they need a stoichiometric ratio of 14.7:1). Not surprisingly, emissions of VOCs are high as large amounts of hydrocarbons pass through unburnt. Attempts have been made to market a cheap computerised device to attach to carburettors to increase the air–fuel mixture closer to the stoichiometric ratio without reducing vehicle performance. This device is claimed to improve fuel efficiency and reduce

---

39 'Mexico City pollution reaches new high', *The Environmental Digest*, 57, Mar 1992, p 11; Darling, J (1992) 'Mexico City chokes on crisis-level smog', *International Herald Tribune*, 24–25 Dec, p 1. Peak hourly ozone levels exceeding 600 ppb (1200 μg/m^3) which were recorded in Mexico City in 1992 have not been experienced in Los Angeles since the mid-1950s.

40 World Bank (1992) *The World Bank and the Environment: Fiscal 1992*, World Bank, Washington, DC, p 72

41 Jauregui, E (1989) 'The dust storms of Mexico City', *International Journal of Climatology*, vol 9, pp 169–180.

42 Faiz, A, Sinha, K, Walsh, M and Varma, A (1990) *Automotive Air Pollution: Issues and Options for Developing Countries*, Working Paper Transport WPS 492, World Bank, Washington, DC.; GEMS (1992) *Urban Air Pollution in Megacities of the World*, Blackwell for WHO/UNEP, New York, pp 27, 155–164; Murley, L (1991) *Clean Air Around the World*, second edition, International Union of Air Pollution Prevention Associations, Brighton, pp 289–307; World Bank (1992) *World Development Report 1992: Development and the Environment*, Oxford University Press, New York, pp 74–75. The number of cars in Mexico City has grown dramatically: there were about 48,000 cars in 1940, 680,000 in 1970, 1.1 million in 1975 and 2.6 million in 1989. In addition to the 2.6 million cars there are 56,500 taxicabs, 7500 buses, 54,500 microbuses, 196,000 petrol-fuelled trucks and 60,000 diesel-fuelled trucks.

emissions of hydrocarbons, nitrogen oxides and carbon monoxide.[43] Carbon monoxide levels are currently very high because of so many old and inefficient vehicles and because of the limitations of the city's oxygen-deficient atmosphere. The scale of the carbon monoxide problem may explain why its eight-hour air quality standard for carbon monoxide is only 13 ppm (15 mg/m^3) compared with the WHO guideline and US standard of 9 ppm (10 mg/m^3).

In November 1989, the authorities launched a four-month traffic restriction experiment aimed at reducing traffic volume and cutting down vehicle emissions. The scheme subsequently became permanent. All private vehicles registered in the city must display one of five colour-coded permits in which each colour represents a weekday on which the vehicle is not to be used ('Hoy No Circula' – no circulation today). Violators are fined $600 and may have their vehicle confiscated. The scheme ('Un dia sin auto' – a day without the car) is claimed to reduce the number of vehicles each day by 400,000, to lessen congestion a little, and to improve air quality by 10–15 per cent. The air quality improvements were less than expected because within a few months of the restrictions being introduced, an additional 190,000 cars were registered in the city. Some were new but many were older vehicles purchased for use on days when a driver's other car was banned. Taxis were initially not covered by the scheme but were recently included.[44]

Ozone smog alerts have been regularly called since the late 1980s. A phase 1 alert is called at 125 ppb (250 μg/m^3, called 250 points by the news media), and requires a 30-40 per cent cut in industrial emissions, a 50 per cent reduction in the use of government vehicles, the halting of street repairs in an attempt to minimise traffic jams, and drivers are requested not to use cars. Phase 2 alert operates at 175 ppb (350 μg/m^3) and increases the cut-back required in industrial emissions to 50–75 per cent, schools are closed (to reduce the number of vehicles taking children to school, or school opening times are delayed until the temperature inversion has lifted during late morning and the air quality improved), and the one day a week ban on vehicles is extended to two days a week to try to reduce vehicle use by 40 per cent (Table 9.5). In January 1989 schoolchildren were given the whole month off. Phase 3 (210 ppb or 420 μg/m^3) is an emergency situation, such as called from 7 to 10 March 1991, when industry has to be closed and many other activities curtailed.[45]

Mexico's massive foreign debt (more than $100 billion) limits the strategies that can be introduced to improve air quality, but several

---

43 Beard, J (1993) 'A cleaner burn for Mexico's cars', *New Scientist*, 20 Nov, p 21

44 Collins, C O and Scott, S L (1994) *Environmental Hazards in the Valley of Mexico: Slide Set*, National Council for Geographic Education, Lincoln, Nebraska

45 Comision Metropolitana Para la Prevencion y Control de la Contaminacion Ambiental (1992) *Manual para la Aplicacion del Programa de Contingencias Ambientales*, Comision Metropolitana Para la Prevencion y Control de la Contaminacion Ambiental en al Valle de Mexico; Fraser, D (1992) 'Mexico tries new plan to beat smog', *Financial Times*, 26 November

Table 9.5 *Extended vehicle restrictions (hoy no circula) during stage 2 smog alerts in Mexico City*

Days when cars are banned	Colour of permit
Monday	Yellow and pink
Tuesday	Pink and blue
Wednesday	Red and green
Thursday	Green and red
Friday	Blue and yellow

important pollution control policies have been introduced in recent years. They rely on financial backing from the World Bank, the US and Japan.[46] Emission standards were tightened significantly for cars in circulation and for new cars from 1993. Twice-yearly vehicle exhaust emissions testing has become mandatory. All new cars sold since 1991 have had to be equipped with catalytic converters. In 1992, 147,000 vehicles were scrapped and replaced with vehicles fitted with catalytic converters, including the older taxis. This followed an announcement in December 1991 that all taxis built before 1984 – about half the city's total fleet – had to be replaced to restrict the maximum age of taxis eventually to ten years. The government offered grants to taxi divers to buy new replacements. Attempts are being made to reduce the use of government vehicles by 30 per cent during the winter. Plans are underway to convert 144,000 public transport and goods vehicles to run on compressed natural gas or liquid petroleum gas. The radical long-term plan requires about one-third of the trucks and 20 per cent of the city's buses to be using alternative fuels by the year 2010.[47]

The amount of lead in leaded petrol was reduced in 1991 from 0.18 to 0.09 g/l (compared with 0.30 g/l in 1983). There is now greater availability of unleaded petrol (it contains 5 per cent MTBE by weight in place of lead), first introduced in July 1990. Leaded petrol still accounted for 85 per cent

46 Investors may provide policy assessments to the Mexican government. For example, the World Bank estimates that to reduce current vehicle emissions by more than 50 per cent using enforcement of tighter emission and fuel standards would cost $560 million. In contrast, a petrol tax, which would reduce demand and stimulate a shift towards less fuel-intensive modes of transport, would achieve the same reduction with a cost saving of about 20 per cent. Moreover the tax would also generate about $300 million in public revenue. World Bank (1992) *World Development Report 1992: Development and the Environment*, Oxford University Press, New York, pp 74–75

47 Garfia, J and Gonzalez, R (1992) 'Air quality in Mexico City', in Dunnett, D A and O'Brien, R J (eds) *The Science of Global Change*, American Chemical Society, Washington, DC, pp 149–161; 'Mexico City – heightening stringency', *Acid News*, No 4, Oct 1992, p 10; 'Mexican vehicles to convert to cleaner fuel', *The Environmental Digest*, no 56, Feb 1992, p 12

of consumption in 1993 but this is expected to fall steadily as the proportion of catalytic cars, running on unleaded petrol, rises. Airborne lead concentrations and blood lead levels in residents can still be high in some parts of the city, especially near metal foundries in the northern industrialised area. A rise in the price of both unleaded and leaded petrol by 35 per cent in March 1995 may lead to a slight reduction in vehicle emissions as motorists look to use their vehicles less, but this measure was really aimed at tackling the country's economic crises rather than improving air quality.[48]

Industry adds significantly to the pollution loading of the city's atmosphere from sources such as petrochemicals (eg PEMEX, the state-owned oil company), power plants, cement plants (supplying the rapidly expanding city with concrete for roads, bridges and buildings), metal foundries and paper manufacturing. Heavy fuel oil, which is used by half the industry, has a high sulphur content. Although the sulphur content was reduced from 4 to 3 per cent recently it remains too high. About 226 temporary or partial closures of industrial plants for pollution violations in 1991 indicate a commitment on the government's part to tackle the pollution problem even if it affects the economy. Even the badly maintained PEMEX oil refinery in the city was closed with the loss of 5400 jobs.[49] Industry is to be consolidated in the northern districts although, unfortunately, this is upwind of the city centre and residential areas (daytime airflow is typically northeast to southwest).[50]

It has recently been suggested that domestic emissions of hydrocarbons may be contributing significant amounts of the hydrocarbons which lead to ozone being formed. Liquid petroleum gas is used widely for cooking and heating in homes, supplying as much energy in Mexico City's homes as electricity. As the city is prone to earthquakes, gas is not piped to homes but is distributed in portable pressurised tanks which people connect to

---

48 Bustani, A and Cobas, E (1993) 'The impacts of fuel substitution policies on air pollutants emissions in Mexico', in Zanetti, P, Brebbia, C A, Garcia Gardea, J E and Ayala Milian, G (eds) *Air Pollution*, Computational Mechanics, Southampton, pp 637–648; Driscoll, W, Mushak, P, Garfia, J and Rothenberg, S J (1992) 'Reducing lead in gasoline: Mexico's experience', *Environmental Science and Technology*, vol 26, pp 1702–1705; Jauregui, E (1989) 'Variaciones espaciales y temporales del plomo atmosferico en la cuidad de Mexico', *Geografia y Desarrollo*, vol 2, pp 15–21; Romieu, I, Palazuelos, E, Meneses, F and Hernandez-Avila, M (1992) 'Vehicular traffic as a determinant of blood-lead levels in children: a pilot study in Mexico City', *Archives of Environmental Health*, vol 47, pp 246–249

49 Mumme, S P and Sanchez, R A (1992) 'New directions in Mexican environmental policy', *Environmental Management*, vol 16, pp 465–474

50 The need to separate potentially dangerous industrial plants from the population was highlighted on 19 November 1984 when a PEMEX liquid petroleum gas storage plant suffered a series of explosions and fires lasting 18 hours in a slum district northwest of Mexico City. More than 500 people were killed, 7000 injured and 39,000 made homeless or evacuated during this disaster; Marshall, V C (1987) *Major Chemical Hazards*, Ellis Horwood, Chichester

their cooking stoves and heaters. It is claimed that large amounts of unburnt liquid petroleum gas are leaking from poor connections adding butene, a hydrocarbon with a high ozone-producing potential, to the atmosphere. In response to this claim, the authorities are planning to educate people to take more care in installing their tanks properly and to reduce the butene content of liquid petroleum gas (removed routinely in the US and Europe).[51]

Mexico City extends over a very wide area due to its huge population and partly due to the prevalence of low-rise buildings in this earthquake-prone and unstable soil area. This urban sprawl encourages lengthy travel times and when vehicles reach the city centre, its old downtown, which was not designed for high traffic volumes, congestion is inevitable. The metro, which began in 1968, has nine lines serving much of the metropolitan area. Fares are subsidised and it helps enormously to reduce the use of private cars by carrying 5.5 million passengers a day in its crowded carriages. There are plans to expand it but, to some extent, expansion of the metro reinforces the trend for the metropolitan area to grow even larger such that those who do choose to travel by car are undertaking longer journeys, adding even more vehicle emissions. One radical consideration was to alter the pattern of working hours in the city to alter the time of the early morning rush hour peak of vehicle emissions, but modelling suggests this is unlikely to lead to any significant improvement in maximum ozone concentrations.[52]

Future progress in tackling the severe air quality problems in Mexico City will depend on many factors, not least the state of the economy, the support of the public in the pursuit of better air quality and the level of international investment and pollution control technology transfer. What is of greatest concern is that population growth, partly the result of 3000 migrants arriving in the city every day, may mean that curbing the emissions per vehicle or per industrial plant will simply be offset or outweighed by the growth in numbers of vehicles and industrial plants. The problems confronting Mexico City now may well be what other rapidly developing megacities in Latin and South America, southeast Asia and even Africa have to face in the future.

---

51 Blake, D R and Rowland, F S (1995) 'Urban leakage of liquified petroleum gas and its impact on Mexico City air quality', *Science*, 269, pp 953–956; Cohen, P (1995) 'Leaky stoves fuel Mexico's pollution problem', *New Scientist*, 26 Aug, p 8

52 Modelling suggests that advancing the emissions peak by an hour may lead to a small increase in the ozone peak due to more ozone precursors being available for photochemical reactions soon after sunrise (and at a time when the temperature inversion is still strong). Delaying the emissions peak by an hour may decrease the ozone peak slightly. The changes to the ozone peak are significant only when the ratio of hydrocarbons to nitrogen oxides in the atmosphere is low. Unfortunately, Mexico City's atmosphere has a high HC/NO_x ratio such that the changes to the ozone peak are not significant according to Ruiz Santoyo, M E G and Cruz Nunez, X (1993) 'Mexico City air quality simulation', in Zanetti, P, Brebbia, C A, Garcia Gardea, J E and Ayala Milian, G (eds) *Air Pollution*, Computational Mechanics, Southampton, pp 293–304

Conclusions: More Similarities than Differences

The air pollution problems facing Los Angeles, London, Athens and Mexico City all differ in some ways, as do the topographical location and the meteorological conditions to which they are subjected. However, the similarities are greater than the differences. This arises because their pollution problems are the consequence of a rapid growth in numbers of motor vehicles and, to a varying degree, growth in the manufacturing, utility and service industries attempting to provide the needs and desires of their large urban populations. The financial resources available to each city, and country within which each is located, vary greatly but wealth is not necessarily a good indicator of the success of pollution control policies in achieving acceptable air quality, as highlighted by Los Angeles. Indeed, affluence brings its own pollution problems, as does poverty. Limited financial resources do not prevent pollution control policies from being advocated, as in Mexico City, but they do preclude the full and effective implementation of the policies and whether they can be sustained in the face of national debt crises. Clearly, rapidly expanding cities in Southern countries need international financial assistance if pollution control policies are to be eventually successful. Regardless of the problems any city experiences during its pursuit of acceptable air quality, it is sustaining the commitment to the goal of healthy urban air quality that really matters. Achieving that goal may take a long time even with the most radical of policies, but this should not be allowed to detract from implementing policies that will eventually achieve healthy air quality, as discussed in the final chapter.

Chapter 10

Achieving and Sustaining Healthy Urban Air Quality in the Twenty-First Century

Current Pollution Threat to Health

The health of as many as 1.6 billion people living in urban areas throughout the world may be at risk from poor air quality. Without the effective implementation of pollution control policies and measures this number may rise as pollution emissions from motor vehicles, industry and households escalate and the population expands (due to urban migration as well as high birth rates in Southern countries). The composition and concentrations of the cocktail of pollutants enveloping urban areas and the severity of the health threat confronting residents vary between cities, but there are common aspects that can be identified. Hundreds of thousands of motor vehicles used by commuters and for transporting goods stream in and out of the city, creating narrow belts of intensely polluted air which criss-cross the city. Pollutant emissions at road junctions, traffic lights and bottlenecks produce pollution hot-spots. Emissions from power stations, oil refineries, chemical and metal processing plants, waste incinerators, and manufacturing plants scattered across a city or grouped into industrial estates produce localised areas of toxic pollution, while the tall stacks characteristic of many industrial plants send narrow plumes of pollutants sweeping across the city. Each household is a tiny pinpoint of pollutant emissions, but collectively these emission specks merge to blanket the city's residential districts with a veil of pollution. Emissions from household cookers and heaters not only pollute the urban atmosphere, but pollute the air inside people's homes as well.

The warmth and buoyancy of industrial, vehicle and household emissions, together with low-level atmospheric turbulence and local breezes (generated by urban heat islands), ensure that the pollutants drift away from their immediate sources, mix and combine to shroud the entire city in polluted air. The consequence is that urban residents breathe a cocktail of pollutants derived from diverse sources. People's exposure to a wide range of pollutants is accentuated as they move from one part of the city to another while commuting to work, shopping and pursuing leisure interests. The worst areas for pollution are often the city centre, alongside the city's primary transport corridors and around industrial complexes.

Assessing the Health Risks Posed by Pollutants

The sooner the city authorities recognise that air pollution threatens the health of its residents, the greater the opportunity for achieving acceptable air quality in a short time and at low cost. An early commitment by the city authorities to the goal of healthy air quality is important.[1] State and national governments may have to be involved because of the legislative powers and/ or resources needed to implement air quality management. However, it is the city authorities who are best placed to understand and resolve their air pollution problems. They should be given the legislative powers and resources to tackle what is essentially a local problem. In other words, the principle of subsidiarity should be applied. However, the support of international bodies (eg the World Bank) and governments may be needed in respect of financial assistance, especially for cities in Southern countries, as well as when agreeing policies which tackle transfrontier pollutants affecting a city.

City authorities first need to assess the health and environmental risks posed by pollutants in their city. Many of the health implications of individual pollutants and combinations of pollutants (leading to synergistic effects) have been known for many years from international studies. This means that health-based air quality guidelines and standards are already defined, although new research may identify new threats such as, for example, in the recognition of the carcinogenic nature of a pollutant or in redefining the threshold level at which a pollutant is considered to pose a risk (eg there may be no safe threshold for PM_{10}). Such findings may require the setting of new or modified air quality standards.

Having assessed the health risks facing a city by measuring the spatial and temporal patterns of pollutants and relating ambient pollution concentrations to health-based air quality standards, the next step is to determine the sources of the pollutants (ie compile emission inventories). Authorities can then begin to devise alternative pollution control policies

1 Ideally, pollution problems should be anticipated as it is easier and less costly to prevent problems rather than to attempt to solve them once they exist. However, there are few examples where air pollution problems have been fully considered in the early stages of urban development. Most cities have to experience serious pollution problems before the political and public will exists to do something about them.

and measures that may be expected to achieve acceptable air quality by a target date. The setting of interim targets to be met on the way to meeting the ultimate goal will enable progress towards the final target to be monitored and policies modified or strengthened if necessary. Targets should not be limited to achieving specific air quality levels, but need to include the means to achieve them. For example, a target may specify the date when all cars must be fitted with catalytic converters, the percentage of commuter journeys that should be undertaken by public transport, walking or cycling, the percentage of sales of ZEVs or the coverage of the city by public transport systems (eg ensuring that everyone has access to a public transport boarding place within a set distance). Formulating and testing the likely air quality effectiveness of various policies and measures using numerical prediction models as well as pilot studies is time consuming and resource intensive, but it is an essential part of urban air quality management. It is intended to ensure that the policies and measures will not be ineffective, misdirected or wasteful of the limited financial resources available to the authorities.

Choosing and Implementing Pollution Control Policies

There are a wide range of pollution control policies and measures currently being implemented in cities across the world with varying degrees of success. New policies and measures may have to be conceived, especially in the case of pollution threats not recognised previously. Each city can learn lessons from the experience of other cities, although the industrial, transport and residential characteristics as well as the topographic and meteorological conditions of each city are unique. The response of each city's population to specific pollution control policies and measures will also vary due to social, cultural and economic differences. Support from the public is vital to the likely success of any pollution control strategy, so educational and publicity campaigns to win the support of residents are an important part of urban air quality management.

The health threat posed by high pollution concentrations during smogs is more readily recognised by the public than the insidious threat posed by sustained levels of pollutants above the threshold at which adverse health effects occur. This often leads to strong pressure being exerted on the city authorities by some groups, especially those already suffering from heart and respiratory disease, to take short-term actions to curb emissions during smogs.[2] In contrast, there is often less pressure from the public to introduce

2 Sensitive groups at risk include people with asthma, those with pre-existing heart and lung diseases, the elderly, infants and pregnant women (and their unborn babies). These groups may amount to one-fifth of the population in cities in The North. If the undernourished in The South are added to this list of vulnerable groups, the proportion of people at high risk from poor air quality increases markedly. The health effects caused by smogs (short-term episodes of high pollution concentrations) can be recognised readily by the public and publicised

measures which reduce the baseline of emissions over the longer term. Whereas there is a certain willingness for residents to accept the inconvenience or cost of temporary measures to tackle smogs lasting a few days, there is often widespread resistance to accepting long-term pollution control policies and measures as they may involve fundamental changes to existing lifestyles (eg having to switch from cars to public transport for commuting to work). Nevertheless, it is the sustained pursuit of policies which will deliver healthy urban air quality that needs to be the priority: actions taken during smogs are not a substitute. Actions taken during smogs reduce the health risk only temporarily, they cannot remove it permanently. Urban residents need to be encouraged to recognise that implementing long-term pollution control policies will lead to the reduced frequency and severity of smogs. In some cities pollution concentrations are so high that what would be deemed short-lived smogs in another city occur for months on end. In such situations, adopting temporary measures is not really appropriate. Dividing resources between implementing short-term (smog) and long-term pollution control measures does not necessarily mean making the choice between one or the other. Smog alerts can reduce morbidity and save lives so they have a part to play in reducing the pollution threat to residents if resources are available. However, they should not be implemented in place of a full commitment to long-term measures. Far more lives will be saved and the health of millions of people in a city improved the sooner that healthy air quality is experienced permanently by urban populations.

Choosing the most cost-effective policies and measures to achieve and sustain acceptable air quality is difficult. Economic and political factors clearly influence the choice of policies such that the most air quality effective are not necessarily those selected, being replaced by policies that are thought to improve air quality without too much cost and sometimes without much conviction that they will lead to acceptable air quality once fully implemented. Mistaken choices of pollution control policies and measures have been made.

Policies may be implemented without considering the full pollution implications. A recent example relates to changing the fuel composition to tackle the health threat posed by high levels of airborne lead. Lead has been added traditionally to petrol to raise its octane level. Removing the lead from petrol would eliminate the largest source of lead in cities. In unleaded petrol, the octane boosting formerly achieved using lead may be produced by increasing levels of aromatic hydrocarbons and alkenes instead (typically to around 4 per cent in the UK compared with 2 per cent in unleaded petrol). The combustion of aromatic hydrocarbons results in emissions of benzene, a genotoxic carcinogen linked with leukaemia, whereas alkenes lead to emissions of butadiene. In 1994 UK premium unleaded (95 octane) petrol

---

by the mass media (eg large numbers of people with pre-existing disease suffering a worsening of symptoms, increased hospital admissions and increased deaths).

accounted for around 55 per cent of sales and super-unleaded (98 octane), containing more aromatics (about 5 per cent benzene), for 6 per cent of sales. Super-unleaded petrol is used by drivers of pre-1990 high-performance cars which have been converted to unleaded fuel and by other drivers who mistakenly believe it will increase vehicle performance and power compared with premium unleaded petrol. Although only cars fitted with catalytic converters (all new cars since 1993) remove the benzene, only 15 per cent of cars were fitted with catalysts in 1995 in the UK. Those cars not fitted with catalysts but using unleaded petrol are emitting aromatics such as benzene without any restraint (even though they are helping to reduce lead emissions by not using leaded petrol). In other words, changing the fuel composition has exchanged one health threat (airborne lead) for another (benzene). The situation could become even worse if reductions in the volatility of petrol during summer months, aimed at tackling ozone problems, result in a 5 per cent increase in the amount of aromatic hydrocarbons in unleaded petrol. Such a situation highlights that air quality management measures based on fuel composition may not be as effective as many people expect. This applies particularly when pollution control policies target individual pollutants in isolation rather than considering the risks posed by all the pollutants involved. The need for a full and detailed assessment of policy decisions before they are taken is clearly indicated.[3]

Improving Urban Air Quality

Technological improvements offer a relatively quick and convenient means of reducing emissions and improving air quality: technological solutions being applied to what many people consider is a technological problem. In this way, a reduction in the emissions of some pollutants can be achieved without fundamental changes in the processes and activities producing the pollutants (a 'business as usual' approach). Policies advocating the introduction of pollution abatement equipment are widespread. Vehicle emissions are reduced by fitting catalytic converters, particulate traps and carbon canisters. Emissions from petrol stations can be reduced by fitting vapour recovery systems to petrol pumps. Flue gas emissions from fossil-fuelled power stations and industrial plants can be reduced by fitting electrostatic precipitators and scrubbers. There is little doubt that pollution

3 'MPs hear conflicting evidence on vehicle emissions and health', *ENDS Report*, 234, 1994, pp 28–29; Hamer, M (1993) 'Green petrol a hazard to health', *New Scientist*, 13 November, p 5; House of Commons Transport Committee (1994) *Transport-related Atmospheric Pollution in London*, Sixth Report, vols 1 and 2, HMSO, London; Royal Commission on Environmental Pollution (1994) *Eighteenth Report: Transport and the Environment*, HMSO, London. Benzene exhaust emissions are proportional to the total aromatic content of the fuel. This is because toluene, xylenes and ethyl benzene undergo dealkylation reactions during the combustion process, leading to benzene formation. Similarly, the higher the alkene content of the fuel, the greater the butadiene emissions.

abatement measures can reduce emissions and that many cities, especially in The South, could benefit greatly from applying some abatement measures. For example, in many Chinese cities even the most basic pollution control equipment for particulate and gaseous emissions from industry and power stations is absent. Reducing emissions by changing the fuel composition is another approach attempted with some success (eg lowering the sulphur content of diesel fuel and the lead and benzene content in petrol or by adding oxygenates to petrol). Technological innovations for vehicles include the development of lean-burn engines which can reduce vehicle emissions. All these pollution control measures can be achieved without fundamental changes to transport modes, industrial activities and the lifestyles of inhabitants (ie they can continue to use their cars).

City authorities (or national government) can encourage the adoption of abatement measures through financial incentives (eg grants, loans) and disincentives (eg fines). Technological improvements can be encouraged by strengthening emission standards for vehicles and industrial plants. Weak monitoring and enforcement of standards occurs in many cities in The South and needs to be rectified (the process can become self-funding through fines imposed on those exceeding standards). A faster replacement of older more polluting vehicles with new vehicles fitted with pollution control equipment can be encouraged by offering grants for those buying new vehicles and/or willing to scrap older ones. Implementing regular annual vehicle emissions inspections and random roadside testing can target the gross polluters who contribute disproportionately to total vehicle emissions. Because local circumstances vary between cities, each city needs to evaluate the measures and market incentives which can deliver the greatest improvements in air quality. A successful measure in one city will not necessarily bring equal success when applied to another city. However, good practice can be recognised and if necessary modified to suit local circumstances.

Technological developments extending beyond simple abatement measures are those which reduce emissions by replacement or substitution technologies. Petrol and diesel vehicles can be modified to use methanol, biofuels, liquid petroleum gas, compressed natural gas and rapeseed methyl ester. A more radical policy would be to require vehicles to be powered by electric batteries, hydrogen fuel cells or solar photovoltaic cells. Alternative fuels and technologies can be used to reduce emissions from households (eg heating systems to use smokeless fuels) and power stations (switching electricity generation in power stations from coal or oil to natural gas and eventually to renewable power sources such as water, wind, geothermal and biomass). However, using alternative fuels, even renewables, can cause other environmental problems. For example, extensive areas of land are needed for wind turbines which may intrude visually on valued landscapes. Electric vehicles are ZEVs only where they operate: they give rise to emissions of pollutants where the electricity to recharge their batteries is generated (eg a coal-fired power station). Stemming the rise in petrol- and diesel-powered vehicles by a gradual replacement with electric vehicles does not prevent traffic growth and worsening road congestion. Abatement measures can sometimes simply exchange one pollution problem for another (eg catalytic converters increase carbon dioxide emissions, adding to global warming) or even shift the pollutants from one environmental medium to another (eg power station electrostatic precipitations increase the amount of solid waste to be disposed, whereas sulphur dioxide scrubbers may lead to increased quarrying of limestone).

Traffic management policies can reduce pollutant emissions as, for example, using speed limits and laws requiring vehicles to switch off their engines when stationary for more than 30 seconds in traffic jams, at traffic light queues and at delivery or collection points. Optimising the efficiency at which vehicles operate can be attempted through smoothing traffic flows and reducing congestion during which engine-idling vehicles produce high emissions. Measures include using co-ordinated traffic lights, Priority Red Routes, variable speed limits on motorways, traffic calming and staggered working hours. However, measures which reduce travel times are not a substitute for measures that reduce the need to travel or the need to travel long distances within urban areas. Similarly, building major new roads or adding more lanes to motorways in and around cities is not the long-term solution to pollution problems as such measures simply generate more traffic (because existing congestion deters some motorists from using their cars).

Sustainable Urban Development

Achieving and maintaining healthy air quality is the pressing challenge that the world's cities face. Pollution control policies and measures need to be selected on the basis of whether they can deliver and sustain the clean air that all urban residents have a right to expect. Motor vehicles have become the principal source of pollutants in cities. Without effective action to curb vehicle emissions, the world's cities will continue to experience poor air quality. Yet many of the policies currently being applied based on abatement, replacement and substitution measures fail to suggest that they can ensure cities will eventually meet health-based air quality standards, let alone sustain them. For example, abatement measures for vehicles, such as fitting equipment to reduce exhaust emissions, can not be fully be effective while the numbers of vehicles and the distances they are driven continue to increase. This highlights the fact that such policies are not addressing the root cause of the air quality problem. What is needed is the adoption of policies that not only reverse the growth in traffic, but also reduce traffic levels throughout the urban area. The current use of motor vehicles, and the infrastructure associated with vehicles, is not only causing serious harm to human health or the quality of life through air pollution, but it is consuming finite resources of energy (especially fossil fuels), materials and land (with roads, car parks and petrol stations, reducing the stock of natural and semi-natural habitats and areas with amenity or cultural value), and it is contributing to irreversible changes in climate (through emissions of greenhouse gases). In addition, it promotes patterns of land use which depend for their viability on motor vehicles and which lead to one or more of these adverse effects. Such a situation is unsustainable in the long term.[4]

The selection of policies needs to be placed in the context of sustainable economic development. Sustainable development is development that meets the needs of the present without compromising the ability of future generations to meet their own needs. It means a process of change in which the exploitation of resources, the direction of investments, the orientation of technological development and institutional changes are consistent with future as well as present needs.[5] It is intended to meet the inhabitants' developing needs without imposing unsustainable demands on local or global natural resources and systems.[6] The challenge of sustainable urban development is to remove the air pollution (and other environmental) problems experienced within cities and those caused by cities without shifting them to other areas, other environmental media or passing them on to future generations while, at the same time, recognising the benefits brought by urban areas and seeking to meet the social and economic needs of residents.[7] The emphasis is on the sustainable city in process terms rather than as an end point.[8]

---

4 Royal Commission on Environmental Pollution (1994) op cit, p 3; Commission of European Communities (1990) *Green Paper on the Urban Environment*, Report COM(90)218, CEC, Brussels

5 World Commission on Environment and Development (1987) *Our Common Future*, Oxford University Press, Oxford (known as the Brundtland Report), pp 8 and 46. Support for the pursuit of sustainable development has been widespread and adopted in many national and international policy statements, eg Agenda 21 drawn up at the United Nations Environment Programme Conference on Environment and Development held at Rio de Janeiro in June 1992 (and the obligations that Local Agenda 21 imposes on local authorities, especially sustainable urban development); Quarrie, J (1992) *Earth Summit '92: the United Nations Conference on Environment and Development*, Regency Press, London. The European Union's Fifth Environment Action Programme entitled *Towards Sustainability* sets out the environmental agenda for the period 1993–2000 period and urges tackling of the root causes of the problems rather than the symptoms – that is, promoting sustainable development; Blowers, A (1993) *Planning for a Sustainable Environment*, London, Earthscan

6 Douglass, M (1992) 'Sustainable cities', *Environment and Urbanization*, vol 4(2), 2–8

7 Sustainable cities are cities where socio-economic interests are brought together in harmony (co-evolution) with environmental and energy concerns to ensure continuity in change. Nijkamp, P and Perrels, A (1994) *Sustainable Cities in Europe*, Earthscan, London, p 4–5; Haughton, G and Hunter, C (1994) *Sustainable Cities*, Regional Policy and Development Series Number 7, Jessica Kingsley, London; Stren, R, White, R and Whitney, J (1992) *Sustainable Cities*, Westview Press, Boulder

8 New urban concepts have been advocated such as the green city, the eco-city, the liveable city, the resourceful city, the compact city and the environmental city. Elkin, T, Maclaren, D and Hillman, M (1990) *Reviving the City: Towards Sustainable Urban Development*, Policy Studies Institute, London

Achieving Healthy Urban Air Quality

In terms of air pollution problems, sustainable urban development means reducing emissions by changing the consumption and production patterns within cities which give rise to pollution. For transport, this can be achieved by adopting planning and land use policies which reduce the distances people need to travel and enable journeys to be undertaken by energy efficient public transport systems rather than cars. The size of the urban area is less critical than its form in that cities need to provide residents good access to workplaces and services using energy efficient public transport systems. Minimising the need for mobility in urban areas requires planning policies that reduce the distances between where people work, live, shop, are educated (eg schools, colleges), participate in leisure activities (eg sports centres, social clubs, cinemas, theatres, libraries) and seek medical treatment (ie hospitals, health centres). This is a radical reversal of the traditional policies most cities and countries have long practised. These policies have favoured cars at the expense of public transport. They are based on predicting seemingly endless traffic growth and responding by building the roads to try to keep up. By building more roads more traffic is generated, which ensures that the predicted rates of traffic growth are realised.

Future policies should aim to achieve sustainable urban mobility through integrating land use, transport and environmental planning. Environmental planning needs to consider water, land and noise pollution as much as air pollution. Residential areas should be developed at a density sufficient to support a transport system which does not rely on the use of the private car.[9] Proposed and existing commercial developments need to be guided towards areas well served by public transport. The potential impact of this policy together with promoting the use of public transport is highlighted by an example from the Netherlands. The Ministry of Housing, Physical Planning and Environment moved its administration from the suburbs to a central railway station in the city centre. Employees now have to pay for the use of a car parking space, whereas those choosing to go by public transport are subsidised by the ministry. Before the relocation, 40 per cent went by car. Now only 4 per cent use a car, 20–30 per cent use bicycles and 65–70 go by public transport.[10] High density development should be restricted to locations of maximum public transport accessibility. Public transport capacities in various parts of the city should be used as indicators (checks) of the size and nature of new developments (eg resulting in limits being placed on the number of parking spaces). New and existing major employers need to be required to take action to reduce the number of single-

9 Fudge, C (1995) 'Settlement and commercial development planning – the influence of Europe', *paper presented to the National Society for Clean Air and Environmental Protection (NSCA) Seminar on Planning and Air Quality, Birmingham, June*, NSCA, Brighton, p 13

10 'Advantage of location', *Acid News*, 3, Jun 1995, p 14

occupant journeys by their employees to meet targets set by the city authorities (ie submit trip reduction plans). Greater consideration should be given to new information and telecommunication technology (eg reducing the need for journeys, working from home). New developments which are significant point sources of emissions, in addition to the traffic emissions they might generate, need to consider the existing air quality in a proposed location. Approval for developments should consider air quality levels in an area in relation to the health-based air quality standards. New developments in non-attainment areas may be permitted through offsets (ie the proposed developers funding emission reductions in existing sources in that area in excess of the pollution levels they will generate). Alternatively, emissions trading, requiring new developments to buy emissions trading permits, is another market-based strategy that can be adopted.

A close examination of lifestyles, especially in the energy consuming cities of The North, is needed with a view to introducing energy saving measures wherever possible. Greater emphasis is needed on recycling, re-use and repair. Recycling of glass, metal, paper and plastics saves energy and materials and so reduces pollution emissions. Reducing wastage, decreasing energy consumption and improving energy efficiency not only reduce emissions of pollutants, but are important for economic development. The use of insulation and conservation measures can reduce energy consumption by as much as 30 per cent in buildings. The choice of building materials and heating systems can affect air quality both inside and outside buildings. More efficient systems include combined heat and power systems and district heating. Improvements in the energy efficiency of industrial furnaces (including power stations), vehicles (setting minimum fuel consumption levels) and household appliances (eg refrigerators, washing machines) and fittings (eg energy-saving light bulbs) can be undertaken. Urban solid waste, if it cannot be recycled, can be incinerated to produce electricity (for industrial plants) and heat (for district heating), which reduces the need to transport it out of the city for disposal in distant landfill sites. The authorities can speed progress towards the adoption of pollution control measures by offering grants, loans and taxes. The adoption of increasingly stringent regulations, codes and standards needs to be considered and those polluters failing to comply need to face fines or other penalties.

Public transport systems consume many times less energy and pollutant emissions per passenger kilometre than private cars. For public transport to gain dominance over the car it will require substantial investment in bus, rail, light rail and metro systems, creating integrated public transport networks. Public transport needs to gain popularity over using private cars by becoming convenient, safe, comfortable, reliable and inexpensive to use. Public transport has to be given priority over cars (eg bus lanes, guideways, bus-only streets, priority at traffic lights and junctions). A mixture of 'push' and 'pull' measures is needed. The public have to be 'pulled' out of their cars by offering improved public transport as well as safe, direct and attractive pedestrian and cycling routes. They have to be 'pushed' towards public transport services by imposing certain restrictions on cars.[11] It may be that banning cars from city centres, which can then be pedestrianised, is inevitable to ensure that public transport, cycling and walking gain dominance over the car.

Public information and promotional campaigns (supported by demonstration or pilot projects) can encourage change. Public support and active participation in the policies and measures concerned with air quality management is essential but will, in part, depend on socio-economic factors. Those groups with low living standards are more concerned with the immediate needs and priorities of day to day living such as adequate water, food and shelter. Such people often have to live in the most polluted parts of the cities (eg near industrial complexes, major roads, inner city areas) and have much to gain from an improvement in urban air quality and environmental quality in general. They will benefit from the development of improved public transport systems offering low fares. Their limited participation in air quality management policies and measures may be less significant when it is recognised that they contribute less to the pollution problems of the city than the more affluent households who own one or more cars (or benefit from a company car) and use them frequently as well as consuming large amounts of energy in their homes and workplaces. In cities in The South poverty affects a larger proportion of the population than in The North, such that the city authorities will be hard pressed to offer sufficient incentives for the poor to participate fully in pollution control policies and measures. Similarly, the financial resources available to city authorities or national governments of Southern nations (eg because of large national debt repayments) may be insufficient for the effective implementation of air quality management policies. This points to the need for the involvement of international organisations to help to initiate and sustain pollution control policies and measures in those cities. Another role for international organisations is to promote accountable and democratic decision-making within cities which empower all inhabitants to participate in decisions concerning the choice of sustainable pollution control policies that their city should follow.

---

11 Some policies aimed at discouraging the use of cars have been found to be less effective than expected. For example, attempting to halve the number of cars in city centres by restricting entry to cars with odd and even licence plates on alternate days can be undermined by commuters purchasing a second car. Reducing the number of parking spaces available in city centres fails to persuade some drivers to switch to use park and ride: they would rather drive further distances in search of one of the elusive parking spaces that may still remain. Park and ride schemes can encourage some longer distance commuters, who would otherwise use public transport for their entire journey, to switch to using cars to drive to the convenient (free) parking facilities provided by such schemes and use their frequent bus services (with subsidised fares).

An example indicating the elements of a successful integration of transport and land use planning in achieving good air quality as well as higher standards of living is that of Curitiba (population 1.8 million) in Brazil. In 1974 it began the development of an innovative public transport system using express buses on exclusive bus lanes operating on five axes, each with a 'trinary' road system. The central road has two exclusive bus lanes in the centre for express buses and is flanked by two local roads. Each side of this central road, one block away, are high capacity, free-flowing, one-way roads – one for traffic going into the city and one going out. In the areas adjacent to each axis, land use legislation has encouraged high-density residential developments, along with services and commerce. The whole city is zoned according to the type of development and the density permitted is related to the distance from public transport. The express buses (coloured red) running along these axes are served by circular inter-district buses (green) and conventional feeder buses (yellow), with connections between different buses organised in a series of bus terminals. One single fare is valid for all buses on the 514 km (321 miles) bus network. Automatic fare collection, articulated buses (including 33 buses each with a capacity of 270 passengers) and traffic lights which give buses priority all help to create an efficient 'surface metro'. Curitiba's public transport system is used by more than 1.3 million passengers each day. Even though Curitiba has 0.5 million cars, the highest rate of car ownership in Brazil, owners use them less frequently because they use the buses (about 28 per cent of express bus users previously travelled by cars). Sustainable urban development is evident in many other aspects of city life. Since 1989, a 'garbage that is not garbage' recycling scheme, involving 70 per cent of the community, has operated. The income earned through the sale of the garbage is reinvested in local social programmes. Those living in the favelas (shantytowns) can sell their bags of garbage for bus fares and basic foods. This highlights that the development needs of the poor can begin to be met while improving environmental quality.[12]

A strategic approach to sustainable urban development means setting clear goals as well as interim targets, specifying what is to be achieved and by what dates. Such explicit statements help to focus people's attention on the end result and enable progress towards the ultimate goal to be assessed. Specific land use and transport policies and measures can be tested to see whether they can fulfil these targets and, if so, at what cost. Given the seriousness of air pollution problems in many cities in the world, sustainable policies which will result in healthy air pollution for all known pollutants, rather than just some, may take 20–30 years. This highlights the importance of setting interim targets (eg quantifying the reduction of urban journeys undertaken by car or levels of reductions in vehicle emissions to be achieved

12 Pearce, F (1992) 'Brazil's sustainable city', *New Scientist*, 13 Jun, pp 52–53; Rabinovitch, J (1992) 'Curitiba: towards sustainable urban development', *Environment and Urbanization*, vol 4 (2), pp 62–73

over five-year periods). Interim targets can provide encouragement towards the ultimate goal of healthy air quality, which to some people may seem daunting and distant.

Sustaining Healthy Urban Air Quality

Sustaining acceptable air quality during the twenty-first century – once it has been attained – may be as difficult as achieving it in the first place. The changing nature and pattern of pollutant emissions in urban areas means that vigilance is needed in the form of an extensive air quality monitoring network and the application of models which project forward expected changes in the urban activities and lifestyles of its residents and their associated emissions. Careful scrutiny of pollution control policies is needed to ensure that they do not solve one pollution problem at the expense of triggering another, perhaps worse, problem. Emphasis needs to be given to preventing new pollution problems occurring. The experience of London has shown that even after ridding the city of life-threatening sulphurous smogs (pea soupers) by the mid-1960s, within two decades it was experiencing serious and worsening air pollution problems in the form of photochemical pollutants, which are more complex and difficult to eliminate. In some cases a pollution threat may have been present for a long time, but the seriousness of the threat only belatedly recognised. For example, reassessments of the health effects of suspended particulates have shown that most cities have underestimated the problem posed by fine particulates (PM_{10}, especially $PM_{2.5}$). This points to city authorities needing to reconsider their choice of pollution control policies and measures.

Clearly, progress towards achieving and then sustaining healthy air quality during the twenty-first century will be marked by successes and setbacks concerning different pollutants. What must be borne in mind throughout this costly and difficult struggle towards achieving that ultimate goal are the benefits that healthy air can bring to the 1.6 billion people currently breathing polluted air in the world's cities. The costs of implementing effective urban air quality management may be substantial, but the consequences of not doing so are even greater.

Index